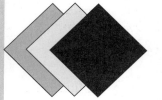

# Procedures Manual
to accompany
# Fundamentals
of Nursing
F i f t h   E d i t i o n

Barbara Kozier, RN, MN

Glenora Erb, RN, BSN

Suzanne C. Beyea, RN, CS, PhD
Saint Anselm College
Manchester, New Hampshire

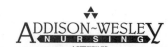
A DIVISION OF
THE BENJAMIN/CUMMINGS PUBLISHING COMPANY, INC.

Redwood City, California • Menlo Park, California
Reading, Massachusetts • New York • Don Mills, Ontario
Wokingham, U.K. • Amsterdam • Bonn • Sydney
Tokyo • Madrid • San Juan

executive editor: *Patricia L. Cleary*

managing editor: *Wendy Earl*

production editor: *Eleanor Renner Brown*

procedure checklists editor: *Cari Boatright Cagle*

cover design: *Yvo Riezebos Design*

compositor: *Jonathan Peck Typographers*

Care has been taken to confirm the accuracy of information presented in this book. The authors, editors, and the publisher, however, cannot accept responsibility for errors or omissions or for consequences from application of the information in this book, and make no warranty, expressed or implied, with respect to its contents.

The authors and publisher have exerted every effort to ensure that drug selection and dosages set forth in this text are in accord with current recommendations and practice at the time of publication. However, in view of ongoing research, changes in government regulations, and the constant flow of information relating to drug therapy and drug reactions, the reader is urged to check the package inserts of all drugs for any change in indications or dosage and for added warnings and precautions. This is particularly important when the recommended agent is a new and/or infrequently employed drug.

Library of Congress Cataloging-in-Publication Data

Kozier, Barbara.
   Procedures manual to accompany Fundamentals of nursing, fifth
   edition / Barbara Kozier, Glenora Erb, Suzanne C. Beyea.
      p.    cm.
   Includes bibliographical references.
   ISBN 0-8053-3503-X
   1. Nursing. I. Erb, Glenora Lea, 1937-   . II. Beyea, Suzanne
C. III. Kozier, Barbara. Fundamentals of nursing. 5th ed.
IV. Title.
RT41.K72   1995 Suppl.
610.73--dc20                                        94-23453
                                                       CIP


ISBN 0-8053-3503-X

1  2  3  4  5  6  7  8  9  10-VG-98  97  96  95  94

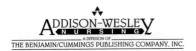

ADDISON-WESLEY
NURSING
A DIVISION OF
THE BENJAMIN/CUMMINGS PUBLISHING COMPANY, INC.

390 Bridge Parkway, Redwood City, CA 94065

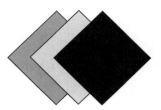

# Preface

When *Fundamentals of Nursing* was first published, instructors said they liked the combination of theory and procedures in a single comprehensive source. Their response led us to include more procedures in the subsequent editions. This *Procedures Manual* has been developed to offer instructors an even more complete range of procedures.

This supplement does not duplicate any procedures in *Fundamentals of Nursing*. The chapter numbers of the supplement coincide with the corresponding chapter numbers in *Fundamentals*. Several chapters do not have any supplementary procedures.

The procedures in this supplement are organized in the same framework as those in the text: Purposes, Assessment Focus, Equipment, Intervention, Evaluation Focus, and Sample Recording.

This book represents our continuing commitment and the commitment of the publisher to provide nurse educators with a variety of teaching materials in nursing fundamentals that can be adapted to almost any curriculum. We hope that the students and instructors using *Fundamentals of Nursing, Fifth Edition*, will find this supplement helpful and will continue to offer suggestions to improve its effectiveness.

*Barbara Kozier*
*Glenora Erb*
*Suzanne Beyea*

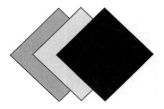

# Contents

*There are no procedures in this supplement for Chapters 1–20*

# 44 Wound Care

# 45 Perioperative Nursing

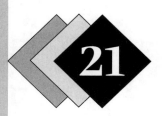

# Assessing Vital Signs

## PROCEDURES

# Fetal Heart Assessment

The fetal heart rate (FHR) is audible as early as the tenth week of pregnancy, using the Doppler stethoscope with ultrasound. At about 18 to 20 weeks, the FHR can be heard by fetoscope or other stethoscope.

The FHR is usually about 140 beats per minute (BPM) with a normal range of 120 to 160 BPM. It can be detected during the early months of pregnancy at the midline of the abdomen over the mother's symphysis pubis (above the pubic hairline); later in the pregnancy, the location varies with the position of the fetus (Figure 21–1).

FHRs are taken under these circumstances:

- If there is any concern about the health of the fetus

- On the client's admission

- Every hour during the onset of regular contractions of the uterus

- Every 30 minutes during cervical dilation

- Every 5 minutes or continually during the second stage of labor

- Immediately after the rupture of the uterine membranes

Because fetal heartbeats are most clearly transmitted through the back of the fetus, locations of maximum FHR intensity vary according to the position of the fetus (Figure 21–2).

The following kinds of stethoscopes are used in assessing FHRs:

- A fetal heart stethoscope (fetoscope) with a large weighted bell designed specifically for fetal heart auscultation (Figure 21–3). The weighted bell negates the need to hold the stethoscope in place, thus avoiding the noise of finger movement, which can interfere with auscultation. Some fetal heart stethoscopes can be adapted to monitor the mother's heart rate and blood pressure by substituting a smaller bell.

- A head stethoscope, which augments the fetal heart sounds; sounds are transmitted not only to the nurse's eardrums but also by bone conduction through the headpiece the nurse wears.

- A Doppler ultrasound stethoscope with probe (transducer) and transmission gel. The DUS is a more sensitive and reliable instrument than other

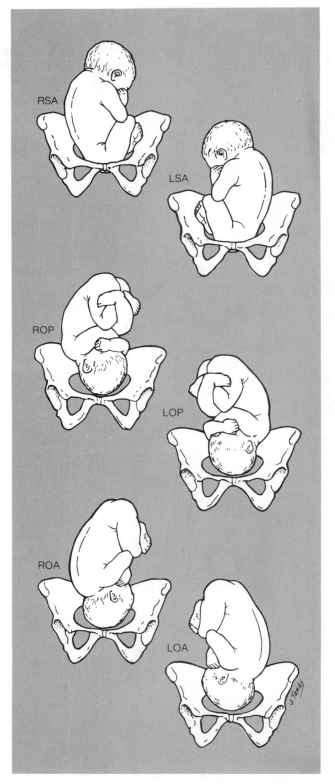

**FIGURE 21–1** Six positions of the fetus: right sacrum anterior (RSA), right occiput posterior (ROP), right occiput anterior (ROA), left sacrum anterior (LSA), left occiput posterior (LOP), and left occiput anterior (LOA).

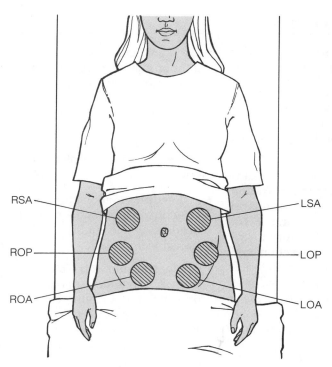

RSA
ROP
ROA
LSA
LOP
LOA

**FIGURE 21–2** Locations of maximum FHR intensity according to the position of the fetus.

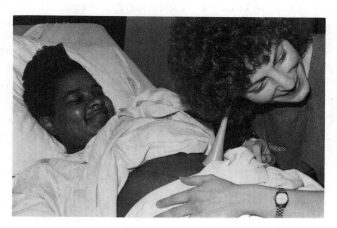

**FIGURE 21–3** A fetoscope.

fetoscopes. The transducer is applied to the woman's abdomen in lieu of the bell of other fetoscopes.

Procedure 21–1 describes how to assess the fetal heart.

## 21-1   Assessing a Fetal Heart

**PURPOSES**
- To establish baseline data in the initial assessment of the client
- To determine whether the rate is within normal range, the rhythm regular, and the beat strong
- To determine any change from previous measurements

**ASSESSMENT FOCUS**

| Varies with gestation period. |
| --- |

### EQUIPMENT

- Fetoscope, head stethoscope, or a Doppler ultrasound stethoscope
- Soft tissues and aqueous solution, if Doppler equipment is used
- Watch with second hand

### INTERVENTION

**1. Position the client appropriately.**

- Assist the woman to a supine position, and expose the abdomen.

**2. Locate the maximum FHR intensity.**

- Determine whether the area of maximum intensity is recorded

on the client's chart or marked on the client's abdomen.
*or*
Perform Leopold's maneuvers to

▶

► **Procedure 21–1  Assessing a Fetal Heart** CONTINUED

determine fetal position and locate its back.

**3. Auscultate and count the FHR.**

- Warm the hands and the head of the fetoscope before touching the client's abdomen.

- Place the bell of the fetoscope or the head stethoscope firmly on the maternal abdomen over the area of maximum intensity of the FHR in accordance with the identified fetal position: right sacrum anterior (RSA), right occiput posterior (ROP), right occiput anterior (ROA), left sacrum anterior (LSA), left occiput posterior (LOP), and left occiput anterior (LOA) (Figure 21–2). *The FHR is best heard when sounds are transmitted through the fetus's back.*

- Listen to and identify the fetal heart tone.

- Differentiate the fetal heart tone from the uterine souffle by simultaneously taking the maternal radial pulse. The *uterine souffle* is the soft blowing sound made when the maternal heart propels the blood through the large blood vessels of the uterus. It synchronizes with the maternal heart rate and can be heard distinctly upon auscultation of the lower portion of the uterus.

- Differentiate the fetal heart tone from the *funic* (umbilical cord) *souffle*, a sharp hissing sound caused by blood rushing through the umbilical cord. It is equivalent to the fetal heart rate, that is, about 140 beats per minute.

- Count the FHR for at least 15 seconds whenever it is monitored during the gestation period before labor.

- During labor, count the FHR for 60 seconds during the relaxation period between contractions to determine the baseline FHR. Then count the FHR for 60 seconds during a contraction and for 30 seconds immediately following a contraction. *Signs of fetal distress may occur during a contraction but most often occur immediately after it. More than 160 or fewer than 120 beats per minute may indicate fetal distress.*

**4. Assess the rhythm and the strength of the heartbeat.**

- Assess the rhythm of the heartbeat by noting the pattern of intervals between the beats. A normal FHR has equal time periods between beats.

- Assess the strength (volume) of the heartbeat. Normally, the heartbeats are equal in strength and can be described as strong or weak.

- Assist the woman to listen to the FHR if she wishes.

**5. Document and report pertinent assessment data.**

- Record the FHR, including the rhythm and strength, on the appropriate record.

- If the fetal heart rate or strength is abnormal, report this immediately to the nurse in charge or physician, and initiate electronic fetal monitoring if appropriate.

**VARIATION: Using a Doppler Stethoscope**

- Follow the manufacturer's instructions about attaching the headset to the audio unit and transducer.

- Apply transmission gel to the woman's abdomen over the area on which the transducer is to be placed. *Gel creates an airtight seal between the skin and the transducer and promotes optimal ultrasound wave transmission.*

- In the early months of pregnancy, ask the client to drink plenty of fluids before the procedure to fill the bladder and improve ultrasound transmission. Later in the pregnancy, this may cause discomfort to the client.

- Place the earpieces of the headset in your ears, adjust the volume of the audio unit, hold that unit in one hand, and place the transducer on the mother's abdomen.

- After determining the FHR, remove the excess gel from the mother's abdomen and from the transducer with soft tissues.

- Clean the transducer with aqueous solutions. *Alcohol or other disinfectants may damage the face of the transducer.*

| EVALUATION FOCUS | FHR in relation to baseline data and normal range; heartbeat rhythm and volume in relation to baseline data and health status. |
|---|---|

**SAMPLE RECORDING**

| Date | Time | Notes |
|---|---|---|
| 9/14/95 | 1300 | FHR 136 over right lower quadrant. Beats regular and strong. ———————————— Eva L. Mendez, SN |

# An Infant's Blood Pressure

The blood pressure of an infant can be measured by auscultation, palpation, ultrasound (Doppler technique), or flush technique. Auscultation is often difficult on infants under age 3, because Korotkoff's sounds are relatively inaudible, but it is the method of choice for children over 3 years of age. When the blood pressure cannot be auscultated, it can be palpated or measured by the flush technique. Both of these methods reveal only a mean pressure between the systolic and diastolic pressures when the blood returns to the limb. The flush technique is largely being replaced by use of an ultrasound device. Some ultrasound models measure only systolic pressures; others measure both systolic and diastolic pressures.

When measuring an infant's blood pressure, the systolic pressure (phase 1) is noted when the first clear tapping sound is heard. Both phase 4 (muffling of sounds) and phase 5 (disappearance of sounds) are recorded for the diastolic pressure. They are recorded in the form "118/78/68." If only phases 1 and 4 can be identified, they are recorded "118/78/0." This indicates that sounds were heard to the 0 point on the manometer.

When a cuff of the appropriate size is not available for an infant or child, it is preferable (a) to use an oversized cuff rather than an undersized one (wide cuffs apparently do not cause the low readings noted in adults [Whaley and Wong 1989, p. 138]) or (b) to use a different site that will accomodate the cuff size. For example, a radial pressure may be taken if the cuff is too small, or a thigh blood pressure may be taken if only a large cuff is available. Systolic blood pressure in the radial artery is usually 10 mm Hg lower than in the brachial artery; it is usually 10 mm Hg higher in the popliteal artery than in the brachial artery in children over age 1 year. Arm and thigh pressures are equal in children under age 1.

---

 **21-2**   # Assessing an Infant's Blood Pressure

| | |
|---|---|
| **PURPOSES** | • To establish a baseline in the initial assessment of the infant<br>• To determine any change from previous measurements<br>• To determine the adequacy of the arterial blood pressure |
| **ASSESSMENT FOCUS** | Signs and symptoms of hypertension and hypotension; factors affecting blood pressure. |

---

## EQUIPMENT

- ☐ Blood pressure cuff of a suitable size
- ☐ Sphygmomanometer (auscultatory method)
- ☐ Stethoscope (auscultatory method) or DUS
- ☐ Elastic bandage of suitable width to cover the limb distal to the cuff (flush method)

---

## INTERVENTION

**1. Prepare the infant/child appropriately.**

- Explain each step of the procedure to children of preschool age and above, e.g., tell them how the cuff will feel (tight or like an arm hug) and to "watch the silver rise in the tube." When possible, demonstrate the procedure on a toy or your own arm.

- Be sure that the environment in which the blood pressure measurement is to take place is quiet and reassuring to the infant. *Frightening sounds or sights can contribute to error in measurement, since anxiety and restlessness increase the blood pressure.*

- Allow time for the infant to recover from any activity or apprehension.

- Assist the child to a comfortable position. Infants and small children may be more quiet if placed in a sitting position on the parent's lap.

- Expose the arm fully, if used, and then support it comfortably at the child's heart level.

**2. Use the auscultation method for a child over 3 years of age.**

- The auscultatory method is essentially the same for children as for adults. (See Procedure 21–6 in *Fundamentals of Nursing*.)

►

▶ **Procedure 21–2 Assessing an Infant's Blood Pressure** *CONTINUED*

• Identify the manometer reading at phases 1, 4, and 5 of Korotkoff's sounds. Phase 1 is the systolic pressure and phases 4 and 5 the diastolic pressures.

**3. Use the palpation method, the flush technique, or a Doppler stethoscope when the blood pressure cannot be auscultated.**

**Palpation Method**

• Place the cuff around the limb so that the lower edge is about 1 cm (0.4 in) above the antecubital space (Figure 21–4).

• Palpate the brachial pulse.

• Inflate the cuff to about 30 mm Hg beyond the point where the brachial pulse disappears.

• Release the cuff at the rate of 2 to 3 mm Hg per second, and identify the manometer reading at the point where the pulse returns in the brachial artery. This pressure is a mean pressure between the systolic and diastolic pressures.

**Flush Technique**

This procedure requires two people and a well-lighted room, so that the

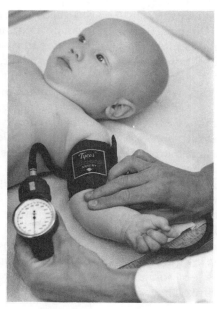

**FIGURE 21–4** Taking an infant's blood pressure by palpation.

pressure at which the flush appears can be accurately determined.

• Place the cuff on the infant's wrist or ankle.

• Elevate the limb. *This promotes venous blood flow to the heart.*

• Wrap the limb distal to the cuff with an elastic bandage. Wrap firmly, starting at the fingers or toes and working up to the blood pressure cuff. *The bandage will force venous blood into the upper part of the limb and restrict arterial blood flow into the lower part of the limb.*

• Lower the extremity to the heart level.

• Inflate the bladder of the cuff rapidly to about 200 mm Hg. *This stops arterial blood flow to the limb.*

• Remove the bandage. The limb should appear pale because of the absence of blood.

• Gradually release the pressure at no more than 5 mm Hg per second.

• Record the pressure at the appearance of a flush as the blood returns in the extremity distal to the cuff. This pressure is a mean blood pressure between the systolic and diastolic pressures.

**EVALUATION FOCUS**

| The blood pressure in relation to baseline data, normal range for age, and heart status; relationship to pulse and respiration. |
| --- |

**SAMPLE RECORDING**

| Date | Time | Notes |
| --- | --- | --- |
| 3/23/95 | 1600 | B/P 116/64 by ultrasound. AP- 120. ——————— Nancy Lopez, SN |

# Assessing Adult Health

## PROCEDURES

## Lumbar Puncture

In a **lumbar puncture** (LP, or spinal tap), cerebrospinal fluid (CSF) is withdrawn through a needle inserted into the **subarachnoid space** of the spinal canal between the third and fourth lumbar vertebrae or between the fourth and fifth lumbar vertebrae. At this level the needle avoids damaging the spinal cord and major nerve roots (Figure 22–1). During a lumbar puncture, the physician frequently takes CSF pressure readings using a **manometer**, a glass or plastic tube calibrated in millimeters. A Queckenstedt-Stookey test may also be done while the manometer is in place. When the veins in the neck are compressed on one or both sides, there is a rapid rise in the pressure of the cerebrospinal fluid of healthy persons, and this

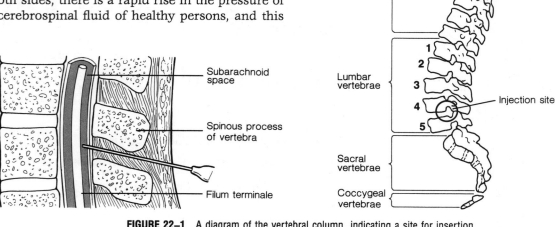

**FIGURE 22–1** A diagram of the vertebral column, indicating a site for insertion of the lumbar puncture needle into the subarachnoid space of the spinal canal.

rise quickly disappears when pressure is taken off the neck. But when there is a block in the vertebral canal the pressure of the cerebrospinal fluid is minimally or not affected by this maneuver. If the nurse is not supporting the client in position, the nurse may be asked to exert digital (finger) pressure on one or both of the internal jugular veins for this test (Figure 22–2).

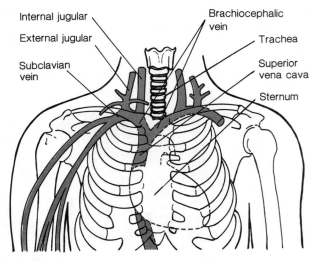

**FIGURE 22–2** Location of the internal jugular vein for the Queckenstedt-Stookey test.

# 22-1  Assisting with a Lumbar Puncture

**PURPOSES**
- To obtain a CSF specimen
- To take CSF pressure readings

**ASSESSMENT FOCUS**

Baseline vital signs; neurologic status; presence of headache; allergies to skin antiseptics or anesthetic agents.

## EQUIPMENT

- Sterile lumbar puncture set containing
  Sterile sponges or gauze squares
  Skin antiseptic
  Drapes (one may be fenestrated)
  Syringe and needle to administer the local anesthetic (A 2-ml syringe and #24 and #22 needles are often provided)

Spinal needle 5 to 12.5 cm (2 to 5 in) long, with stylet. The shorter needles are used for infants.
Manometer
Three-way stopcock (a valve between the spinal needle and the manometer that regulates the flow of CSF by shutting off the CSF drainage, allowing the CSF to flow either into the manometer or out into a receptacle)

Specimen containers and labels
Local anesthetic, e.g., 1% procaine (if not included in preassembled set, a vial or ampule of it must be obtained)
Small dressing
- Face masks (optional)
- Sterile gloves
- Examining light, if needed

## INTERVENTION

### Preprocedure

**1. Explain the procedure to the client and support persons.**

- Tell the client
  a. That the physican will be taking a small sample of spinal fluid from the lower spine.
  b. That a local anesthetic will be given so that the client will feel little pain.
  c. When and where the procedure will occur, e.g., at the bedside or in the treatment room.
  d. Who will be present, i.e., the physician and the nurse.
  e. How much time is involved, e.g., about 15 minutes.

- In addition, tell the client what to expect during the procedure. The client may feel slight discomfort (like a pinprick) when the local anesthetic is injected

and a sensation of pressure when the spinal needle (Figure 22–3) is being inserted. Remind the client that it is important to remain still and in one position throughout the procedure. A restless client or a child will need to be held to prevent movement.

**2. Prepare the client.**

- Have the client empty the bladder and bowels prior to the procedure. *This prevents unnecessary discomfort.*

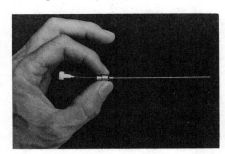

**FIGURE 22–3** A spinal needle with the stylet protruding from the hub.

- Position the client laterally with the head bent toward the chest, the knees flexed onto the abdomen, and the back at the edge of the bed or examining table (Figure 22–4). Place a very small pillow under the client's head to maintain the horizontal alignment of the spine. *In this position the back is arched, increasing the spaces between the vertebrae so that the spinal needle can be inserted readily.*

- Drape the client to expose only the lumbar spine.

- Open the lumbar puncture set (Figure 22–5) if requested to do so by the physician.

### During the Procedure

**3. Support and monitor the client throughout.**

- Stand in front of the client, and support the back of the neck and

▶

▶ **Procedure 22–1  Assisting with a Lumbar Puncture** *CONTINUED*

knees if the client needs help remaining still (Figure 22–4).

- Reassure the client throughout the procedure by explaining what is happening. Encourage the client to breathe normally and to relax as much as possible. *Excessive muscle tension, coughing, or changes in breathing can increase CSF pressure, giving a false reading.*

- Observe the client's color, respirations, and pulse during the lumbar procedure.

**4. Handle specimen tubes appropriately**.

- Don gloves before handling test tubes. *The outside may have been in contact with the CSF.*

- Label the specimen tubes in sequence if they are not already labeled. While handling the tubes, take care to prevent contamination of the physician's sterile gloves, the sterile field, and yourself. *The CSF may contain virulent microorganisms, e.g., organisms that cause meningitis.*

**5. Place a small sterile dressing over the puncture site**. *This helps prevent infection after the needle is removed.*

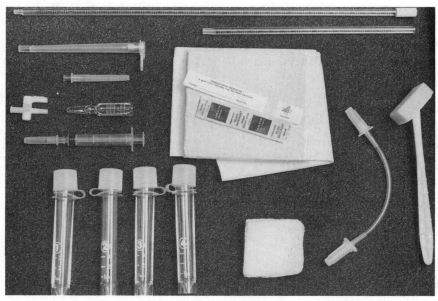

**FIGURE 22–5**  A preassembled lumbar puncture set. Note the manometer at the top of the set.

### Postprocedure

**6. Ensure the client's comfort and safety**.

- Assist the client to a dorsal recumbent position with only one head pillow. The client remains lying down for 8 to 24 hours, until the spinal fluid is replaced. Determine the recommended time this position should be maintained. *Some clients experience a headache following a lumbar puncture, and the dorsal recumbent position tends to prevent or alleviate it.*

- Determine whether analgesics are ordered and can be given for headaches.

**7. Monitor the client**.

- Observe for swelling or bleeding at the puncture site.

- Determine whether the client feels faint.

- Monitor changes in neurologic status.

- Determine whether the client is experiencing any numbness, tingling, or pain radiating down the legs. *This may be due to nerve irritation.*

**8. Transport the specimens to the laboratory**.

**9. Document the procedure on the client's chart**. Include the date and time it was performed; the name of the physician; the color, character, and amount of CSF obtained; the pressure readings; the number of specimens obtained; and the nurse's assessments and interventions.

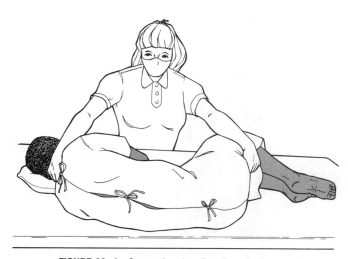

**FIGURE 22–4**  Supporting the client for a lumbar puncture.

▶ **Procedure 22–1** *CONTINUED*

| **EVALUATION FOCUS** | Vital signs; neurologic status; status of puncture site; complaints of discomfort or feelings of numbness or tingling in the lower extremities. |
|---|---|

**SAMPLE RECORDING**

| Date | Time | Notes |
|---|---|---|
| 5/24/95 | 1500 | Lumbar puncture performed by Dr Guido. Four 2 ml specimens of cloudy serous CSF sent to lab. Initial pressure 130 mm. Closing pressure 100 mm. No apparent discomfort. Resting. ——————— Sarah D. Nicols, NS |

## Abdominal Paracentesis

Normally the peritoneum creates just enough peritoneal fluid for lubrication. The fluid is continuously formed and absorbed into the lymphatic system. However, in some disease processes, a large amount of fluid accumulates in the cavity; this condition is called **ascites**. Normal ascitic fluid is serous, clear, and light yellow in color. An **abdominal paracentesis** is carried out to obtain a fluid specimen for laboratory study and to relieve pressure on the abdominal organs due to the presence of excess fluid.

The procedure is carried out by a physician with the assistance of a nurse. Strict sterile technique is followed. A common site for abdominal paracentesis is midway between the umbilicus and the symphysis pubis on the midline (Figure 22–6). The physician makes a small incision with a scalpel, inserts the **trocar** (a sharp, pointed instrument) and **cannula** (tube), and then withdraws the trocar, which is inside the cannula (Figure 22–7). Tubing is attached to the cannula and the fluid flows through the tubing into a receptacle. If the purpose of the paracentesis is to obtain a specimen, the physician may use a long aspirating needle attached to a syringe rather than making an incision and using a trocar and cannula. Normally about 1500 ml is the maximum amount of fluid drained at one time, to avoid hypovolemic shock. The fluid is drained very slowly for the same reason. Some fluid is placed in the specimen container before the cannula is withdrawn. The small incision may or may not be sutured; in either case, it is covered with a small sterile bandage.

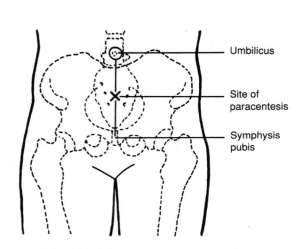

**FIGURE 22–6** A common site for an abdominal paracentesis.

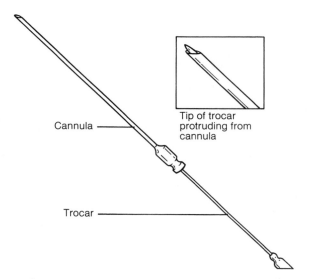

**FIGURE 22–7** A trocar and cannula may be used for an abdominal paracentesis.

## 22-2 Assisting with an Abdominal Paracentesis

**PURPOSES**
- To obtain a fluid specimen
- To relieve abdominal pressure due to excess fluid

▶ **Procedure 22–2** *CONTINUED*

<table>
<tr><td>ASSESSMENT<br>FOCUS</td><td>Baseline vital signs; degree of ascites in the abdomen (weigh the client and measure the abdominal girth at the level of the umbilicus); general appearance and health status; allergies to skin antiseptic or anesthetic agents.</td></tr>
</table>

## EQUIPMENT

- Sterile set containing
  Sterile sponges or gauze squares with an antiseptic solution
  Drape or drapes (one may be fenestrated)

  2-ml syringe and #24 and #22 needles
  Small scalpel, needle holder, and sutures
  Receptacle for the fluid
  Aspirating set or aspirating needle

  Local anesthetic
- Specimen containers and labels
- Masks (optional)
- Sterile gloves
- Nonsterile disposable gloves for the nurse

## INTERVENTION

### Preprocedure

**1. Prepare the client.**

- Explain the procedure to the client. Normally, an abdominal paracentesis is not painful, and, when a client has considerable ascites, the procedure can relieve discomfort caused by the fluid. The procedure to remove ascitic fluid usually takes 30 to 60 minutes. Obtaining a specimen usually takes about 15 minutes. Emphasize the importance of remaining still during the procedure. Include in your explanation when and where the procedure will occur and who will be present.
- Have the client void just before the paracentesis. *This lessens the possibility of puncturing the urinary bladder.* Notify the physician if the client cannot void.
- Help the client assume a sitting position in bed or in a chair. *This allows the fluid to accumulate in the lower abdominal cavity, and the force of gravity and the pressure of the abdominal organs will help the flow of the fluid from the cavity.* Some clients may be able

to sit on the edge of the bed with pillows to support the back.

- Cover the client to expose only the necessary area. If using a fenestrated drape, place the opening at the site where the fluid will be removed.

### During the Procedure

**2. Assist and monitor the client.**

- Support the client verbally, and describe the steps of the procedure as needed.
- Observe the client closely for signs of distress, e.g., abnormal pulse rate, skin color, and blood pressure. Observe for signs of hypovolemic shock induced by the loss of fluid: pallor, dyspnea, diaphoresis (profuse perspiration), and a drop in blood pressure.
- Place a small sterile dressing over the site of the incision after the cannula or aspirating needle is withdrawn. *This prevents bleeding or leakage of fluid.*

### Postprocedure

**3. Monitor the client closely.**

- Observe for hypovolemic shock (see step 2).
- Observe the puncture site regularly for leakage.
- Observe the client for any scrotal edema.
- Monitor vital signs, urine output, and drainage from the puncture site every 15 minutes for at least 2 hours and every hour for four hours thereafter, or as the client's condition indicates.
- Measure the abdominal girth with a tape measure in the same place it was measured preprocedure.

**4. Document all relevant information.**

- Record the procedure on the client's chart, including the date and time; the name of the physician; the girth of the client's abdomen before and after the procedure; the color, clarity, and amount of drained fluid; and any nursing assessments and interventions.

**5. Transport the correctly labeled specimens to the laboratory.**

▶

▶ **Procedure 22–2　Assisting with an Abdominal Paracentesis** *CONTINUED*

| | |
|---|---|
| **EVALUATION FOCUS** | Abdominal girth; weight; vital signs; urine output; drainage from puncture area; signs of infection (elevated body temperature); signs of internal hemorrhage (lowered blood pressure, accelerated pulse, hard, boardlike abdomen). |

**SAMPLE RECORDING**

| Date | Time | Notes |
|---|---|---|
| 7/18/95 | 1400 | Paracentesis performed by Dr Johnson, 300 ml clear serosanguinous fluid obtained. Abdominal girth at umbilical level 114 cm before, 109 cm after. Specimen sent to laboratory. P 72, BP 120/85. Slight pallor. Resting comfortably. ————————————————————— Roxanne J. Tuttle, NS |

## Thoracentesis

Normally, only sufficient fluid to lubricate the pleura is present in the pleural cavity. However excessive fluid can accumulate as a result of injury, infection, or other pathology. In such a case or in a case of pneumothorax, a physician may perform a **thoracentesis** to remove the excess fluid or air to ease breathing. Thoracentesis is also performed to introduce chemotherapeutic drugs intrapleurally.

The physician and the assisting nurse follow strict sterile technique. The physician attaches a syringe and/or stopcock to the aspirating needle. The stopcock must be in the closed position so that no air will enter the pleural space. The physician inserts the needle through the intercostal space to the pleural cavity. In some instances, the physician threads a small plastic tube through the needle and then withdraws the needle. (The tubing is less likely to puncture the pleura.)

If a syringe is used to receive the fluid, the plunger is pulled out to draw out the pleural fluid as the stopcock is opened. If a large container is used to receive the fluid, the tubing is attached from the stopcock to the adapter on the receiving bottle. When the adapter and stopcock are opened, negative pressure in the container created by a pump or suction machine will draw the fluid from the pleural cavity. After the fluid has been withdrawn, the physician removes the needle or plastic tubing.

## 22-3  Assisting with a Thoracentesis

Before the thoracentesis, note any orders for medication. A cough suppressant is sometimes ordered to be given 30 minutes before the procedure. An analgesic may also be ordered.

**PURPOSES**
- To remove excess fluid or air from the pleural cavity
- To introduce chemotherapeutic drugs intrapleurally

**ASSESSMENT FOCUS**

| |
|---|
| Baseline vital signs; respirations for bilateral depth and chest movement during inspiration; any differences in chest expansion between the sides; dyspnea, abnormal breath sounds, coughing, or chest pain; character and amount of sputum if cough is productive; allergies to skin antiseptics or anesthetic agents. |

## EQUIPMENT

- Sterile set containing
  Sterile sponges or gauze
    squares
  Skin antiseptic
  Drape or drapes (one may be
    fenestrated)
  2-ml syringe and #24 and #22
    needles
  Receptacle for the fluid (50-ml
  syringe and #16 needle or an
  airtight container)
  Three-way stopcock
  Two-way stopcock with
    connecting tubing
  Thoracentesis needle, usually a
    #15 needle about 5 to 7.5 cm
    (2 to 3 in) long
  Specimen container and label
  Local anesthetic
  Specimen containers and labels
- Sterile gloves
- Disposable gloves for the nurse
- Masks (optional)

## INTERVENTION

### Preprocedure

**1. Prepare the client.**

- Explain the procedure to the client. Normally, a thoracentesis is not painful, although the client may experience a feeling of pressure when the needle is inserted. The procedure may bring considerable relief if breathing has been difficult. The procedure takes only a few minutes, depending primarily on the time it takes for the fluid to drain from the pleural cavity. To avoid punc-

▶

▶ **Procedure 22–3 Assisting with a Thoracentesis** CONTINUED

⚠️ turing the lungs, <u>it is important for the client not to cough while the needle is inserted.</u> Include in your explanation when and where the procedure will occur and who will be present.

- Help the client assume a comfortable position. This is usually a sitting position with the arms above the head, which spreads the ribs and enlarges the intercostal space. Two positions commonly used are one in which the arm is elevated and stretched forward (Figure 22–8, *A*) and one in which the client leans forward over a pillow (Figure 22–8, *B*). To make sure that the needle is inserted below the fluid level when fluid is to be removed (or above any fluid if air is to be removed), the physician will palpate the chest and select the exact site for insertion of the needle. A site on the lower posterior chest is often used to remove fluid, and a site on the upper anterior chest is used to remove air.

- Cover the client as needed with a bath blanket. If using a fenestrated drape, place the opening at the site of the thoracentesis.

**During the Procedure**

**2. Support and monitor the client throughout.**

- Support the client verbally, and describe the steps of the procedure as needed.

- Observe the client for signs of distress, such as dyspnea, pallor, and coughing. If the client becomes distressed or has to cough, the procedure is halted briefly.

**3. Place a small sterile dressing over the site of the puncture.**

**Postprocedure**

**4. Monitor the client**.

- Assess pulse rate and respiratory rate and skin color. *A shift in the mediastinum (e.g., heart and large blood vessels) can occur with removal of large amounts of fluid.* Signs of mediastinal shift include pallor, accelerated pulse rate, dyspnea, accelerated respiration rate, and dizziness.

- Observe changes in the client's cough, sputum, respiratory depth, breath sounds, and note complaints of chest pain.

**5. Position the client appropriately**.

- Some agency protocols recommend that the client lie on the unaffected side with the head of the bed elevated 30° for at least 30 minutes. *This position facilitates expansion of the affected lung and eases respirations.*

**6. Document all relevant information**.

- Record the thoracentesis on the client's chart, including the date and time; the name of the physician; the amount, color, and clarity of fluid drained; and nursing assessments and interventions provided.

**7. Transport the specimens to the laboratory**.

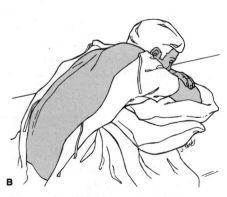

**FIGURE 22–8** Two positions commonly used for a thoracentesis: *A*, sitting on one side with the arm held to the front and up; *B*, sitting and leaning forward over a pillow.

| **EVALUATION FOCUS** | Respiratory rate, depth, and bilateral chest movement; bilateral breath sounds; vital signs; evidence of cyanosis or dyspnea; complaints of chest pain. |
| --- | --- |

**SAMPLE RECORDING**

| Date | Time | Notes |
| --- | --- | --- |
| 4/18/95 | 1500 | Thoracentesis performed by Dr Sargent. 275 ml of cloudy serosanguineous fluid removed. Specimen sent to laboratory. R 32, shallow and wet. P 76. Skin pale. Coughing occasionally. Small amount of thick white sputum. Resting more comfortably. —————————————— Ron L. Landry, NS |

## Bone Marrow Biopsy

A bone marrow biopsy is the removal of a specimen of bone marrow for laboratory study. The biopsy is used to detect specific diseases of the blood, e.g., pernicious anemia and leukemia. The bones of the body commonly used for a bone marrow biopsy are the sternum and the iliac crests (Figure 22–9).

The physician introduces a bone marrow needle with stylet through the skin and bone into the red marrow of the spongy bone (Figure 22–10). Once the needle is in the marrow space, the stylet is removed and a 10-ml syringe is attached to the needle. The plunger is withdrawn until 1 to 2 ml of marrow has been obtained. The physician replaces the stylet in the needle, withdraws the needle, and places the specimen in test tubes and/or on glass slides.

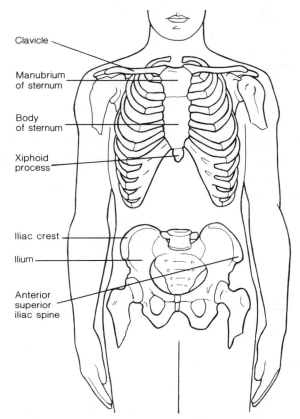

**FIGURE 22–9**  The sternum and the iliac crests are common sites for a bone marrow biopsy.

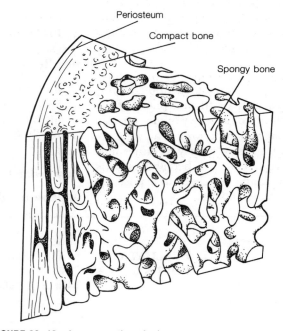

**FIGURE 22–10**  A cross section of a bone.

 **22-4**  **Assisting with a Bone Marrow Biopsy**

**PURPOSE**
• To obtain a bone marrow sample to check for abnormal blood cell development

**ASSESSMENT FOCUS**
Baseline vital signs; allergies to skin antiseptics or anesthetic agents.

## EQUIPMENT

- A sterile set containing
  Drape or drapes (one is often fenestrated)
  Antiseptic
  Local anesthetic

2-ml syringe and #25 needle
10-ml syringe
Bone marrow needle with stylet
Sterile gauze squares
Test tubes and/or glass slides

- Masks (optional)
- Sterile gloves
- Disposable, nonsterile gloves for the nurse
- Specimen containers and labels

▶

▶ **Procedure 22–4  Assisting with a Bone Marrow Biopsy** *CONTINUED*

## INTERVENTION

### Preprocedure

### 1. Prepare the client.

- Explain the procedure. The client may experience pain when the marrow is aspirated. There may be a crunching sound when the needle is pushed through the cortex of the bone. The entire procedure usually takes 15 to 30 minutes. Include in your explanation when and where the procedure will occur and who will be present.

- Help the client assume a supine position (with one pillow if desired) for a biopsy of the sternum (sternal puncture) or a prone position for a biopsy of either iliac crest. Fold the bedclothes back or drape the client to expose the area.

### During the Procedure

### 2. Monitor and support the client throughout.

- Describe the steps of the procedure as needed, and provide verbal support.

- Observe the client for pallor, diaphoresis, and faintness due to bleeding or pain.

### 3. Place a small dressing over the site of the puncture after the needle is withdrawn.

- Some agency protocols recommend direct pressure over the site for 5 to 10 minutes to prevent bleeding.

### Postprocedure

### 4. Monitor the client.

- Assess for discomfort and bleeding from the site. The client may experience some tenderness in the area. Bleeding and hematoma formation need to be assessed for several days. Report any bleeding or pain to the nurse in charge.

- Provide an analgesic as needed and ordered.

### 5. Document all relevant information.

- Record the procedure, including the date and time of the procedure, the name of the physician, and any nursing assessments and interventions.

### 6. Transport the specimens to the laboratory.

---

**EVALUATION FOCUS**

| Vital signs and puncture site for bleeding. |
| --- |

**SAMPLE RECORDING**

| Date | Time | Notes |
| --- | --- | --- |
| 8/19/95 | 0900 | Bone marrow biopsy from right iliac crest performed by Dr Rosenthal. Site dry, no apparent bleeding. No complaints of discomfort. Specimen sent to the laboratory. —————————————————— Donna S. Lambert, NS |

## Liver Biopsy

A liver biopsy is a short procedure, generally performed at the client's bedside, in which a sample of liver tissue is aspirated. A physician inserts a needle in the intercostal space between two of the right lower ribs and into the liver (Figure 22–11) or through the abdomen below the right rib cage (subcostally). The client exhales and stops breathing while the physician inserts the biopsy needle, injects a small amount of sterile normal saline to clear the needle of blood or particles of tissue picked up during insertion, and aspirates liver tissue by drawing back on the plunger of the syringe. After the needle is withdrawn, the nurse applies pressure to the site to prevent bleeding, often by positioning the client on the biopsy site.

Because many clients with liver disease have blood clotting defects and are prone to bleeding, prothrombin time and platelet count are normally taken well in advance of the test. If the test results are abnormal, the biopsy may be contraindicated.

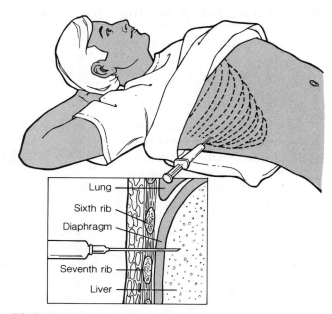

**FIGURE 22–11** A common site for a liver biopsy.

---

 **22-5** ## Assisting with a Liver Biopsy

**PURPOSES**
- To obtain data about the nature of liver disease
- To facilitate diagnosis
- To gain information about specific changes in liver tissue

**ASSESSMENT FOCUS**

> Client's ability to hold the breath for up to 10 seconds and remain still while the biopsy needle is inserted; prothrombin time and platelet count; allergies to skin antiseptics and anesthetic agents.

---

### EQUIPMENT

☐ Sterile liver biopsy set containing

    Sterile sponges or gauze squares with an antiseptic solution

    2-ml syringe and a #22 and #25 needle (6 in)

Large biopsy syringe and needle

Drapes

Local anesthetic

Sterile normal saline

Specimen container with formalin

☐ Face masks (optional)
☐ Sterile gloves
☐ Disposable gloves for the nurse
☐ Specimen containers and labels

---

### INTERVENTION

**Preprocedure**

**1. Prepare the client.**

- Give preprocedural medications as ordered. *Vitamin K may be given for several days before the biopsy to reduce the risk of hemorrhage. Vitamin K may be lacking in some clients with liver disease. It is essential for the production of prothrombin, which is required for blood clotting.*

- Explain the procedure. Tell the client

    **a.** What the physician will do,

i.e., take a small sample of liver tissue by putting a needle into the client's side or abdomen.

    **b.** That a sedative and local anesthetic will be given, so the client will feel no pain.

▶

► **Procedure 22–5 Assisting with a Liver Biopsy** *CONTINUED*

**c.** When and where the procedure will occur.

**d.** Who will be present.

**e.** The time required.

**f.** What to expect as the procedure is being performed; e.g., the client may experience mild discomfort when the local anesthetic is injected and slight pressure when the biopsy needle is inserted.

- Ensure that the client fasts for at least 2 hours before the procedure.

- Administer the appropriate sedative about 30 minutes beforehand or at the specified time.

- Help the client assume a supine position, with the upper right quadrant of the abdomen exposed. Cover the client with the bedclothes so that only the abdominal area is exposed.

**During the Procedure**

**2. Monitor and support the client throughout**.

- Support the client in a supine position.

- Instruct the client to take a few deep inhalations and exhalations and to hold the breath after the final exhalation for up to 10 seconds as the needle is inserted, the biopsy obtained, and the needle withdrawn. *Holding the breath after exhalation immobilizes the chest wall and liver and keeps the diaphragm in its highest position, avoiding injury to the diaphragm and laceration of the liver.*

- Instruct the client to resume breathing when the needle is withdrawn.

- Apply pressure to the site of the puncture. *Pressure will help stop any bleeding.*

**3. Apply a small dressing to the site of the puncture**.

**Postprocedure**

**4. Position the client appropriately**.

- Assist the client to a right side-lying position with a small pillow or folded towel under the biopsy site (Figure 22–12). Instruct the client to remain in this position for several hours. *The right lateral position compresses the biopsy site of the liver against the chest wall and minimizes the escape of blood or bile through the puncture site by applying pressure to the area.*

**5. Monitor the client**.

- Assess the client's vital signs— i.e., pulse, respirations, blood pressure—every 15 minutes for the first hour following the test or until the signs are stable. Then monitor vital signs every hour for 24 hours or as needed. *Complications of a liver biopsy are rare, but hemorrhage from a perforated blood vessel can occur.*

- Determine whether the client is experiencing abdominal pain. *Severe abdominal pain may indicate bile peritonitis (an inflammation of the peritoneal lining of the abdomen caused by bile leaking from a perforated bile duct).*

- Check the biopsy site for localized bleeding. Pressure dressings may be required if bleeding does occur.

**6. Document all relevant information**.

- Record the procedure, including the date and time it was performed, the name of the physician, and all nursing assessments and interventions.

**7. Transport the specimens to the laboratory**.

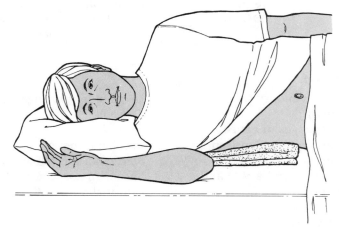

**FIGURE 22–12** The position to provide pressure on a liver biopsy site.

| EVALUATION FOCUS | Vital signs; bleeding from puncture site; complaints of abdominal pain. |
|---|---|

▶ **Procedure 22–5** *CONTINUED*

**SAMPLE RECORDING**

| Date | Time | Notes |
|------|------|-------|
| 2/13/95 | 1000 | Liver biopsy performed by Dr Martinez. Specimen sent to laboratory. P 86, R 16 and regular, BP 110/76/70. Small amount bleeding at site (0.3 cm diameter). Resting comfortably in right lateral position. ———————<br>——————————————————————————— Theresa A. Milligan, NS |

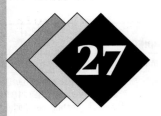

# Preventing the Transfer of Microorganisms

## PROCEDURE

# 27-1 Performing a Surgical Hand Scrub

**PURPOSES**

- To render the hands and forearms as free as possible of microorganisms
- To apply an antimicrobial residue on the skin and reduce the growth of microorganisms for several hours

## EQUIPMENT

- Antimicrobial solution
- Deep sink with foot, knee, or elbow controls
- Towels for drying the hands
- Nail-cleaning tool, such as a file or orange stick
- Two surgical scrub brushes
- Mask and cap

## INTERVENTION

**1. Prepare for the surgical hand scrub.**

- Remove wristwatch and all rings, unless plain bands are allowed by agency protocol. Ensure that fingernails are trimmed. *A wristwatch and rings can harbor microorganisms and be damaged by water.*

- Make sure that sleeves are above the elbows.

- Ensure that the uniform is well-tucked in at the waist. *A loose-fitting uniform can contaminate the hands if it touches them.*

- Apply cap and face mask.

- Turn on the water, and adjust the temperature to lukewarm. *Warm water removes less protective oil from the skin than hot water. Soap irritates the skin more when hot water is used.*

**2. Scrub the hands.**

- Wet the hands and forearms under running water, holding the hands above the level of the elbows so that the water runs from the fingertips to the elbows (Figure 27–1). *The hands will become cleaner than the elbows. The water should run from the least contaminated to the most contaminated area.*

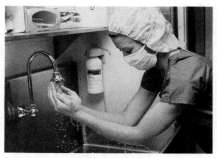

**FIGURE 27–1** The hands are held higher than the elbows during a hand wash before sterile technique.

- Apply 2 to 4 ml (1 tsp) antimicrobial solution to the hands. Most agencies supply a liquid antimicrobial beside the sink. In some agencies, antimicrobial soap wafers are available.

- Use firm, rubbing, and circular movements to wash the palms and backs of the hands, the wrists, and the forearms. Interlace the fingers and thumbs, and move the hands back and forth. Continue washing for 20 to 25 seconds. *Circular strokes clean most effectively, and rubbing ensures a thorough and mechanical cleaning action. (Other areas of the hands still need to be cleaned, however.)*

- Hold the hands and arms under the running water to rinse thor-oughly, keeping the hands higher than the elbows. *The nurse rinses from the cleanest to the least clean area.*

- Check the nails, and clean them with a file or orange stick if necessary. Rinse the nail tool after each nail is cleaned. *Sediment under the nails is removed more readily when the hands are moist. Rinsing the nail tool prevents the transmission of sediment from one nail to another.*

- Apply antimicrobial solution and lather the hands again. Using a scrub brush, scrub each hand for 45 seconds. Scrub each side of all fingers, including the skin between each of the fingers and the thumb, and the back and the palm of the hand. *Scrubbing loosens bacteria, including those in the creases of the hands.*

- Using the scrub brush, scrub from the wrists to 5 cm (2 in) above each elbow. Scrub all parts of the arms: lower forearm (15 seconds), upper forearm (15 seconds), and antecubital space to marginal area above elbows (15 seconds). Continue to hold the hands higher than the elbows. *Scrubbing thus proceeds from the*

▶

▶ **Procedure 27–1 Performing a Surgical Hand Scrub** CONTINUED

*cleanest area (hands) to the least clean area (upper arm).*

- Discard the brush.

- Rinse hands and arms thoroughly so that the water flows from the hands to the elbows. *Rinsing removes resident and transient bacteria and sediment.*

- If a longer scrub is required, use a second brush and scrub each hand and arm with soap for the recommended time (e.g., each hand for 30 seconds, forearms for 45 seconds).

- Discard second brush, and rinse hands and arms thoroughly.

- Turn off the water with the foot or knee pedal.

**3. Dry the hands and arms.**

- Use a sterile towel to dry one hand thoroughly from the fingers to the elbow. Use a rotating motion. Use a second sterile towel to dry the second hand in the same manner. In some agencies towels are of a sufficient size that one half can be used to dry one hand and arm and the second half for the second hand and arm. *Moist skin readily becomes chapped and subject to open sores. Thorough drying also makes it easier to don sterile gloves. The nurse dries the hands from the cleanest to the least clean area.*

- Discard the towels.

- Keep the hands in front and above the waist. *This position maintains the cleanliness of the hands and prevents accidental contamination.*

# Assisting with Hygiene

## PROCEDURES

# Infant Hygiene Care

Practices in the hygienic care of infants vary considerably. For example, in some agencies the nurse bathes the newborn when it is first admitted to the nursery; in others, the nurse simply removes any birth debris from the infant's face, for aesthetic reasons, and then diapers and wraps the baby warmly in a blanket. Some agencies require that the nurse remove the **vernix caseosa** (the whitish, cheesy, greasy protective material found on the skin at birth), whereas others do not. When the newborn's status is stabilized, daily hygienic care often includes a sponge bath until the umbilical cord stump falls off. Cord care and, for some male infants, circumcision care

are also required. The cord stump usually falls off spontaneously in 5 to 8 days, but it may remain up to 2 weeks. Procedure 29–1 explains how to give an infant sponge bath.

After the cord stump has separated and the umbilicus is healed, the infant's body can be immersed in a tub of water. New parents need information from the nurse about this basic hygienic care. Many agencies provide bath demonstrations and opportunities for new parents to ask questions before they leave the hospital. Procedure 29–2 describes how to give an infant tub bath. Procedure 29–3 describes how to change a diaper.

---

## 29-1   Giving an Infant Sponge Bath

 Before commencing the infant's sponge bath, determine (a) whether the infant requires a complete or partial bath, (b) whether the baby's weight is to be taken in conjunction with the bath; and (c) whether the infant's temperature is to be taken after the bath. Wear gloves when having contact with a baby's mucous membranes, non-intact skin, body fluids, and blood. Also wear gloves during the period after delivery until the first bath is completed and during diapering.

**PURPOSES**
- To remove the vernix caseosa that covers the skin of the fetus, particularly from creases and folds, such as under the foreskin of the glans penis in male babies and between the labia in female babies, if required
- To clean the skin, including the scalp, genitals, and buttocks
- To provide care for the umbilical cord stump
- To assess the skin, healing of the cord stump and circumcision incision, and general physical growth and functioning

**ASSESSMENT FOCUS**
> Dry, cracked, or peeling skin areas; cradle cap on the scalp; signs of redness at the cord stump or a foul-smelling discharge around the umbilicus; diaper rash, healing of circumcision, overall color of skin.

---

## EQUIPMENT

- Basin with water at 38° to 40° C (100° to 105° F)
- Gloves
- Towel to place under the baby during the bath
- Disposable cups
- Soft washcloth or absorbent pad

- Cotton balls
- Moisture-resistant bag
- Mild, nonperfumed soap in a container
- Soft-bristled brush or baby comb
- Isopropyl alcohol

- Bath blanket or towel to cover the infant
- Mild lotion or baby oil if needed for dry skin
- Shirt and/or nightgown
- Diaper

▶ **Procedure 29–1** *CONTINUED*

**INTERVENTION**

**1. Prepare the environment.**

- Wash hands before handling a newborn, because infants have few defenses against unfamiliar microorganisms.

- Ensure that the room is warm and free of drafts. *This is particularly important when caring for newborns, because their temperature-regulating mechanisms are not completely developed.*

- Measure the temperature of the water with a bath thermometer, or test it against the inside of your wrist or elbow.

- Don gloves, if necessary.

**2. Prepare the infant.**

- Remove the infant's diaper, and wipe away any feces on the baby's perineum with tissues.

- Reassure the infant before and during the bath by talking in soothing tones, and hold the infant firmly but gently.

- Undress the infant, and bundle it in a supine position in a towel.

- Place small articles such as safety pins out of the infant's reach.

- Ascertain the infant's weight and vital signs. They are often measured in conjunction with a bath.

**3. Wash the infant's head.**

- Clean the baby's eyes with water only, using a washcloth or cotton balls. Use a separate corner of the washcloth or a separate ball for each eye. Wipe from the inner to the outer canthus. Some nurses prefer to wash the infant's eyes, face, and scalp *before* the infant is undressed. Dispose of cotton balls in moisture-resistant bag. *Using a separate corner or ball prevents the transmission of mircoorganisms from one eye to the other. Wiping away from the*

inner canthus avoids wiping debris into the nasolacrimal duct.

- Wash and dry the baby's face using water only. Soap may be used to clean the ears. *Soap can be very irritating to the eyes.*

- Pick the baby up using the football hold; that is, hold the baby against your side, supporting the body with your forearm and the head with the palm of your hand (Figure 29–1). Position the baby's head over the washbasin, and lather the scalp with a mild soap. Massage the lather over the scalp using the soft-bristled brush, the baby comb, or your fingertips. *This loosens any dry scales from the scalp and helps to prevent cradle cap.* If cradle cap is present, it may be treated with baby oil, a dandruff shampoo, or ointment prescribed by the physician.

- Rinse and dry the scalp well. Place the baby supine again.

**4. Wash the infant's body.**

- Wash, rinse, and dry each arm and hand, paying particular attention to the axilla. Avoid excessive rubbing. Dry thoroughly. *Rubbing can cause skin irritation, and moisture can cause excoriation of the skin.*

- Wash, rinse, and dry the baby's chest and abdomen.

- Keep the baby covered with the bath blanket or towel between washing and rinsing. *Covering the infant prevents chilling.*

- Clean the base of the umbilical cord with a cotton ball dipped in 70% isopropyl alcohol. Other antiseptics, such as povidone-iodine (Betadine) are also used. *Using alcohol promotes drying and prevents infection.*

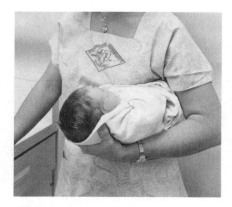

**FIGURE 29–1** Using a football hold to carry an infant.

- Wash, rinse, and dry the baby's legs and feet. Expose only one leg and foot at a time. Give special attention to the areas between the toes. *Keeping exposure to a minimum maintains the baby's warmth.*

- Turn the baby on the stomach or side. Wash, rinse, and dry the back.

**5. Clean the genitals and anterior perineum.**

- Place the baby on the back. Clean and dry the genitals and anterior perineal area from front to back. *The rectal area is cleaned last because it is the most contaminated.*

- Clean the folds of the groin.

- For females, separate the labia, and clean between them. Clean the genital area from front to back, using moistened cotton balls. Use a clean swab for each stroke. *The smegma that collects between the folds of the labia (and under the foreskin in males) facilitates bacterial growth and should be removed. Lotions, powders, and so on, can also accumulate between the labia and need to be removed. Clean swabs are used to avoid spreading microorganisms from the rectal area to the urethra.*

▶

▶ **Procedure 29–1 Giving an Infant Sponge Bath** *CONTINUED*

- If a male infant is uncircumcised, retract the foreskin if possible, and clean the glans penis, using a moistened cotton ball. If the foreskin is tight, do not forcibly retract it. Gentle pressure on a tight foreskin over a period of days or weeks may accomplish eventual retraction. **Phimosis** (narrowness of the opening of the foreskin) may require correction by circumcision. After swabbing, replace the foreskin to prevent edema (swelling) of the glans penis. Clean the shaft of the penis and the scrotum. In some agencies, the foreskin is not retracted.

- If a male infant has been recently circumcised, clean the glans penis by gently squeezing a cotton ball moistened with clear water over the site. Note any signs of bleeding or infection. In some agencies, petroleum jelly or a bactericidal ointment is applied to the circumcision site. Avoid applying excessive quantities of ointment. *Excess ointment may obstruct the urinary meatus.*

- Apply A and D Ointment (lanolin and petrolatum) to the perineum according to agency protocol. *This helps prevent diaper rash.*

6. **Clean the posterior perineum and buttocks.**

- Grasp both of the baby's ankles, raise the feet, and elevate the buttocks.

- Wash and rinse the area with the washcloth.

- Dry the area, and apply ointment, according to agency policy. Do not apply powder. *The baby may inhale particles of powder, which can irritate the respiratory tract.*

7. **Check for dry, cracked, or peeling skin, and apply a mild baby oil or lotion as required.**

8. **Dress and position the infant.**

- Clothe the baby in a shirt (if the temperature of the environment

warrants it) and/or nightgown and a diaper. Place the diaper below the cord site. *Exposing the cord site to the air will promote healing.*

- Until the umbilicus and circumcision are healed, position the baby on its side in the crib with a rolled towel or diaper behind the back for support. *This position allows more air to circulate around the cord site, facilitates drainage of mucus from the mouth, and is more comfortable for circumcised babies.*

- After the umbilicus and circumcision are healed, place the baby in a safe position.

- Cover and bundle the baby with a blanket, if the environmental temperature permits. *This gives the baby a sense of security as well as providing warmth.*

9. **Record any significant assessments.**

---

**EVALUATION FOCUS**

| Reddened areas or skin rashes; color and consistency of stool; state of cord stump; state of circumcision incision. |
| --- |

**SAMPLE RECORDING**

| Date | Time | Notes |
| --- | --- | --- |
| 3/3/95 | 0900 | Bathed infant. Skin moist, slightly jaundiced. Umbilicus healing well, no discharge. Responsive to tactile stimulation ——————— Laurie Law, SN |

# 29-2   Giving an Infant Tub Bath

 Before commencing an infant tub bath, determine (a) whether the baby's weight and temperature are to be measured in conjunction with the bath, and (b) any skin problems and other progress assessments that need to be made.

**PURPOSES**
- To clean and deodorize the skin
- To stimulate circulation to the skin
- To provide a sense of well-being
- To assess the skin, reflexes, and so on

**ASSESSMENT FOCUS**

| Skin color, texture, turgor, and temperature; presence of lesions or skin breakdown. |
|---|

## EQUIPMENT
- Tub with bath water at 38° to 40° C (100° to 105° F)
- Towel to place under the baby before and after the bath and to dry the infant
- Soft washcloth or absorbent pad
- Cotton balls
- Bag in which to dispose of used cotton balls
- Mild, nonperfumed soap in a container
- Soft-bristled brush
- Bath blanket or towel to cover the infant before and after the bath
- Mild lotion or baby oil if needed for dry skin
- Shirt and/or nightgown
- Diaper
- Gloves if indicated

## INTERVENTION

### 1. Prepare the bath area.

- Prepare a flat, padded surface in the bath area on which to dress and undress the infant. It should be high enough so that you or the parent can avoid stooping, which can produce back strain. Usually parents use a counter or table top in the bathroom or kitchen, unless a bathinette is available. Cover the surface with a towel.

- Assemble all supplies needed so that they are within easy reach. *A baby left unattended or out of sight for even a few seconds can move or fall from the bath area.* Keep supplies out of reach of the infant, however. *Small articles, such as safety pins, can be hazardous to an active and curious infant.*

- For small infants, use a wash basin.

- Place the tub or basin near the dressing surface to prevent exposure and chilling when transferring the baby in and out of the tub. Be sure the room is warm and free from drafts.

- Measure the temperature of the water with a bath thermometer, or test it against the inside of your wrist or elbow.

### 2. Clean the infant's eyes and face before placing the infant in the tub.

- Follow Procedure 29–1, step 3.

### 3. Pick up and place the infant in the tub.

- Pick up and hold the baby securely, with the head and shoulders supported on one forearm and the hips and buttocks supported on the other hand (Figure 29–2). *Young infants have not de-* *veloped sufficiently to hold their heads up alone.*

- Gradually immerse the baby into the tub. *This gives the infant time to adjust to the water.*

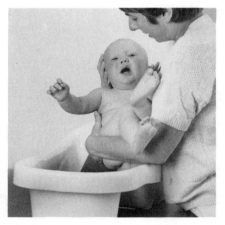

**FIGURE 29–2**   Holding an infant while placing him in a tub.

▶

▶ **Procedure 29–2  Giving an Infant Tub Bath** *CONTINUED*

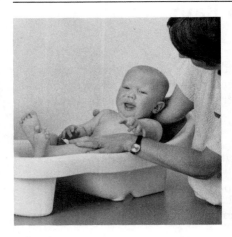

**FIGURE 29–3** Keeping the infant's head and back supported during a tub bath.

**4. Wash the infant.**

- Keeping the baby's head and back supported on your forearm (Figure 29–3), lather the scalp with a mild soap. Massage the lather over the scalp, using the soft-bristled brush or your fingertips. Rinse the scalp well. *This loosens any dry scales from the scalp and helps prevent cradle cap.* If cradle cap is present, it may be treated with mineral oil, a dandruff shampoo, or ointment prescribed by the physician.

- Soap and rinse the baby's trunk, extremities, genitals, and perineal area with your free hand. Hold the baby as shown in Figure 29–3 throughout. If the baby enjoys the bath, this can be done in a leisurely manner.

**5. Remove the infant from the tub, and dry the infant well.**

- Remove the baby from the tub by the hold shown in Figure 29–2, and quickly bundle the baby in a towel. *It is important to avoid chilling the infant.*

- Gently pat the baby dry, giving special attention to the body creases and folds. *Rubbing can cause skin irritation.*

- Apply baby oil or lotion to dry, cracked, or peeling areas.

**6. Ensure the infant's comfort and safety.**

- Clothe the baby in a shirt (if the temperature of the environment warrants it) and/or a nightgown and a diaper.

- Place the baby in a side-lying position in the crib. *This position facilitates the drainage of mucus from the mouth.*

- Cover and bundle the baby with a blanket, if the environmental temperature permits. *This gives the baby a sense of security as well as providing warmth.*

**7. Document all pertinent information.**

- Record any significant observations, such as reddened areas or skin rashes, and the color and consistency of the stool.

**EVALUATION FOCUS**

| See Assessment Focus. |
| --- |

**SAMPLE RECORDING**

| Date | Time | Notes |
| --- | --- | --- |
| 3/5/95 | 1010 | Tub bath given. Skin clear, moist, warm. No reddened areas. ——————— Laurie Law, SN |

**Changing a Diaper**

When a diaper becomes soiled with either urine or feces, it should be changed promptly so that the baby's skin does not become irritated by the waste products. The infant's perineal–genital area is washed and thoroughly dried before a clean diaper is applied.

 Before commencing to change the diaper, determine (a) type of diaper required and (b) any special precautions, e.g., not elevating buttocks by lifting legs, need for a stool specimen.

**PURPOSES**
- To maintain the infant's comfort and cleanliness
- To maintain the integrity of the skin by preventing irritation from urine and/or feces

**ASSESSMENT FOCUS**

Condition of the skin around the perineum and buttocks; amount, color, and odor of the urine and feces; state and progress of circumcision.

## EQUIPMENT
- Clean disposable or cloth diaper
- Receptacle for the soiled diaper
- Commercially prepared wipes
- or a basin with warm water, 38° to 40° C (100° to 105° F)
- Soap
- Washcloth
- Towel
- Mild lotion or protective ointment, e.g., zinc oxide
- Gloves

## INTERVENTION

**1. Fold a clean diaper, if using a cloth diaper.**

- Three methods can be used to fold diapers: rectangular, triangular, or kite (Figures 29–4 to 29–6). When using the rectangular method, provide an extra thickness of material either at the front (for boys) or the back (for girls) for additional absorbency. It may also be placed at the front for girls who are positioned on their stomachs for sleep (so that the urine runs to the front).

**2. Position and handle the infant appropriately.**

- Place the infant in a supine position on a clean, flat surface near the assembled supplies.
- Handle the infant slowly and securely, and speak in soothing tones. *Slow movements and soothing voice tones will help calm any of the infant's fears.*

**3. Remove the soiled diaper.**

-  Place your fingers between the baby's skin and the diaper, and unpin the diaper on each side. Close the pins, and place them out of reach of the infant. *The fingers protect the baby from being pricked as the pins are removed. Babies may grab the pins and place them in their mouths if the pins are within reach.*
- Pull the front of the diaper down between the infant's legs.
- Grasp the infant's ankles with one hand, and lift the buttocks (Figure 29–7).
- Use the clean portion of the diaper to wipe any excess urine or feces from the buttocks. Wipe from anterior to posterior. *Wiping toward the posterior of the infant wipes away the urethral orifice and decreases the possibility of transferring microorganisms to the urinary tract.*
- Remove the diaper. Lower the baby's buttocks. Dispose of the diaper. Do not let the infant out of your sight or reach. *The infant could roll over and off the changing surface.*

**4. Clean the buttocks and anal-genital area.**

- Use warm water and soap or commercial cleansing tissues.
- Clean toward the posterior as in step 3, above. *Cleaning removes remaining urine and feces, which can irritate the skin.*

► **Procedure 29–3 Changing a Diaper** *CONTINUED*

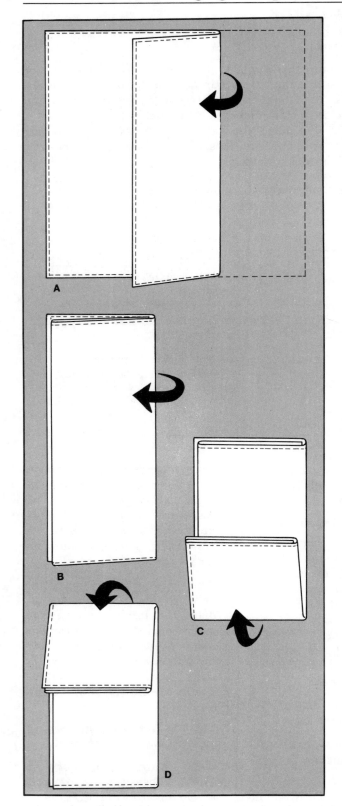

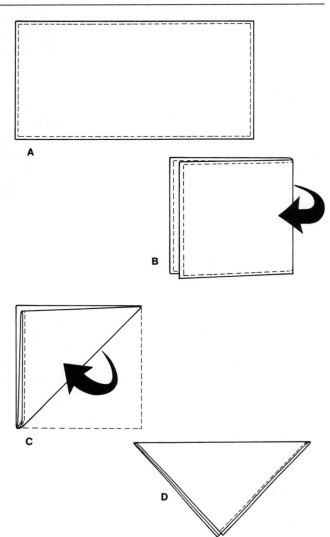

**FIGURE 29–5** The triangular method of folding a diaper: *A*, Fold a square cloth to a rectangular shape; *B*, fold the cloth again to form a square; *C*, bring opposite corners together to form a triangle; *D*, apply the triangle with the fold at the waist.

**FIGURE 29–4** The rectangular method of folding a diaper: *A, B*, Fold the diaper into a rectangle by bringing the sides over; *C*, fold the bottom edge up to provide the thickness in front; or *D*, fold the top edge down to provide the thickness at the back.

► **Procedure 29–3** *CONTINUED*

- Rinse and dry the area well with the towel. *Drying well prevents irritation of the skin by moisture.*

- Apply a protective ointment or lotion to the perineum and buttocks, especially to the skin creases.

**5. Apply the clean diaper, and fasten it securely.**

- Lay the diaper flat on a clean surface with the folded edges up,

and place the baby on the center of the diaper width so that the back edge of the diaper is at waist level.

*or*

Grasp the baby's ankles with one hand and raise the baby's legs and buttocks. Place the diaper under the baby so that the back edge is at waist level.

- Draw the diaper up between the baby's legs to the waist in front.

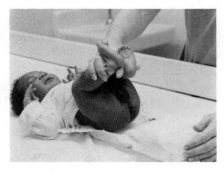

**FIGURE 29–7** Lifting the infant's buttocks to remove a soiled diaper.

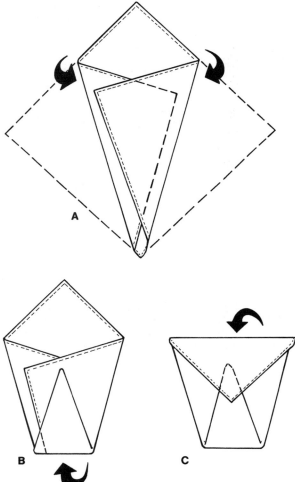

**FIGURE 29–6** The kite method of folding a diaper: *A,* Make a triangle by folding the side corners to the center; *B,* bring the bottom corner up to the center; *C,* fold down the top corner.

- Fold the diaper below the umbilicus until the infant's cord stump has healed. *This promotes drying and healing of the stump site and minimizes possible infection from wet diapers.*

- Fasten the diaper at the waist with tape provided so that it fits snugly. If using safety pins for cloth diapers, hold your fingers between the baby and the diaper while pinning. *The fingers protect the baby from being pricked with the pins.*

- Position the pins either vertically or horizontally. *The horizontal position is suggested when the child is old enough to sit. The pins are then less likely to poke the body. The vertical position is suggested for diapers pinned at the sides rather than at the front, if the infant does not yet sit up.*

- Insert the diaper pins so that they face upward or outward. *If a pin opens inadvertently, it will not puncture the baby's thigh or abdomen.*

**6. Ensure infant comfort and safety.**

- Dress the infant with additional clothes as required.

▶ **Procedure 29–3  Changing a Diaper** *CONTINUED*

- Return the infant to the crib.

**7. Document all pertinent information.**

- Record stool and/or urine observations on the record sheet and/or the infant's chart.

- Record other pertinent observations, such as skin redness, on the patient's record.

| | |
|---|---|
| **EVALUATION FOCUS** | See Assessment Focus. |

**SAMPLE RECORDING**

| Date | Time | Notes |
|---|---|---|
| 10/3/95 | 1800 | Father assisted with diaper change. Demonstrated procedure without difficulty. Small amount of yellow stool noted. ———————— Amy Mulcahay, RN |

**29-4**   # Care of the Client with Pediculosis

| | |
|---|---|
| **PURPOSE** | • To destroy and remove lice |
| **ASSESSMENT FOCUS** | Presence of skin abrasions from scratching; location of lice (head, body, or pubic area); presence of lice on other family members or other close contacts. |

## EQUIPMENT

### For Head Lice
- Shampoo containing gamma benzene hexachloride (or lindane) or similar acting medications, e.g., Kwell, GBH, Scabine
- Fine-toothed comb and brush

### For Body and Pubic Lice
- Cream, lotion, or powder containing a medication, e.g., Kwell
- Topical ointment for the skin as ordered, e.g., antibiotic, antipruritic, or steroid cream

### For All Types
- Gown and gloves
- Surgical cap (as recommended by agency)
- Bath towels
- Impervious isolation bag
- Clean gown and bed linens

## INTERVENTION

### 1. Remove head lice.
- Don gown, gloves, and (if agency recommends) surgical cap before the procedure. *These prevent spread to the nurse's clothing and skin and subsequent transmission to others.*

- Place a small damp or dry washcloth over the client's eyes to protect them from the shampoo. *The medication in the shampoo is irritating to the eyes.*

- Apply the medicated shampoo according to the manufacturer's directions. Some shampoos may be left in place for 5 minutes.

- Shampoo the hair and scalp thoroughly. Be careful to keep the medicated shampoo out of the client's eyes.

- Rinse the hair and scalp thoroughly. *Thorough rinsing removes dead lice and the medicated shampoo and prevents scalp irritation.*

- If necessary, remove dead lice and nits with a fine-toothed comb or brush dipped in hot vinegar (optional). *A comb or brush dipped in hot vinegar tends to loosen nit cement and facilitates removal of nits.*

- Disinfect the comb and brush with the medicated shampoo. Repeat the shampoo if indicated.

### 2. Remove body and pubic lice.
- Have the client bathe in soap and water.

- Don gown and gloves.

- Apply medicated topical cream or lotion to infested areas—e.g., axillae, chest, and pubic areas—and allow it to remain for the prescribed time period, according to the manufacturer's directions.

- Clean the treated areas with soap and water to remove dead lice and medication and prevent skin irritation.

- If eyelashes are involved, use a prescribed ophthalmic ointment as ordered and directed. Remove nits manually.

### 3. Dispose of linens and clothing appropriately.
- Place any used towels and the client's soiled gown and bed linen into a labeled isolation bag.

- Provide a clean gown and bed linens for the client.

- Dispose of your gown and gloves appropriately, and wash your hands.

### 4. Document any pertinent information.
- Include the date and time of treatment, area of the body treated, and all nursing assessments and interventions.

| | |
|---|---|
| **EVALUATION FOCUS** | Client's knowledge of preventive and control measures and presence of pediculi. |

►

▶ **Procedure 29–4 Care of the Client with Pediculosis** *CONTINUED*

**SAMPLE RECORDING**

| Date | Time | Notes |
|------|------|-------|
| 11/9/95 | 1030 | Hair shampooed with Kwell soap as ordered for pediculosis. Pustules present behind ears and at hairline. Instructed to shower and apply Kwell lotion. Infested clothing bagged for family to clean at home. ——————————————————————— Michelle M. Nutter, RN |

## 29-5 Braiding the Hair

Braiding is a method of entwining hair. For young children who have long hair, two braids can provide a particularly neat and attractive appearance. Braids (except cornrows) need to be undone daily, and the hair needs to be brushed and combed.

**PURPOSE**

• To maintain a neat appearance

**ASSESSMENT FOCUS**

Does the client desire a braid or braids?

## EQUIPMENT

□ Towel
□ Brush
□ Comb

□ Ribbon(s) or covered elastic band(s)

## INTERVENTION

**1. Brush and comb the hair, and remove any tangles.**

• For short hair, brush and comb one side at a time. Divide long hair into two sections by parting it down the middle from the front to the back. If the hair is very thick, divide each section into front and back subsections or into several layers.

• Holding one section at a time with one hand, brush from the scalp toward the ends. Rotate the wrist in such a way that the brush massages the scalp. Then comb that section of hair. *Massaging stimulates blood circulation in the scalp and thus nourishment of the hair.*

• Brush and comb each section, moving from one side of the head to the other.

• Brush and comb each layer, working from the ends toward the scalp. Mats can usually be pulled apart with fingers or worked out with repeated brushings.

• If the hair is very tangled, rub alcohol or an oil, such as mineral oil, on the strands to help loosen the tangles.

**2. Braid the hair.**

• To make one braid, divide the hair into three even sections (strands). For two braids, part the hair down the middle, and then divide each side into three strands. Two braids are usually more comfortable for clients lying in bed. *This avoids the need to lie on the bulk of one braid.*

• Hold the left strand in the left hand, the center strand by the second finger and thumb of the left hand, and the right strand in the right hand (Figure 29–8). Hold the strands firmly and tautly, but do not pull. *Pulling can damage the hair and cause pain.*

• Lay the right strand (3) over the middle strand (2). Transfer strand 3 to the left hand and strand 2 to the right hand (Figure 29–9). Strand 3 is now the middle strand, and strand 2 is the right strand.

• Still holding the strands of hair tautly, cross the left strand (1)

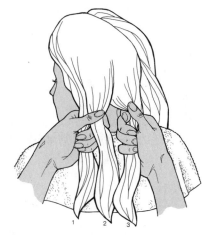

**FIGURE 29–8** Beginning step for braiding hair: dividing the hair into three even strands.

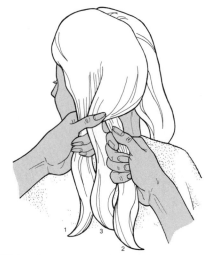

**FIGURE 29–9** Crossing the right outside strand over the middle strand.

►

▶ **Procedure 29–5 Braiding the Hair** *CONTINUED*

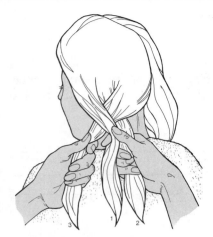

**FIGURE 29–10** Crossing the left outside strand over the new middle strand.

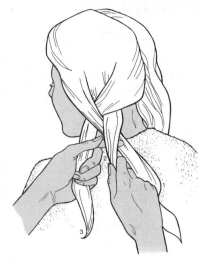

**FIGURE 29–11** Continuing to cross alternate side strands over the center strand.

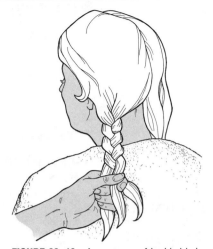

**FIGURE 29–12** Appearance of braided hair.

over the middle strand (3) (Figure 29–10). Strand 1 is now the middle strand, and strand 3 is the left strand. The left hand holds strand 3, the right fingers hold strand 1, and the right hand holds strand 2.

• Cross the right strand (2) over the center strand (1) (Figure 29–11). Then cross the left strand (3) over the middle strand (2).

• Continue crossing the side strands over the center strand, alternating right and left sides until you reach the ends of the strands (Figure 29–12).

• When all the hair has been braided, firmly secure the end of the braid with a covered elastic band or a ribbon so that the strands cannot come undone.

• Braid the other side of the hair if a second braid is needed.

# 29-6   Inserting Contact Lenses (Hard and Soft)

Before inserting contact lenses, determine (a) the client's own practices regarding cleaning and inserting the lenses, and (b) any reasons for not inserting the lenses.

| | |
|---|---|
| **PURPOSE** | • To enhance the client's visual acuity |
| **ASSESSMENT FOCUS** | Presence of eye inflammation, infection, discomfort, or excessive tearing; when lenses were last worn and cleaned; cleanliness of the lenses; any scratches on the lenses. |

## EQUIPMENT

☐ Client's lens storage case
☐ Gloves (optional)
☐ Wetting agent

## INTERVENTION

**1. Take the client's lens storage case, and select the correct lens for the eye.** *Each lens is ground to fit the individual eye and correct its visual defect.*

• Start with the right eye. *Always starting with the right eye establishes a habit so that incorrect placement of each lens is avoided.*

• Don gloves, if desired.

*To Insert Hard Lenses*

**2. Lubricate the lens.**

• Put a few drops of sterile wetting solution on the right lens. Solutions of saline, methyl cellulose, or polyvinyl alcohol are frequently used. *Wetting solution helps the lens to glide over the cornea, thus reducing the risk of injury.*

• Spread the wetting solution on both surfaces of the lens by using your thumb and index finger or an absorbent applicator, or place the lens in the palm of your hand and spread the solution with your index finger.

**3. Insert the lens.**

• Ask the client to tilt the head backward.

• Place the lens convex side down on the tip of your dominant index finger (the right, if you are righthanded; Figure 29–13).

• Separate the upper and lower eyelids of the right eye with the thumb and index finger of your nondominant hand (Figure 29–13). When separating the eyelids, exert gentle pressure with your fingers over the supraorbital and infraorbital bony prominences. *This prevents direct pressure, discomfort, and injury to the eyeball.*

• Place the lens as gently as possible on the cornea, directly over the iris and the pupil.

• Repeat the above steps for the other lens.

**4. If the lens is off center, center the lens.**

• Separate the eyelids, using the index or middle finger of the left hand to lift the upper lid and the index or middle finger of the right hand to depress the lower lid.

• Locate the lens, and ask the client to gaze in the opposite direction (Figure 29–14).

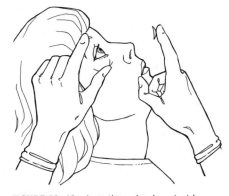

**FIGURE 29–13**   Inserting a hard contact lens.

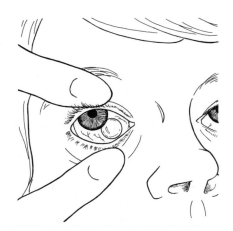

**FIGURE 29–14**   Locating a lens that is off center by separating the eyelids and asking the client to gaze in the opposite direction.

# ▶ Procedure 29–6 Inserting Contact Lenses *CONTINUED*

- Gently push the lens in the direction of the cornea, using a finger or the eyelid margins.
- Ask the client to look slowly toward the lens. The lens will slide easily onto the cornea as the client looks toward it.

*To Insert Soft Lenses*

### 5. Keep the dominant finger dry for insertion.

- Remove the lens from its saline-filled storage case with your nondominant hand. *Because "water-loving" soft contact lenses have a natural attraction to wet surfaces, the lens will adhere more readily to the moist eye if the finger is dry.*

### 6. Position the lens correctly for insertion.

*For A Regular Soft Lens*

- Hold the lens at the edge between your thumb and your index finger.
- Flex the lens slightly. The lens is in the correct position if the edges point inward. If the edges point outward, it is in the wrong position (i.e., inside out) and must be reversed (Figure 29–15). *A lens placed on the eye inside out is less comfortable (an edge sensation may be felt), tends to fold on the eye, can drop to a lower position on the eye, and may move excessively on blinking.*

*For an Ultrathin Soft Lens*

- Do not flex an ultrathin lens. Instead, put the lens on your placement finger and allow it to dry slightly for a few seconds.
- Closely inspect the lens to see whether the edges turn upward (Figure 29–16, *A*). If they turn downward (Figure 29–16, *B*), the lens is inside out and must be reversed. *Flexing an ultrathin lens may cause the lens to fold and stick together.*

### 7. Wet the lens with saline so-

lution using your nondominant fingers.

- See step 2 for hard lenses.

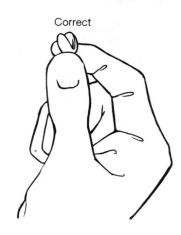

Correct

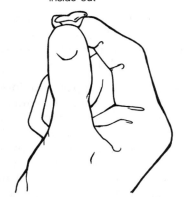

Inside out

**FIGURE 29–15** Checking the position of a soft contact lens before insertion.

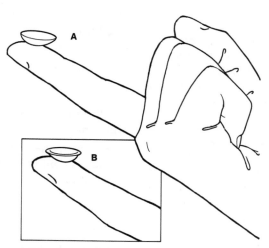

**FIGURE 29–16** Checking the position of an ultrathin contact lens before insertion: *A*, position is correct, i.e., edges are turned upward; *B*, lens is inside out and must be reversed.

### 8. Insert the lens.

- Ensure that your placement finger is dry. This is particularly important for ultrathin soft lenses.
- Place the lens convex side down on the tip of your dominant index finger.
- Insert the lens in the same manner as a hard contact lens.

### 9. Store lens equipment appropriately.

- Replace the lens container, lens cleaner, and wetting solution in the drawer of the bedside table.

### 10. Document pertinent information.

- Record insertion of the contact lenses if a nurse is required to remove them; otherwise, this is not normally recorded (consult agency protocol).
- Record all assessments, and report to the nurse in charge any problems observed in the eyes or the lenses.
- Record on the nursing care plan the time for the lenses to be removed.

► **Procedure 29–6** *CONTINUED*

**EVALUATION FOCUS**

> Discharge from eyes; color and clarity of conjunctiva; discomfort; tearing; client's perception of sight.

**SAMPLE RECORDING**

| Date | Time | Notes |
|------|------|-------|
| 10/10/95 | 2100 | Contact lenses inserted in both eyes. Slight white discharge from inner canthus R eye. Upper eyelid R eye reddened. No discomfort. States can read now. ———————————— Marilyn S. McLean, SN |

# 29-7 Removing Contact Lenses (Hard and Soft)

| PURPOSES | • To prevent eye damage from prolonged lens wearing<br>• To prevent loss of the lenses |
| --- | --- |
| ASSESSMENT FOCUS | Any eye irritation; length of time lens has been in place. |

## EQUIPMENT

- □ Gloves (optional)
- □ Flashlight (optional)
- □ Cotton applicator dipped in saline (optional)

- □ Lens storage case; or, if not available, two small medicine cups or specimen containers partially filled with normal saline solution and marked "L lens" and "R lens."

## INTERVENTION

**1. Locate the position of the lens.** *The lens must be positioned directly over the cornea for proper removal.*

- Don gloves, if needed.

- Ask the client to tilt the head backward.

- Retract the upper eyelid with your index finger, and ask the client to look up, down, and from side to side.

- Retract the lower eyelid with your index finger, and ask the client to look up and down and from side to side.

- Use a flashlight if necessary to find a colorless soft lens.

**2. Reposition a displaced lens.**

- Ask the client to look straight ahead.

- Using your index fingers, gently exert pressure on the inner margins of the upper and lower lids, and move the lens back onto the cornea.
  *or*
  Using a cotton-tipped applicator dipped in saline, gently move the lens into place.

*To Remove Hard Lenses*

**3. Separate the upper and lower eyelids.**

- Use both thumbs or index fingers to separate the upper and lower eyelids of one eye until they are beyond the edges of the lens (Figure 29–17). Exert pressure toward the bony orbit above and below the eye. *Retraction of the eyelids against the bony orbit prevents direct pressure, discomfort, and injury to the eyeball.*
  *or*
  Use the middle finger to retract the upper eyelid and the thumb of the same hand to retract the lower lid. *Using one hand for retraction keeps the other hand free to receive the lens.*

**4. Remove the lens.**

- Gently move the margins of both the lower eyelid and the upper eyelid toward the lens. *The margins of the lids trap the edges of the lens.*

- Hold the top eyelid stationary at the edge of the lens, and lift the bottom edge of the contact lens by pressing the lower lid at its margin firmly under the lens (Figure 29–18). *Pressure exerted under the edge of the lens interrupts the suction of the lens on the cornea.*

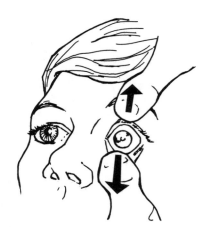

**FIGURE 29–17** Separating the eyelids until they are beyond the edges of a hard lens.

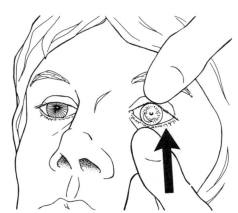

**FIGURE 29–18** Holding the top lid stationary at the edge of a hard lens and lifting the bottom edge of the lens by pressing the lower lid at its margin.

▶ **Procedure 29–7** *CONTINUED*

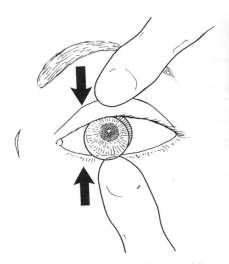

**FIGURE 29–19** Sliding a hard lens out of the eye by moving both eyelids toward each other.

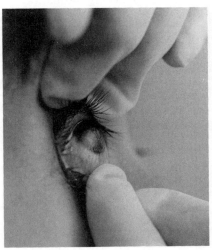

**FIGURE 29–20** Moving a soft lens down to the inferior part of the sclera.

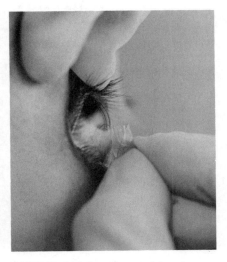

**FIGURE 29–21** Removing a soft lens by pinching it between the pads of the thumb and index finger.

- After the lens is slightly tipped, slide the lens off and out of the eye by moving both eyelids toward each other (Figure 29–19).

- Grasp the lens with your index finger and thumb, and place it in the palm of your hand.

- To avoid lens mixups, place the first lens in its designated cup in the storage case before removing the second lens.

- Repeat the above steps for the other lens.

*To Remove Soft Lenses*

**5. Separate the eyelids.**

- Ask the client to look upward at the ceiling and keep the eye opened wide.

- Retract the lower or upper lid with one or two fingers of your *nondominant* hand.

- Using the index finger of your dominant hand, move the lens down to the inferior part of the sclera (Figure 29–20). *Moving the lens onto the sclera reduces the risk of damage to the cornea.*

**6. Remove the lens.**

- Gently pinch the lens between the pads of the thumb and index finger of your dominant hand (Figure 29–21). *Pinching causes the lens to double up, so that air enters underneath the lens, breaking the suction and allowing removal. The pads of the fingers are used to prevent scratching the eye or the lens with the fingernails.*

- Place the lens in the palm of your hand.

- For *ultrathin* lenses, open the lens with the thumb and index finger *immediately* on removal. *This keeps the edges from sticking together.*

- Repeat the above steps for the other lens.

**7. Clean and store the lenses appropriately.**

- Clean the lenses according to manufacturer's instructions.

- Place the lens in the correct slot in its storage case. The slots are labeled for right and left lenses.

- Be sure each lens is centered in the storage case. *If the lens is not centered, it may crack, chip, or tear.* Tighten or close the cover.

- Place the contact lens container in the drawer of the bedside table. *The lenses and the case should never be exposed to direct sunlight or extreme heat, because these can dry or warp them.*

**8. Document all relevant information.**

- Document the removal of the lenses prior to surgery or when this is a nursing responsibility.

- Document all assessments and problems, such as redness of the conjunctiva, and report problems to the nurse in charge.

▶

► **Procedure 29–7  Removing Contact Lenses** CONTINUED

EVALUATION
FOCUS

Absence of eye inflammation; adequacy of visual acuity with lenses inserted; integrity of lenses; eye comfort.

**SAMPLE RECORDING**

| Date | Time | Notes |
|------|------|-------|
| 3/22/95 | 2100 | Contact lenses removed. No redness of eyelids or conjunctiva noted. Both lenses intact. ——————————————————— Anita R. Rodriguez, SN |

## 29-8   Removing, Cleaning, and Inserting an Artificial Eye

Before removing, cleaning, and inserting an artificial eye, determine the client's routine eye care practices.

**PURPOSES**
- To maintain the integrity of the eye socket and eyelids
- To prevent infection of the eye socket and surrounding tissues
- To assess the tissues and sockets for irritation or infection
- To maintain the client's self-esteem

**ASSESSMENT FOCUS**

Client's care regimen; inflammation of surrounding tissues; drainage from the eye socket; crusting of the eyelashes.

### EQUIPMENT

- Small labeled storage container, such as a denture or specimen container
- Gloves (optional)

- Small rubber bulb, a syringe bulb, or a medicine dropper bulb (optional)

- Soft gauze or cotton wipe
- Bowl of warm normal saline

### INTERVENTION

**1. Remove the eye.**

- Make sure that the container in which the prosthesis will be stored has been lined to cushion the eye and prevent scratches. Also, be sure to use sterile supplies. (This is not a sterile procedure, however.)

- Assist the client to a sitting or supine position, if the client's health permits.

- Identify the eye to be removed, and don gloves, if indicated.

- If the client has an effective method for removing the eye, follow that method. *Most people can remove their own eyes under normal circumstances, and they may have a convenient method.*

- Otherwise:

   **a.** Pull the lower eyelid down over the infraorbital bone with your dominant thumb, and exert slight pressure

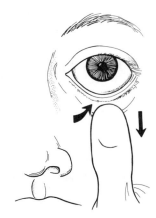

**FIGURE 29–22** Removing an artificial eye by retracting the lower eyelid and exerting slight pressure below the eyelid.

below the eyelid (Figure 29–22).
   *or*

   **b.** Compress a small rubber bulb, and apply the tip directly on the eye. Gradually decrease the finger pressure on the bulb, and draw the eye out of the socket. *Com-

*pression squeezes the air out of the bulb, causing a negative pressure inside the bulb. When the finger pressure is released, the suction of the bulb counteracts the suction holding the eye in the socket.*

- Receive the eye with the other hand, and place it carefully in the container. Do not scratch or drop the eye.

**2. Clean the eye and the socket.**

- Expose the socket by raising the upper lid with the index finger and pulling the lower lid down with the thumb.

- Clean the socket with soft gauze or cotton wipes and normal saline. Pat dry.

- Wash the tissue around the eye, stroking from the inner to the outer canthus using a fresh gauze for each wipe. *This direction of stroking avoids washing any debris down the lacrimal can-*

▶ **Procedure 29–8  Artificial Eyes** *CONTINUED*

*aliculi, if they are still intact.* Be sure to wash crusts off the upper and lower lids and eyelashes.

- Dry the tissues gently, in the direction described in the step above, using dry wipes.

- Wash the artificial eye gently with the warm normal saline, and dry it with dry wipes.

- If the eye is not to be inserted, place it in the lined container filled with water or saline solution, close the lid, label the container with the client's name and room number, and place it in the drawer of the bedside table.

**3. Reinsert the eye.**

- Ensure that the eye is moistened with water or saline. *Moisture facilitates insertion by reducing friction.*

- Using the thumb and index finger of one hand, retract the eyelids, exerting pressure on the supraorbital and infraorbital bones (Figure 29–23).

- With the thumb and index finger of the other hand, hold the eye so that the front of it is toward

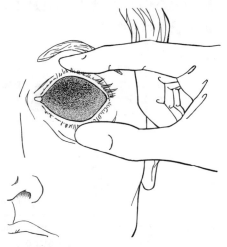

**FIGURE 29–23** Exposing the socket by retracting the upper and lower eyelids.

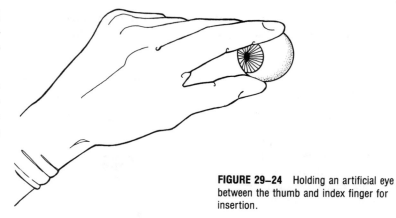

**FIGURE 29–24** Holding an artificial eye between the thumb and index finger for insertion.

the palm of your hand (Figure 29–24). Slip the eye gently into the socket, and release the lids. The eye should fit securely under the lids.

**4. Document pertinent information.**

- Record the removal, cleaning, and/or insertion of an artificial eye prior to surgery or for a helpless person. Otherwise, these procedures are not usually recorded.

- Document any assessments and problems, and report them to the nurse in charge.

| | |
|---|---|
| **EVALUATION FOCUS** | Clean appearance and uniform pale pink color of tissues in the eye socket; absence of encrustations on the eyelids; scratches or rough areas on eye. |

**SAMPLE RECORDING**

| Date | Time | Notes |
|---|---|---|
| 1/8/95 | 1200 | Client safely and correctly replaced artificial eye. No redness or drainage noted in socket. ——————————————————— Elizabeth Corwin, SN |

32

# Stress and Coping

## PROCEDURES

**32-1** # Teaching Progressive Relaxation

**PURPOSES**
- To reduce stress
- To control chronic pain
- To ease tension
- To obtain maximum benefits from rest and sleep periods
- To enable the client to gain control over body responses to stress and pain

**ASSESSMENT FOCUS**

Willingness to participate in the relaxation exercises; the nature and location of any pain; vital signs; signs of stress.

## INTERVENTION

**1. Ensure that the environment is quiet, peaceful, and at a temperature that promotes comfort to the client.** *Interruptions or distractions and a room that is too cool interfere with the client's ability to achieve full relaxation.*

**2. Tell the client how progressive relaxation works.**

- Provide a rationale for the procedure. *This enables the client to understand how stress affects the body.*

- Ask the client to identify the stressors operating in the client's life and the reactions to these stressors.

- Demonstrate the method of tensing and relaxing the muscles. *Demonstration enables the client to understand the complete relaxation procedure clearly.*

**3. Assist the client to a comfortable position.**

- Ensure that all body parts are supported and the joints slightly flexed, with no strain or pull on the muscles (e.g., arms and legs should not be crossed). *Assuming a position of comfort facilitates relaxation.*

**4. Encourage the client to rest the mind.**

- Ask the client to gaze slowly around the room, e.g., across the ceiling, down the wall, along a window curtain, around the fabric pattern, and back up the wall. *This exercise focuses the mind outside the body, and creates a second center of concentration, facilitating relaxation.*

**5. Instruct the client to tense and then relax each muscle group.**

- Progress through each muscle group in the following order, starting with the dominant side:

  a. Hand and forearm
  b. Upper arm
  c. Forehead
  d. Central face
  e. Lower face and jaw
  f. Neck
  g. Chest, shoulders, and upper back
  h. Abdomen
  i. Thigh
  j. Calf muscles
  k. Foot

- Encourage the client to breathe slowly and deeply during the en-

tire procedure. *Slow, deep breathing facilitates relaxation.*

- Encourage the client to focus on each muscle group being tensed and relaxed.

- Speak in a soothing voice that encourages relaxation, and coach the client to focus on each muscle group: e.g., "Make a tight fist," "Clench your fist tightly," "Hold the tension for 5 to 7 seconds," "Let all the tension go," and "Enjoy the feelings as your muscles become relaxed and loose."

**6. Ask the client to state whether any tension remains after all muscle groups have been tensed and relaxed.**

- Repeat the procedure for muscle groups that are not relaxed.

**7. Terminate the relaxation exercise slowly by counting backward from 4 to 1.**

- Ask the client to move the body slowly: first the hands and feet; then arms and legs; and finally the head and neck.

**8. Document the client's response to the exercise.**

**EVALUATION FOCUS**

Signs of relaxation (e.g., decreased muscle tension, slowed breathing); the client's feelings regarding success or problems with the technique.

► **Procedure 32–1** *CONTINUED*

**SAMPLE RECORDING**

| Date | Time | Notes |
|------|------|-------|
| 9/10/95 | 1300 | Instruction provided for progressive relaxation technique. States has difficulty relaxing and resting because of worries about recent diagnosis of cancer, work pressures, and financial concerns. During the technique respirations slowed to 14 and facial body tension not evident. Stated felt "more peaceful" following the technique.————————————————— Sharon Stookey, RN |

# 32-2  Assisting with Guided Imagery

**PURPOSES**
- To improve the body's response to therapy
- To control acute and chronic pain
- To reduce muscle tension
- To augment other relaxation techniques

**ASSESSMENT FOCUS**

Willingness to participate in imagery exercises.

## INTERVENTION

**1. Provide a comfortable, quiet environment free of distractions.** *An environment free of distractions is necessary for the client to focus on the selected image.*

**2. Explain the rationale and benefits of imagery.** *The client is an active participant in an imagery exercise and must understand completely what to do and what the expected outcomes are.*

**3. Assist the client to a comfortable position.**

- Assist the client to a reclining position, and ask the client to close the eyes. *A position of comfort can enhance the client's focus during the imagery exercise.*

- Use touch only if this does not threaten the client. For some clients, physical touch may be disturbing because of cultural or religious beliefs.

**4. Implement actions to induce relaxation.**

- Use the client's preferred name. *During imagery exercises, the client is more likely to respond to the preferred name.*

- Speak clearly in a calming and neutral tone of voice. *Positive voice coaching can enhance the effect of imagery. A shrill or loud voice can distract the client from the image.*

- Ask the client to take slow, deep breaths and to relax all muscles.

- Use progressive relaxation exercises as needed to assist the client to achieve total relaxation (see Procedure 32–1).

- For pain or stress management, encourage the client to "go to a place where you have previously felt very peaceful."
  *or*
  For internal imagery, encourage the client to focus on a meaningful image of power and to use it to control the specific problem.

**5. Assist the client to elaborate on the description of the image.**

- Ask the client to use all the senses in describing the image and the environment of the image. Sometimes clients will think only of visual images. *Using all the senses enhances the client's benefit from imagery.*

**6. Ask the client to describe the physical and emotional feelings elicited by the image.**

- Direct the client to explore the response to the image. *This enables the client to modify the image. Negative responses can be redirected by the nurse to provide a more positive outcome. Positive responses can be enhanced by describing them in detail.*

**7. Provide the client with continuous feedback.**

- Comment on signs of relaxation and peacefulness.

**8. Take the client out of the image.**

- Slowly count backward from 5 to 1. Tell the client that the client will feel rested when the eyes are opened.

- Remain until the client is alert.

**9. Following the experience, discuss the client's feelings about the experience.**

- Identify anything that could enhance the experience.

**10. Encourage the client to practice the imagery technique.**

- Imagery is a technique that can be done independently by the client once one knows how.

**EVALUATION FOCUS**

Signs of relaxation and/or decreased pain (e.g., decreased muscle tension; slow, restful breathing; and peaceful affect); the effectiveness of the image selected.

▶ **Procedure 32–2** *CONTINUED*

**SAMPLE RECORDING**

| Date | Time | Notes |
|---|---|---|
| 8/4/95 | 1000 | States inability to get enough rest because of chronic back pain ("I wake up in the middle of the night and can't get back to sleep. During the day I can't sit in a chair for very long either so I have to walk and move to relieve the pain.") Assisted with guided imagery. Needed encouragement to use her senses of smell and hearing as well as the visual image. States would like to try imagery again this afternoon with assistance. ———— Marilyn Morrison, RN |

# Activity and Exercise

## PROCEDURES

# 34-1   Using a Hydraulic Lift

**PURPOSE**
- To facilitate transfer of a totally dependent client to and from bed, wheelchair, tub, or toilet, without strain on the nurse

**ASSESSMENT FOCUS**

> Ability to comprehend instructions; degree of physical disability; weight of the client (to ensure that the lift can safely move the client); presence of orthostatic hypotension and pulse rate before transfer.

---

## EQUIPMENT
- Hoyer lift with slings and canvas straps

---

## INTERVENTION

### 1. Prepare the client.
- Explain the procedure, and demonstrate the lift. *Some clients are afraid of being lifted and will be reassured by a demonstration.*

### 2. Prepare the equipment.
- Lock the wheels of the client's bed.
- Raise the bed to the high position, and adjust the bed gatches so that the mattress is flat.
- Put up the side rail on the opposite side of the bed, and lower the side rail near you.
- Position the lift so that it is close to the client.
- Place the chair that is to receive the client beside the bed. Allow adequate space to maneuver the lift.
- Lock the wheels, if a chair with wheels is used.

### 3. Position the client on the sling.
- Roll the client away from you.
- Place the canvas seat or sling under the client, with the wide lower edge under the client's thighs to the knees and the more narrow upper edge up under the client's shoulders. *This places the sling under the client's center of gravity and greatest part of body weight. Correct placement permits the client to be lifted evenly, with minimal shifting.*
- Raise the bed rail on your side of the bed, and go to the opposite side of the bed. Lower this side rail.
- Roll the client to the opposite side, and pull the canvas sling through.
- Roll the client to the supine position on top of the canvas sling.

### 4. Attach the sling to the swivel bar.
- Wheel the lift into position, with the footbars under the bed on the side where the chair is positioned. Lock the wheels of the lifter.
- Lower the side rail.
- Lower the horizontal bar or mast boom to sling level by releasing the hydraulic valve. Lock the valve.
- Attach the lifter straps or hooks to the corresponding openings in the canvas seat. Check that the hooks are correctly placed and that matching straps or chains are of equal length.

### 5. Lift the client gradually.
- Elevate the head of the bed to place the client in a sitting position.
- Ask the client to remove eyeglasses, and put them in a safe place. *The swivel bar may come close to the face and cause breakage of eyeglasses.*
- Nurse 1: Close the pressure valve, and gradually pump the jack handle until the client is above the bed surface. *Gradual elevation of the lift is less frightening to the client than a rapid rise.*
- Nurse 2: Assume a broad stance, and guide the client with your hands as the client is lifted. *This prepares to hold the client and provide control during the movement.*
- Check the placement of the sling before moving the client away from the bed.

### 6. Move the client over the chair.
- Nurse 1: With the pressure valve securely closed, slowly roll the lift until the client is over the chair. Use the steering handle to maneuver the lift.
- Nurse 2: Guide movement by hand until the client is directly

▶

► **Procedure 34–1 Using a Hydraulic Lift** *CONTINUED*

over the chair (Figure 34–1). *Slow movement decreases swaying and is less frightening. Guidance also decreases swaying and gives a sense of security.*

**7. Lower the client into the chair.**

• Nurse 1: Release the pressure valve very gradually. *Gradual release is less frightening than a quick descent.*

• Nurse 2: Guide the client into the chair.

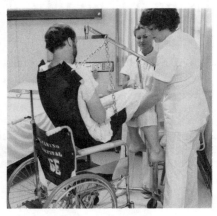

**FIGURE 34–1** Moving the client with a hydraulic lift.

**8. Ensure client comfort and safety.**

• Remove the hooks from the canvas seat. Leave the seat in place. *The seat is left in place in preparation for the lift back to bed.*

• Align the client appropriately in a sitting position.

• Return the client's eyeglasses, if appropriate.

• Apply a seatbelt or other restraint as needed.

• Place the call bell within reach.

| EVALUATION FOCUS | Body alignment in sitting position; vital signs, especially pulse rate and blood pressure to determine response to the transfer; safety precautions required for clients after the transfer. |
|---|---|

**SAMPLE RECORDING**

| Date | Time | Notes |
|---|---|---|
| 11/29/95 | 1100 | Assisted to chair via hydraulic lift. Tolerated well, B/P - 128/86. AP - 82. Alert and oriented. Call bell in place. ———————————— Kristen Morrison, SN |

## 34-2   Providing Passive Range-of-Motion Exercises

**PURPOSES**
- Determine which movements are unsafe for the client because of age or pathology (e.g., adducting the hip of a client who has had hip surgery).
- To maintain joint flexibility for effective daily functioning
- To prevent joint stiffness

**ASSESSMENT FOCUS**

> Degree of range-of-motion of joints needed to ambulate or perform essential ADLs; presence of contractures, joint swelling, redness, or pain.

### INTERVENTION

**1. Prior to initiating the exercises, review any possible restrictions with the physician or physical therapist. Also refer to the agency's protocol.**

**2. Assist the client to a supine position near you, and expose the body parts requiring exercise.**

- Place the client's feet together, place the arms at the sides, and leave space around the head and the feet. *Positioning the client close to you prevents excessive reaching.*

**3. Return to the starting position after each motion. Repeat each motion three times on the affected limb.**

**Shoulder and Elbow Movement**
Begin each exercise with the client's arm at the client's side. Grasp the arm beneath the elbow with one hand and beneath the wrist with the other hand, unless otherwise indicated (Figure 34–2).

**4. Flex, externally rotate, and extend the shoulder.**

- Move the arm up to the ceiling and toward the head of the bed (Figure 34–3). The elbow may need to be flexed if the headboard is in the way.

**5. Abduct and externally rotate the shoulder.**

- Move the arm away from the

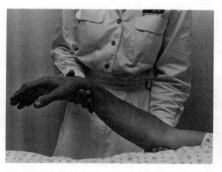

**FIGURE 34–2**  Supporting the client's arm.

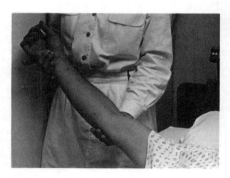

**FIGURE 34–3**  Flexing and extending the shoulder.

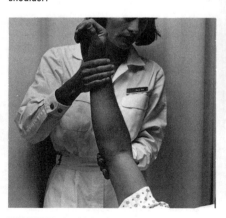

**FIGURE 34–4**  Abducting the shoulder.

body (Figure 34–4) and toward the client's head until the hand is under the head (Figure 34–5).

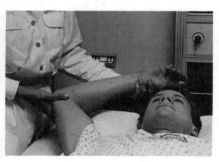

**FIGURE 34–5**  Abducting and externally rotating the shoulder.

**6. Adduct the shoulder.**

- Move the arm over the body (Figure 34–6) until the hand touches the client's other hand.

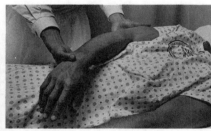

**FIGURE 34–6**  Adducting the shoulder.

**7. Rotate the shoulder internally and externally.**

- Place the arm out to the side at shoulder level (90° abduction), and bend the elbow so that the

▶

## ▶ Procedure 34–2 Providing Passive Range-of-Motion Exercises CONTINUED

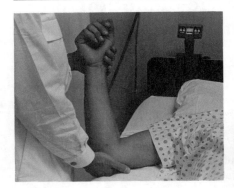

**FIGURE 34–7** Position before rotating the shoulder.

forearm is at a right angle to the mattress (Figure 34–7).

- Move the forearm down until the palm touches the mattress (Figure 34–8) and then up until the

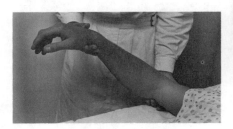

**FIGURE 34–8** Rotating the shoulder.

back of the hand touches the bed.

**8. Flex and extend the elbow.**

- Bend the elbow until the fingers touch the chin, then straighten the arm (Figure 34–9).

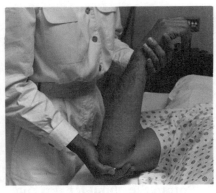

**FIGURE 34–9** Flexing and extending the elbow.

**9. Pronate and supinate the forearm.**

- Grasp the client's hand as for a handshake, and turn the palm downward (Figure 34–10) and upward (Figure 34–11), ensuring that only the forearm (not the shoulder) moves.

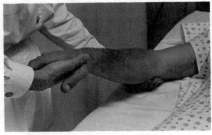

**FIGURE 34–10** Pronating the forearm.

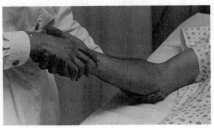

**FIGURE 34–11** Supinating the forearm.

**Wrist and Hand Movement**

For wrist and hand exercises, flex the client's arm at the elbow until the forearm is at a right angle to the mattress. Support the wrist joint with one hand while your other hand manipulates the joint and the fingers (Figure 34–12).

**10. Hyperextend the wrist, and flex the fingers.**

- Bend the wrist backward, and at the same time flex the fingers, moving the tips of the fingers to the palm of the hand (Figure 34–13).

- Align the wrist in a straight line with the arm, and place your fingers over the client's fingers to make a fist.

**11. Flex the wrist, and extend the fingers.**

- Bend the wrist forward, and at the same time extend the fingers (Figure 34–14).

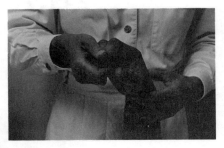

**FIGURE 34–12** Position for wrist and hand movements.

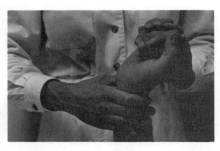

**FIGURE 34–13** Hyperextending the wrist and flexing the fingers.

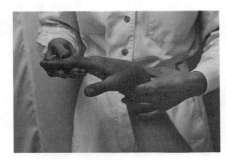

**FIGURE 34–14** Flexing the wrist and extending the fingers.

**12. Abduct and oppose the thumb.**

- Move the thumb away from the fingers and then across the hand toward the base of the little finger (Figure 34–15).

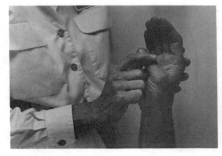

**FIGURE 34–15** Abducting the thumb.

▶ **Procedure 34–2** *CONTINUED*

**Leg and Hip Movement**
To carry out leg and hip exercises, place one hand under the client's knee and the other under the ankle (Figure 34–16).

### 13. Flex and extend the knee and hip.

- Lift the leg and bend the knee, moving the knee up toward the chest as far as possible. Bring the leg down, straighten the knee, and lower the leg to the bed (Figure 34–17).

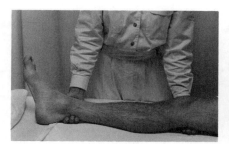

**FIGURE 34–16** Position for knee and hip movements.

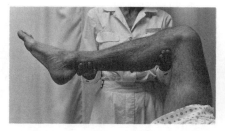

**FIGURE 34–17** Flexing the knee and the hip.

### 14. Abduct and adduct the leg.

- Move the leg to the side, away from the client (Figure 34–18) and back across in front of the other leg (Figure 34–19).

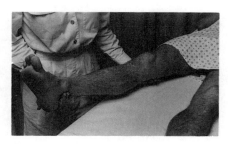

**FIGURE 34–18** Abducting the leg.

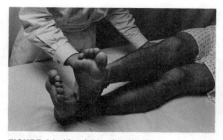

**FIGURE 34–19** Adducting the leg.

### 15. Rotate the hip internally and externally.

- Roll the leg inward (Figure 34–20), then outward (Figure 34–21).

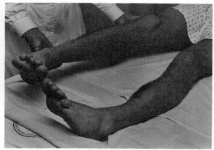

**FIGURE 34–20** Internally rotating the hip.

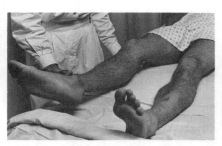

**FIGURE 34–21** Externally rotating the hip.

**Ankle and Foot Movement**
For ankle and foot exercises, place your hands in the positions described, depending on the motion to be achieved.

### 16. Dorsiflex the foot and stretch the Achilles tendon (heel cord).

- Place one hand under the client's heel, resting your inner forearm against the bottom of the client's foot.
- Place the other hand under the knee to support it.

- Press your forearm against the foot to move it upward toward the leg (Figure 34–22).

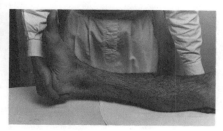

**FIGURE 34–22** Dorsiflexing the foot.

### 17. Invert and evert the foot.

- Place one hand under the client's ankle and the other over the arch of the foot.
- Turn the whole foot inward (Figure 34–23), then turn it outward (Figure 34–24).

### 18. Plantar flex the foot, and extend and flex the toes.

- Place one hand over the arch of the foot to push the foot away from the leg.

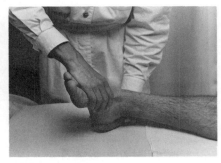

**FIGURE 34–23** Inverting the foot.

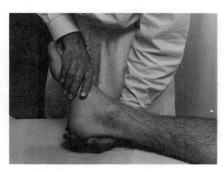

**FIGURE 34–24** Everting the foot.

▶

► **Procedure 34–2 Providing Passive Range-of-Motion Exercises** CONTINUED

- Place the fingers of the other hand under the toes, to bend the toes upward (Figure 34–25), and

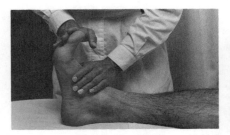

FIGURE 34–25   Extending the toes.

then over the toes, to push the toes downward (Figure 34–26).

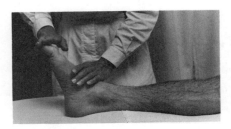

FIGURE 34–26   Plantar flexing the foot and flexing the toes.

**Neck Movement**
Remove the client's pillow.

**19. Flex and extend the neck.**

- Place the palm of one hand under the client's head and the palm of the other hand on the client's chin.

- Move the head forward until the chin rests on the chest, then back to the resting supine position without the head pillow (Figure 34–27).

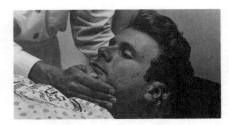

FIGURE 34–27   Flexing the neck.

**20. Laterally flex the neck.**

- Place the heels of the hands on each side of the client's cheeks.

- Move the top of the head to the right and to the left (Figure 34–28).

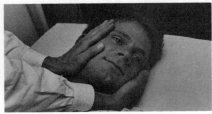

FIGURE 34–28   Laterally flexing the neck.

**Hyperextension Movements**

**21. Assist the client to a prone or lateral position on the side of the bed nearest you but facing away from you.**

**22. Hyperextend the shoulder.**

- Place one hand on the shoulder to keep it from lifting off the bed and the other under the client's elbow.

- Pull the upper arm up and backward (Figure 34–29).

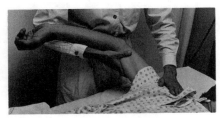

FIGURE 34–29   Hyperextending the shoulder.

**23. Hyperextend the hip.**

- Place one hand on the hip to stabilize it and keep it from lifting off the bed. With the other arm and hand, cradle the lower leg in the forearm, and cup the knee joint with the hand.

- Move the leg backward from the hip joint (Figure 34–30).

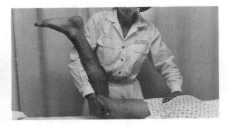

FIGURE 34–30   Hyperextending the hip.

**24. Hyperextend the neck.**
 Ⓢ Avoid hyperextending the neck of the immobilized elderly client, because such movements can cause painful nerve damage (Hogan and Beland 1976, p. 1106).

- Remove the pillow. With the client's face down, place one hand on the forehead and the other on the back of the skull.

- Move the head backward (Figure 34–31).

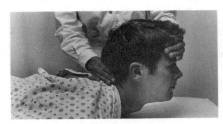

FIGURE 34–31   Hyperextending the neck.

**Following the Exercise**
**25. Assess the client's pulse and endurance of the exercise.**

**26. Report to the nurse in charge any unexpected problems or notable changes in the client's movements, e.g., rigidity or contractures.**

**27. Document the exercises and your assessments.**

▶ **Procedure 34–2** *CONTINUED*

**EVALUATION FOCUS**

Ability to tolerate the exercise; range of motion of the joint; any discomfort during the exercises.

**SAMPLE RECORDING**

| Date | Time | Notes |
|------|------|-------|
| 06/14/95 | 1100 | Passive exercises provided to R leg and foot for 5 minutes with no pain. Full ROM in hip, knee, and ankle. ——————————— Sally S. Ames, SN |

# 34-3 Applying a Continuous Passive Motion Device to the Knee

**PURPOSES**
- To prevent contractures, muscle atrophy, venous stasis, and thromboembolism
- To increase the joint range of motion
- To reduce joint swelling

**ASSESSMENT FOCUS**
Complaints of discomfort; appearance of joint (i.e., size and color); character and amount of drainage.

## EQUIPMENT
- Continuous passive motion device
- Padding for the cradle
- Restraining straps
- Goniometer

## INTERVENTION

**1. Check the safety test date.**
- Note the date the machine was tested for electrical safety, and ensure that it is within the guidelines established at the agency.

**2. Verify the physician's orders and agency protocol.**
- Determine the degrees of flexion, extension, and speed initially prescribed.
- Check agency protocol and physician's orders about increases in degrees and speed for subsequent treatments.

**3. Set up the machine.**
- Place the machine on the bed. Remove an egg crate mattress, if indicated. *This provides a stable surface.*
- Apply a supportive sling to the movable metal cradle.
- Attach the machine to a Balkan frame using traction equipment.
- Connect the control box to the machine.

**4. Set the prescribed levels of flexion and extension and speed.**
- Most postoperative clients are started on 10° to 45° of flexion

and 0° to 10° of extension (Maier 1986, p. 47).
- Flexion is usually increased to 5° to 10° per shift or 20° in 24 hours if tolerated (Maier 1986, p. 47).
- Adjust the speed control to the slow to moderate range for the first postoperative day, and then increase the speed as ordered and tolerated.
- Check that the machine is functioning properly by running it through a complete cycle.

**5. Position the client, and place the leg in the machine.**
- Place the client in a supine position, with the head of the bed slightly elevated.
- Support the leg and, with the client's help, lift the leg and place it in the padded cradle.
- Lengthen or shorten appropriate sections of the frame to fit the machine to the client. The knee and hip should be at the hinged joints of the machine.
- Adjust the footplate so that the foot is supported in a neutral position or slight dorsiflexion (e.g., 20°). Check agency protocol.

- Ensure that the leg is neither internally nor externally rotated.
- Apply restraining straps around the thigh and top of the foot and cradle, allowing enough space to fit several fingers under it.

**6. Start the machine.**
- Ensure the controls are set at the prescribed levels.
- Turn the on/off switch to the "on" position, and press the start button.
- ⚠️S When the machine reaches the fully flexed position, stop the machine, and verify the degree of flexion with a goniometer.
- Restart the machine, and observe a few cycles of flexion and extension to ensure proper functioning.

**7. Ensure continued client safety and comfort.**
- Make sure that the client is comfortable.
- ⚠️S Raise the side rails to keep the machine and client contained.
- ⚠️S Stay with a confused or sedated client while the machine is on.

▶ **Procedure 34–3** *CONTINUED*

- Instruct a mentally alert client how to operate the on/off switch.

- Loosen the straps, and check the client's skin at least twice per shift.

- Wash the perineal area at least once per shift, and keep it dry.

- Drape a towel over the groin of a male client. *This prevents scrotal irritation by contact with the machine.*

**8. Document all relevant information.**

- Record the procedure, the degree of flexion, the degree of extension, the speed, and the duration of the therapy.

<br>

**EVALUATION FOCUS**

> Response to therapy; increase in tolerance and range of motion; degree of discomfort; skin integrity of feet, elbow, sacrum, and groin.

**SAMPLE RECORDING**

| Date | Time | Notes |
|------|------|-------|
| 07/11/95 | 0900 | Continuous passive motion machine applied to knee as ordered for 30 minutes. Flexion control set at 80°; extension at 0°. Procedure tolerated well. <br> — Michaela Nichols, RN |

# 34-4  Assisting a Client to Use a Cane

**PURPOSES**

- To enhance the client's balance and gait alignment
- To provide additional support (e.g., when the client has weakness on one side of the body) even though weight-bearing is possible

**ASSESSMENT FOCUS**

Client's abilities to walk with a cane (i.e., physical strength of the lower extremities and arm and hand holding the cane); ability to bear body weight; ability to keep balance in a standing position on one or both legs; ability to hold the body erect.

## EQUIPMENT

□ Cane of the correct length with rubber tip

## INTERVENTION

### 1. Prepare the client for walking.

- Ask the client to hold the cane on the *stronger* side of the body. *This provides maximum support and appropriate body alignment when walking. The arm opposite the advancing foot normally swings forward when walking, so the hand holding the cane will come forward and the cane will support the weaker leg.*

- Position the tip of a standard cane (and the nearest tip of other canes) about 15 cm (6 in) to the side and 15 cm (6 in) in front of the near foot, so that the elbow is slightly flexed. *This provides the best balance and prevents the person from leaning on the cane. In this position the client stands erect, with the center of gravity within the base of support.*

- Ensure that the client has balance and feels well enough to walk.

### 2. When maximum support is required, instruct the client to move as follows:

- Move the cane forward about 30 cm (1 ft), or a distance that is comfortable while the body weight is on both legs (Figure 34–32, *A*).

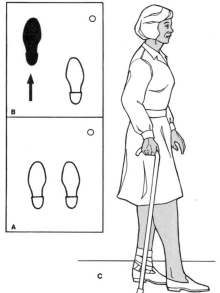

**FIGURE 34–32**  Steps involved in using a cane to provide maximum support.

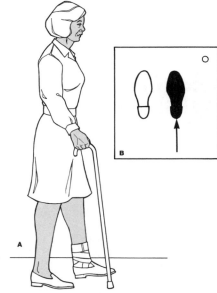

**FIGURE 34–33**  Steps involved in using a cane when less than maximum support is required.

- Then, move the affected (weak) leg forward to the cane while the weight is on the cane and stronger leg (Figure 34–32, *B*).

- Next, move the unaffected (stronger) leg forward ahead of the cane and weak leg while the weight is on the cane and weak leg (Figure 34–32, *C*).

- Repeat the above three steps. This pattern of moving provides

at least two points of support on the floor at all times.

### 3. When the client becomes stronger and requires less support, instruct the client to follow these steps:

- Move the cane and weak leg forward at the same time, while the weight is on the stronger leg (Figure 34–33, *A*).

▶ **Procedure 34–4** *CONTINUED*

- Move the stronger leg forward while the weight is on the cane and the weak leg (Figure 34–33, *B*).

4. **Ensure client safety.**

- Walk beside the client on the affected side. *The client is most likely to fall toward the affected side.*

- Walk the client for the time or distance indicated on the nursing care plan.

- If the client loses balance or strength and is unable to regain it, slide your hand up to the client's axilla, and take a broad stance to provide a base of support. Have the client rest against your hip until assistance arrives, or gently lower yourself and the client to the floor.

| **EVALUATION FOCUS** | Body alignment standing and walking with a cane; gait when walking with the cane. |
|---|---|

**SAMPLE RECORDING**

| Date | Time | Notes |
|------|------|-------|
| 1/25/95 | 1400 | Instructed in use of cane. Safely and correctly demonstrated its use. Ambulated 40 feet—steady on feet with use of cane. ———————— Karyn Neinas, SN |

# 34-5 Assisting a Client to Use Crutches

**PURPOSES**
- To increase the client's sense of independence
- To help the client walk and move with crutches safely and with minimum expenditure of energy

**ASSESSMENT FOCUS**

Leg or foot disability (i.e., whether the client can bear weight on one leg only or partially on the affected leg or foot; ability to maintain balance in an erect standing position; muscle strength, particularly in the arms and unaffected leg; previous experience with crutches; learning needs.

## EQUIPMENT

- Crutches with suction tips, hand bars, and axillary pads
- Walking belt (optional)

## INTERVENTION

1. **Prepare the client.**

- Verify the correct length for the crutches and the correct placement of the handpieces.
- Ensure that the client is wearing supportive, nonskid shoes with laces or Velcro.

2. **Assist the client to assume the tripod (triangle) position, the basic crutch stance used before crutch walking.**

- Ask the client to stand and place the tips of the crutches 15 cm (6 in) in front of the feet and out laterally about 15 cm (6 in). See Figure 34–34. *The tripod position provides a wide base of support and enhances both stability and balance.*
- Make sure the feet are slightly apart. A tall person requires a wider base than a short person.
- Ensure that posture is erect; i.e., the hips and knees are extended, the back is straight, and the head is held straight and high. There should be no hunch to the shoulders and thus no weight borne by the axillae. The elbows should be extended sufficiently to allow weight-bearing on the hands.

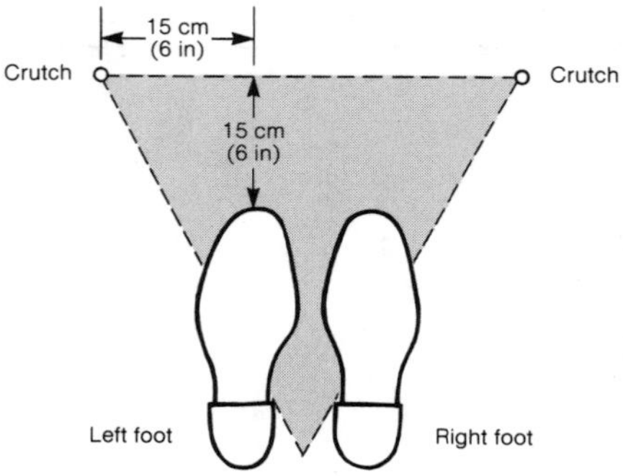

**FIGURE 34–34** The tripod position.

- Stand slightly behind and on the client's affected side. *By standing behind the client and toward the affected side, the nurse can provide support if the client loses balance.*
- If the client is unsteady, place a walking belt around the client's waist, and grasp the belt from above, not from below. *A fall can be prevented more effectively if the belt is held from above.*

3. **Teach the client the appropriate crutch gait.**

**Four-Point Alternate Gait**
This is the most elementary and safest gait, providing at least three points of support at all times, but it requires coordination. It can be used when walking in crowds because it does not require much space. To use this gait, the client has to be able to bear some weight on both legs (Figure 34–35, reading from bottom to top). Ask the client to

- Move the right crutch ahead a suitable distance, e.g., 10 to 15 cm (4 to 6 in).
- Move the left foot forward, preferably to the level of the crutch.
- Move the left crutch forward.
- Move the right foot forward.

**Three-Point Gait**
To use this gait, the person must be able to bear entire body weight on the unaffected leg. The two crutches and the unaffected leg bear weight alternately (Figure 34–36, reading from bottom to top). Ask the client to

- Move both crutches and the weaker leg forward.
- Move the stronger leg forward.

**Two-Point Alternate Gait**
This gait is faster than the four-point gait. It requires more balance, because only two points support the body at one time; it also requires at least partial weight bear-

▶ **Procedure 34–5** *CONTINUED*

ing on each foot. In this gait, arm movements with the crutches are ing normal walking (Figure 34–37, reading from bottom to top). Ask the client to

- Move the left crutch and the right foot forward together.

- Move the right crutch and the left foot ahead together.

**Swing-To Gait**

The swing gaits are used by people with paralysis of the legs and hips. Prolonged use of these gaits results in atrophy of the unused muscles. The swing-to gait is the easier of

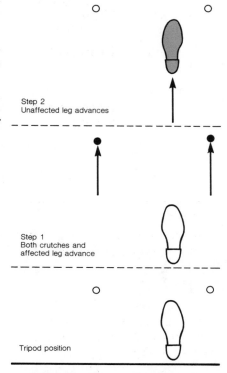

Step 2
Unaffected leg advances

Step 1
Both crutches and affected leg advance

Tripod position

**FIGURE 34–36** The three-point crutch gait.

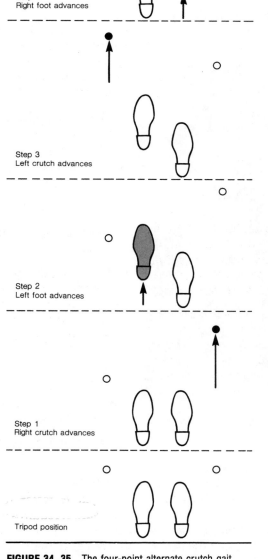

Step 4
Right foot advances

Step 3
Left crutch advances

Step 2
Left foot advances

Step 1
Right crutch advances

Tripod position

**FIGURE 34–35** The four-point alternate crutch gait.

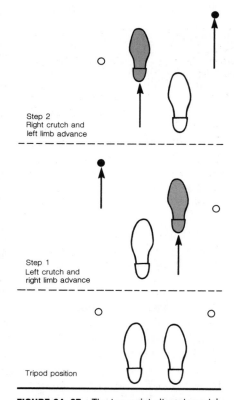

Step 2
Right crutch and left limb advance

Step 1
Left crutch and right limb advance

Tripod position

**FIGURE 34–37** The two-point alternate crutch gait.

▶ **Procedure 34–5 Assisting a Client to Use Crutches** CONTINUED

these two gaits (Figure 34–38). Ask the client to

- Move both crutches ahead together.
- Lift body weight by the arms and swing *to* the crutches.

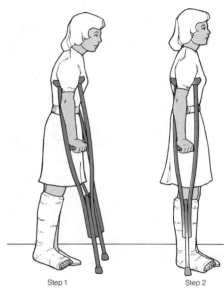

FIGURE 34–38   The swing-to crutch gait.

**Swing-Through Gait**

This gait requires considerable client skill, strength, and coordination (Figure 34–39). Ask the client to

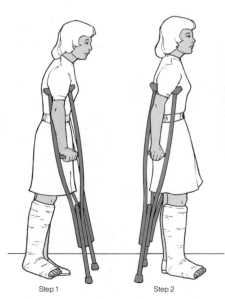

FIGURE 34–39   The swing-through crutch gait.

- Move both crutches forward together.
- Lift body weight by the arms and swing *through and beyond* the crutches.

**4. Teach the client to get into and out of a chair.**

**Getting Into a Chair**

- Ensure that the chair has armrests and is secure or braced against a wall.
- Instruct the client to

  **a.** Stand with the back of the unaffected leg centered against the chair. *The chair helps support the client during the next steps.*

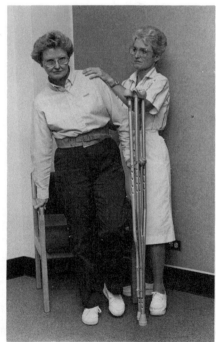

FIGURE 34–40   A client with crutches getting into a chair.

  **b.** Transfer the crutches to the hand on the affected side, hold the crutches by the hand bars, and then grasp the arm of the chair with the hand on the unaffected side (Figure 34–40). *This al-*

*lows the client to support the body weight on the arms and the unaffected leg.*

  **c.** Lean forward, flex the knees and hips, and lower into the chair.

**Getting Out of a Chair**

- Instruct the client to

  **a.** Move forward to the edge of the chair and place the unaffected leg slightly under or at the edge of the chair. *This position helps the client stand up from the chair and achieve balance, because the unaffected leg is supported against the edge of the chair.*

  **b.** Grasp the crutches by the hand bars in the hand on the affected side, and grasp the arm of the chair by the hand on the unaffected side. *The body weight is placed on the crutches and the hand on the armrest to support the unaffected leg when the client rises to stand.*

  **c.** Push down on the crutches and the chair armrest while elevating the body out of the chair.

  **d.** Assume the tripod position before moving.

**5. Teach the client to go up and down stairs.**

**Going Up Stairs**

- Stand behind the client and slightly to the affected side.

- Ask the client to

  **a.** Assume the tripod position at the bottom of the stairs.

  **b.** Transfer the body weight to the crutches and move the unaffected leg onto the step (Figure 34–41).

  **c.** Transfer the body weight to the unaffected leg on the

▶ **Procedure 34–5** CONTINUED

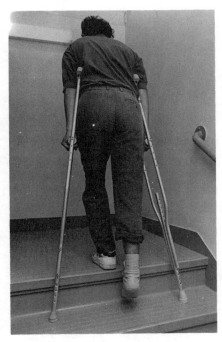

**FIGURE 34–41**  Climbing stairs: placing weight on the crutches while first moving the unaffected leg onto a step.

step and move the crutches and affected leg up to the step. *The affected leg is always supported by the crutches.*

- Repeat steps b and c until the top of the stairs is reached.

**Going Down Stairs**

- Stand one step below the person on the affected side.

- Ask the client to

  **a.** Assume the tripod position at the top of the stairs.

  **b.** Shift the body weight to the unaffected leg, and move the crutches and affected leg down onto the next step (Figure 34–42).

  **c.** Transfer the body weight to the crutches, and move the unaffected leg to that step. *The affected leg is always supported by the crutches.*

  **d.** Repeat steps b and c until the bottom of the stairs is reached.

*or*

- Ask the client to

  **a.** Hold both crutches in the outside hand and grasp the hand rail with the other hand for support.

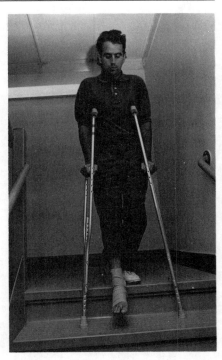

**FIGURE 34–42**  Descending stairs: moving the crutches and affected leg first down to the next step.

  **b.** Move as in steps b and c, above.

**6. Document teaching and all assessments.**

---

**EVALUATION FOCUS**

How well the client achieves stability in gait without falling; correct use of crutch gait taught; ability to get into and out of chairs as taught; ability to go up and down stairs as taught.

**SAMPLE RECORDING**

| Date | Time | Notes |
|------|------|-------|
| 7/17/95 | 1800 | Instructed in use of crutches and three-point gait. Safely and correctly demonstrated use when walking and transferring to chair. ————————————————————— Samantha Dreyfus, SN |

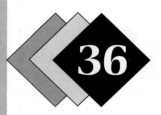

**36**

# Comfort and Pain

## PROCEDURE

# 36-1   Managing Pain with a Transcutaneous Electric Nerve Stimulation Unit

Before applying a TENS unit, determine the presence of factors contraindicating usage (presence of a cardiac pacemaker; history of dysrhythmias, myocardial ischemia, or myocardial infarction; first-trimester pregnancy; confusion; history of peripheral vascular problems altering neurosensory perception).

**PURPOSES**

- To reduce chronic and acute pain (especially postoperative pain)
- To decrease opioid requirements and reduce the chances of depressed respiratory function from narcotic usage
- To facilitate client involvement in managing pain control

**ASSESSMENT FOCUS**

Client's mental status and ability to follow instructions in using the TENS unit; intactness of skin and absence of signs of infection and irritation; appearance of incisional area of postoperative client; characteristics of pain (intensity, location, associated factors, precipitating factors, and alleviating factors); amount of pain medication required before and during treatment.

## EQUIPMENT

- TENS Unit
- Bath basin with warm water
- Soap
- Washcloth
- Towel
- Conduction cream, gel, or water (see manufacturer's instructions)
- Hypoallergenic tape

## INTERVENTION

**1. Explain the purpose and application procedure to the client and family.**

- Explain that the TENS unit may not completely eliminate pain but should reduce pain to a level that allows the client to rest more comfortably and/or carry out everyday activities.

**2. Prepare the equipment.**

- Insert the battery into the TENS unit to test the status of functioning.

- With the TENS unit off, plug the lead wires into the battery-operated unit at one end, leaving the electrodes at the other end.

**3. Clean the application area.**

- Wash, rinse, and dry the designated area with soap and water. *This reduces skin irritation and facilitates adhesion of the electrodes to the skin for a longer period of time.*

**4. Apply the electrodes to the client.**

- If the electrodes are not prejelled, moisten them with a small amount of water or apply conducting gel. (Consult the manufacturer's instructions). *This facilitates electrical conduction.*

- Place the electrodes on a clean, unbroken skin area. Choose the area according to the location, nature, and origin of the pain.

- Ensure that the electrodes make full surface contact with the skin. *This prevents an inadvertent burn.*

- Secure the electrodes with hypoallergenic tape.

**5. Turn the unit on.**

- Ascertain that the amplitude control is set at level 0.

- Slowly increase the intensity of the stimulus (amplitude) until

the client notes a slight increase in discomfort.

- When the client notes discomfort, slowly decrease the amplitude until the client notes a pleasant sensation. Once this has been achieved, keep the TENS unit set at this level to maintain blockage of the pain sensation.

**6. Monitor the client.**

- If the client complains of itching, pricking, or burning, explore the following options:

  a. Turn the pulse-width dial down.

  b. Check that the entire electrode surface is in contact with the skin.

  c. Increase the distance between the electrodes.

  d. Select another type of electrode suitable for the model

►

# ▶ Procedure 36–1 Managing Pain with a TENS Unit *CONTINUED*

of TENS unit in use.

e. Discontinue the TENS, and consider the possibility of another brand of TENS.

- If the sensation of the stimulus is unpleasant, too intense, or distracting, turn down both the amplitude and the pulse-width dial.

- If the client complains of headache or nausea during application or use, turn down both the amplitude and the pulse-width dial. Repositioning of the electrodes may also be helpful.

- If further troubleshooting is not effective, discontinue the use of the TENS unit, and notify the physician.

## 7. Provide client teaching.

- Review with the client instructions for use, and verify that the client understands.

- Have the client demonstrate the use of the TENS unit and verbalize ways to troubleshoot if headache, nausea, or unpleasant sensations occur.

- Instruct the client not to submerge the unit in water but instead to remove and reapply it after bathing.

- Check the manufacturer's instructions for removing electrode gel from the electrodes.

## 8. Document all relevant information.

- Record the date and time TENS therapy was initiated, the location of electrode placement and status of skin in that area, the character and quality of the pain, settings of TENS unit used, any side-effects experienced, and the client's response.

---

| EVALUATION FOCUS | Response of the client in terms of pain relief or side-effects experienced; self-care abilities. |
|---|---|

**SAMPLE RECORDING**

| Date | Time | Notes |
|---|---|---|
| 4/23/95 | 1000 | TENS unit applied near midline abdominal incision for postoperative pain at intensity level given by client of 6–7. Lead 1 and lead 2 settings on 6.0 Verbalized minimum relief of discomfort upon initiation of treatment.——————————————————————— Mark McCormick, SN |

# Nutrition

## PROCEDURES

# 37-1 | Assisting an Adult to Eat

**PURPOSES**
- To maintain the client's nutritional status
- To teach the client required eating skills

**ASSESSMENT FOCUS**

Self-care abilities for eating and assistance required (note hand coordination, level of consciousness, and visual acuity); appetite for and tolerance of food and fluid; difficulty swallowing; anthropometric measurements for baseline data as required; any need for a special diet; any food allergies and food likes and dislikes.

## EQUIPMENT

- Meal tray with the correct food and fluids
- Extra napkin or small towel
- Straw, special drinking cup, weighted glass, or other adaptive feeding aid as required

## INTERVENTION

### 1. Confirm the client's diet order.

- Check the client's chart or Kardex for the diet order and to determine whether the client is fasting for laboratory tests or surgery or whether the physician has ordered "nothing by mouth" (NPO). For clients who are fasting or on NPO, ensure that the appropriate signs are placed on either the room door or the client's bed, according to agency practice.

- If there is a change in the type of food the client is to receive, notify the dietary staff.

### 2. Prepare the client and overbed table.

- Assist the client to the bathroom or onto a bedpan or commode if the client needs to urinate.

- Offer the client assistance in washing the hands prior to a meal. If the client has problems with oral hygiene, brushing the teeth or using a mouthwash can improve the taste in the mouth and hence the appetite.

- Clear the overbed table so that there is space for the tray. If the client must remain in a lying position in bed, arrange the overbed table close to the bedside so that the client can see the food.

### 3. Position the client and yourself appropriately.

- Assist the client to a comfortable position for eating. Most people sit during a meal; if it is permitted, assist the client to sit in bed (Figure 37–1) or in a chair, whichever is appropriate.
  *or*
  If the client is unable to sit, assist the client to a lateral position. *People will swallow more easily in*

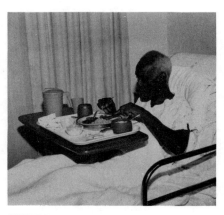

**FIGURE 37–1** A supported sitting position contributes to a client's comfort while eating.

*these positions than in a backlying position.*

- If the client requires assistance with feeding, assume a sitting position, if possible, beside the client. *This position conveys a more relaxed presence, which is more conducive to the client's eating an adequate meal.*

### 4. Assist the client as required.

- Check each tray for the client's name, the type of diet, and completeness. If the diet does not seem to be correct, check it against the client's chart. Confirm the client's name by checking the wristband before leaving the tray. Do *not* leave an incorrect diet for a client to eat.

- Encourage the client to eat independently, assisting as needed. Do not take over the feeding process. *Participation by the client enhances feelings of independence.*

- Remove the food covers, butter the bread, pour the tea, and cut the meat, if needed.

- For a blind person, identify the placement of the food as you

▶ **Procedure 37–1** *CONTINUED*

would describe the time on a clock. For instance, say, "The potatoes are at 8 o'clock; the beef steak at 12 o'clock; and the green beans at 4 o'clock." (Figure 37–2).

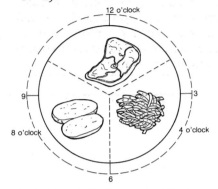

**FIGURE 37–2**  The clock system used to describe the location of food on the plate for a blind client.

- If assistance with feeding is required,

  **a.** Ask in which order the client desires to eat the food.

  **b.** Use normal utensils whenever possible. *Using ordinary utensils enhances self-esteem.*

  **c.** If the client cannot see, tell which food you are giving.

  **d.** Warn the client if the food is hot or cold.

  **e.** Allow ample time for the client to chew and swallow the food before offering more.

  **f.** Provide fluids as requested, or, if the client is unable to tell you, offer fluids after every three or four mouthfuls of solid food.

  **g.** Use a straw or special drinking cup for fluids that would spill from normal containers.

  **h.** Make the time a pleasant one, choosing topics of conversation that are of interest to the client, if the person wants to talk.

**5. After the meal, ensure client comfort.**

- Assist the client to clean the mouth and hands.

- Reposition the client.

- Replace the food covers, and remove the food tray from the bedside.

**6. Document all relevant information.**

- Note how much and what the client has eaten and the amount of fluid taken. Record fluid intake and calorie count as required.

- If the client is on a special diet or is having problems eating, record the amount of food eaten and any pain, fatigue, or nausea experienced.

- If the client is not eating, notify the nurse in charge so that the diet can be changed or other nursing measures can be taken, e.g., rescheduling the meals, providing smaller, more frequent meals, or obtaining special self-feeding aids.

| EVALUATION FOCUS | Appetite; tolerance of food and fluids taken; amount of fluid intake, if being measured; calorie count, if required; any chewing or swallowing difficulties and the need for any adjustments in food consistency (e.g., minced or pureed foods, need for special feeding aids); comparison of anthropometric measurements to baseline data, as required. |
|---|---|

**SAMPLE RECORDING**

| Date | Time | Notes |
|---|---|---|
| 05/13/95 | 0800 | Refused all solid food. Ingested 120 ml milk. Nauseated. Dull crampy pain persists in epigastric region. ——————— Wendy B. Low, SN |

# 37-2  Bottle-Feeding an Infant

**PURPOSES**
- To provide the nutrients required for normal growth and life
- To provide feelings of love and security to the infant for sound psychologic development

**ASSESSMENT FOCUS**

> The infant's general nutritional status; weight gain or loss; development of suck reflex; eagerness to take fluids; family history of allergy. The mother's education level or ability to understand feeding instructions; previous experience with infant feeding.

## EQUIPMENT
- ☐ Sterile bottle
- ☐ Sterile nipple
- ☐ Sterile formula
- ☐ Bib or clean cloth

## INTERVENTION

**1. Obtain essential information before the feeding:**
- The type of formula recommended by the physician
- The amount per feeding, e.g., 4 to 5 oz
- The type of bottle and nipple used
- The frequency of feeding, e.g., every 4 hours, and the specific times of day
- How the formula is prepared, i.e., at what dilution
- What other fluids, e.g., water or apple juice, are given at scheduled times per day and the amounts

**2. Prepare the bottle, nipple, and formula.**
- If the formula is refrigerated, warm it to room temperature. The formula should feel lukewarm to the inner wrist when a few drops are shaken onto it. *Babies digest formula at room temperature more quickly than cold formula and are less likely to develop abdominal cramps.*
- Test the size of the nipple holes by turning the bottle upside down. If a drop of milk appears at the tip of the nipple, the holes are the correct size. If no milk appears or if milk flows out freely, the nipple needs to be changed. *The nipple holes need to be large enough to allow the baby to get formula with normal sucking but not large enough to allow milk to flow freely, which can cause choking and regurgitation. Nipple holes that are too small require too much energy to suck, and too much air is sucked with them.*

**3. Ensure infant comfort.**
- Check whether the infant needs a diaper change. If so, change the diaper. Handle the infant calmly, gently, and unhurriedly. *A clean, dry diaper is conducive to pleasurable feeding. Calm, gentle handling soothes the infant.*
- Arrange a quiet, comfortable environment in which to feed the infant. *A calm environment is conducive to successful feeding.*
- Carry the infant, using the football hold, to the feeding chair (see Figure 29–1). *The football hold supports the infant's head and back yet frees one of the nurse's hands to carry the bib and formula.*
- Sit comfortably in the chair, and relax. *Discomfort and tension can be transmitted to the infant and can interfere with feeding and digestion.*
- Tuck the bib or clean cloth under the infant's chin.

**4. Position the infant appropriately.**
- Cradle the baby in your arms, with the head slightly elevated. Support the head and neck in the bend of your elbow while the buttocks rest on your lap. *Elevating the head facilitates swallowing. Infants need to be held while being fed to feel warm and loved.*
- If the baby cannot be removed from an isolette or crib because of therapy (e.g., an oxygenated croupette or traction), provide as much hand contact as possible, and stay with the infant during the feeding.
- Never leave an infant with a propped bottle. *The infant can suck in excessive air or ingest the formula too quickly. Both circumstances induce regurgitation and possible aspiration of fluid into the lungs, which can cause pneumonia in the baby.*

**5. Insert the nipple, and feed the infant.**

▶ **Procedure 37–2** *CONTINUED*

• Insert the nipple gently along the infant's tongue and hold the bottle at about a 45° angle so that the nipple is filled with formula and not air (Figure 37–3). *Excessive swallowed air causes gas, abdominal distention, discomfort, and possible regurgitation.*

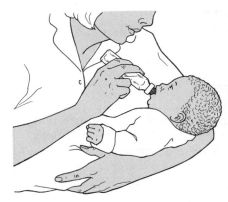

**FIGURE 37–3** Position of infant and bottle when bottle-feeding an infant.

**6. Remove the bottle periodically and burp (bubble) the baby.**

• Small infants may need to be burped after every ounce or at least at the middle and end of the feeding. With some collapsible feeding bottles, infants suck in very little air and may need to be burped only at the end of the feeding. The infant who was crying before the feeding may have swallowed air and may need to be burped before the feeding begins or after taking just enough formula to calm down. *Periodic burping helps the infant expel the swallowed air and therefore consume the maximum amount of formula.*

• Place the baby either

  **a.** Over your shoulder (Figure 37–4).

  **b.** In a supported sitting position on your lap (Figure 37–5). *This position is often preferred because the infant's responses can be observed continuously.*

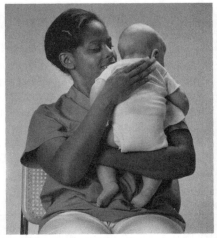

**FIGURE 37–4** Burping an infant over the shoulder.

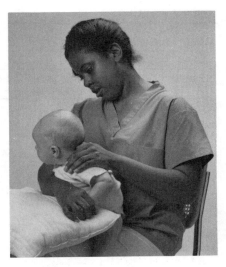

**FIGURE 37–5** Burping an infant in a supported sitting position.

  **c.** In a prone position over your lap (Figure 37–6).

• Place the bib where it will protect your clothing. *Newborns frequently regurgitate small amounts of feedings. This normal occurrence may be due initially to excessive mucus and gastric irritation from foreign substances in the stomach from birth. Later, regurgitation may occur when the infant feeds too rapidly and swallows air or when the infant is overfed and the cardiac sphincter*

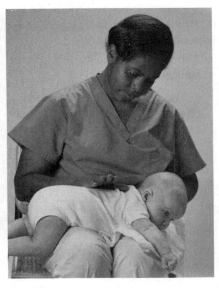

**FIGURE 37–6** Burping an infant in a prone position.

*allows the excess to be regurgitated.*

• Rub or pat the infant's back gently. *Patting encourages relaxation of the cardiac sphincter of the stomach and the expulsion of air.*

**7. Continue with the feeding until the formula is finished and/or the baby is satisfied.**

• An infant feeding generally takes about 30 minutes. *Prolonged feeding times tend to foster lazy eating habits.*

• For newborns who need encouragement to continue sucking during initial feedings, provide gentle tactile stimulation to the feet and hands. *Stimulation helps maintain sucking for a sufficient time to complete a feeding.*

• Once feedings are established, encourage the infant to set the pace.

• Avoid overfeeding or feeding every time the infant cries. *Overfeeding results in infant obesity. A fat baby is not necessarily healthy.*

▶

**Procedure 37–2  Bottle-Feeding an Infant** *CONTINUED*

**8. Ensure infant safety and comfort after the feeding.**

- Return the infant to the crib or isolette.

- Check whether the diaper needs changing, and change it if necessary. *Smaller infants commonly move their bowels while feeding because of the gastrocolic reflex.*

- Position the infant on the side with the head to one side. *In this position, the infant is less likely to aspirate any fluid that may be regurgitated. For infants in whom regurgitation is a problem, a right side-lying position tends to facilitate the explusion of air without regurgitation, since the cardiac sphincter is on the left side of the stomach.*

- Ensure that the crib sides are elevated before leaving the infant.

- Assess the infant for signs of allergic reaction, particularly with initial formula usage or when formula type is changed.

**9. Document all relevant information.**

- Record the type and the amount of the feeding taken and all assessments.

---

**EVALUATION FOCUS**

Responses of the infant (e.g., amount and frequency of regurgitation, whether the infant seems satisfied after the feeding and rests quietly, any allergy), weight gain or loss; color and characteristics of the feces or urine.

**SAMPLE RECORDING**

| Date | Time | Notes |
|------|------|-------|
| 06/06/95 | 0700 | 5 oz Similac taken well. Regurgitated small amount formula × 1. Resting quietly on right side. —————————————— Sally R. Duprez, SN |

# Introduction of Solid Foods

The introduction of solid foods to an infant's diet is based on (a) the infant's need for nutrients that solid foods provide and (b) developmental stage or readiness to handle solid foods. Both of these phenomena occur at about the same time—4 to 7 months of age. See the box below for an infant's developmental abilities relative to feeding.

Infants may be fed solids while being held in the arms, as for bottle-feeding, or while seated and restrained in an infant seat. When old enough to sit unsupported, the infant can sit on the nurse's or another person's lap rather than in an infant seat. Young children progress to a highchair.

---

## The Infant's Developmental Abilities in Relation to Feeding

- The extrusion reflex is normally present for the first 4 months. This reflex causes young infants to spit out solids rather than swallow them. At 4 months, because infants can reach their mouths with their hands, the hands may get in the way during feeding.

- Between 4 and 6 months of age, the infant learns to transfer soft foods from the front of the tongue to the back.

- By 5 to 6 months, infants can sit with support, can grasp objects in a mittenlike fashion, can bring their lips to the rim of a cup and begin drinking, and can begin to chew.

- At 7 months, infants can feed themselves a biscuit, like to play with food and smear it, bang cups and objects on the table, and enjoy finger foods (e.g., pieces of banana).

- At 9 months, infants can hold their bottles, sit erect unsupported in a highchair, and develop finger-to-thumb (pincer) movements to pick up food.

- At 10 months, infants poke at food with their index fingers, reach for food and utensils, and like to hold a spoon and push objects with it.

- Beyond 10 months, infants show an increased desire to feed themselves. They begin to use a spoon and to hold a cup with both hands, but frequently spill food. Between 2 and 3 years of age, self-feeding is completed with only occasional spilling.

---

 **37-3** **Feeding Solid Foods to an Infant**

**PURPOSES**
- To provide nutrients and calories to meet the infant's needs
- To promote muscular development of the mouth and tongue

**ASSESSMENT FOCUS**

Developmental status (e.g., extrusion reflex); appetite; food likes and dislikes; food allergies.

---

**EQUIPMENT**
- ☐ Small feeding spoon and unbreakable dishes
- ☐ Proper food (e.g., pureed or diced) at room temperature
- ☐ Bib
- ☐ Infant seat or high chair, if required

---

**INTERVENTION**

**1. Prepare the infant and yourself for the meal.**
- Change the diaper if damp or soiled.
- Wash hands.

- Approach the infant in a pleasant, relaxed manner, and provide a calm environment. *An infant old enough to eat solids will be well aware of this, because interest in the surroundings is increasing.*

- Put the bib on the infant, and place the infant on your lap or in the infant seat or highchair.

- Seat yourself comfortably, and relax. *Feeding times need to be un-*

▶

► **Procedure 37–3 Feeding Solid Foods to an Infant** *CONTINUED*

*hurried and relaxed to promote good eating habits and good digestion.*

**2. Promote acceptance and digestion of the food.**

- Control the infant's hands with your free hand by giving something to hold or by gently holding the arms (Figure 37–7). *Holding the arms prevents young infants from smearing their food.*

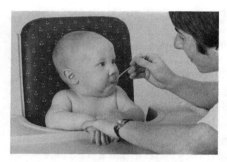

**FIGURE 37–7** Controlling an infant's hands when feeding the infant in a highchair.

- Offer plain foods before sweet ones, e.g., cereal and vegetables before fruits. *Infants may reject plain foods after eating the sweeter tasting ones.*

- Place small spoonfuls of food well back on the infant's tongue. *Putting food well back in the mouth overcomes the extrusion reflex, if it is present.*

- Scrape up any food that is pushed back out of the mouth, and refeed it.

- Continue to feed at a pace appropriate for the infant until the infant is satisfied. Hungry infants tend to eat quickly and show frustration if the food is given too slowly.

- Talk to the infant throughout the meal. *Friendly talk at mealtimes*

*is conducive to digestion and socialization.*

**3. Provide follow-up care as needed.**

- Wash and dry the infant's face and hands.

- Feed a young infant the recommended formula.

- Change the diaper, if required.

- Place the infant in a safe position in the crib. (See Procedure 37–2, step 8). Encourage the child to nap or rest. Ensure that the crib sides are elevated before leaving the infant.

**4. Document all relevant information.**

- Record assessments, the type and amount of feeding taken, and the infant's responses.

| EVALUATION FOCUS | Type and amount of food ingested; weight gain or loss; specific food likes and dislikes. |
|---|---|

**SAMPLE RECORDING**

| Date | Time | Notes |
|---|---|---|
| 5/29/95 | 1000 | Tolerated 30ml of rice cereal mixed with formula well. ———————————————— Corey Newton, SN |

# 38

# Fluid, Electrolyte, and Acid-Base Balance

## PROCEDURES

# 38-1  Using a Dial-A-Flo In-Line Device

| | |
|---|---|
| **PURPOSE** | • To regulate delivery of the correct amount of intravenous fluid |
| **ASSESSMENT FOCUS** | Patency of existing IV line; amount of solution prescribed. |

## EQUIPMENT

- ☐ Dial-A-Flo in-line device
- ☐ Equipment for an intravenous infusion.

## INTERVENTION

**1. Attach the Dial-A-Flo device appropriately.**

- Connect the Dial-A-Flo device to the end of the IV tubing.
- Connect the insertion spike of the IV tubing to the solution container.

**2. Prime the tubing.**

- Adjust the regulator on the Dial-A-Flow to the open position.
- Open all clamps and infusion flow regulators on the IV tubing.
- Remove the protective cap at the end of the tubing, and allow the fluid to run through the tubing.
- Reclamp the tubing to prevent continued flow of fluid.

**3. Establish the infusion.**

- Attach the primed tubing to the venipuncture needle or catheter hub.
- Open the IV tubing flow regulator.
- Align the Dial-A-Flo regulator to the arrow indicating the desired volume of fluid to infuse over 1 hour.

**4. Confirm the appropriate drip rate.**

- Count the drip rate for 15 seconds, and multiply by 4. *This ensures that the rate coincides with the calculated drip rate.*
- Recheck the drip rate after 5 minutes and again after 15 minutes. *This detects potential changes in the rate resulting from expansion or contraction of the tubing.*

- If the drip rate does not coincide with that calculated, it may be necessary to adjust the height of the IV pole. *Elevation of the IV pole facilitates flow by gravity.*

**5. Monitor the infusion flow.**

- Check the volume of fluid infused at least every hour, and compare it with the time tape on the IV container.

**6. Document all relevant information.**

- Record the date and time of starting the infusion, the type and amount of fluid infused, the rate at which the IV is being infused, the infusion device used, the status of the IV insertion site, and any adverse responses of the client.

| | |
|---|---|
| **EVALUATION FOCUS** | Amount of fluid infused in designated time period; status of IV insertion site; any adverse responses of client. |

**SAMPLE RECORDING**

| Date | Time | Notes |
|---|---|---|
| 12/03/95 | 1500 | 1000 ml IV D$_5$W started at 125 ml/hour using Dial-A-Flo. Venipuncture site dry and clean c̄ no signs of infiltration or infection.—— Carola Brown, SN |

## 38-2 Using an Infusion Controller or Pump

**PURPOSES**
- To maintain the prescribed fluid infusion rate
- To prevent fluid overload

**ASSESSMENT FOCUS**

Amount and type of IV fluid prescribed; flow rate.

### EQUIPMENT

- Infusion controller or pump
- The IV solution or medication
- A volume control chamber (Buretrol or Solu-set) for pediatric clients
- An IV pole
- An IV administration set with compatible IV tubing
- Sterile peristaltic tubing or a cassette if required
- Alcohol swabs and tape

### INTERVENTION

**Infusion Controller**

**1. Attach the controller to the IV pole.**

- Attach the controller to the IV pole so that it will be below and in line with the IV container.
- Plug the machine into the electric outlet, unless battery power is used.

**2. Set up the IV infusion.**

- Open the IV container, maintaining the sterility of the port, and spike the container with the administration set.
- Place the IV container on the IV pole, and position the drip chamber 76 cm (30 in) above the venipuncture site. *This provides sufficient gravitational pressure for the fluid to flow into the client.*
- Fill the drip chamber of the IV tubing one-third full. *If the drip chamber is filled more than halfway, the drops may be miscounted.*
- Rotate the drip chamber. *This removes vapor that could make the drop count inaccurate.*
- Prime the tubing, and close the clamp. Nonvolumetric controllers (regulators that measure the infusion in drops/minute) use standard tubing that is gravity-primed. *Priming expels all the air from the tubing.*

**3. Attach the IV drop sensor, and insert the IV tubing into the controller.**

- Attach the IV drop sensor (electronic eye) to the drip chamber so that it is below the drip orifice and above the fluid level in the drip chamber. *This placement ensures an accurate drop count. If the sensor is placed too high, it can miss drops; if placed too low it may mistake splashes for drops.*
- Make sure the sensor is plugged into the controller.
- Insert the tubing into the controller according to the manufacturer's instructions.

**4. Initiate the infusion.**

- Perform a venipuncture or connect the tubing to the primary IV tubing or catheter. Don gloves before performing a venipuncture.
- Open the IV control clamp completely.

**5. Set volume dials for the appropriate volume per hour.**

- Close the door to the controller, and ensure that all tubing clamps are wide open. *This enables the controller to regulate the fluid flow.*
- Set the dials on the front of the controller to the appropriate infusion rate and volume. Set the volume at 50 ml less than the required amount, if the controller counts the volume infused. *This will give you time to attach a new container before the present one runs out completely.*
- Press the power button and the start button.
- Count the drops for 15 seconds, and multiply the result by 4. *This verifies that the rate has been correctly set and the controller is operating accurately.*
- Some nurses recommend that all connections be taped. Count the drop rate again after the taping. *Taping could change the drop rate.*

**6. Set the alarm (optional).** *The alarm notifies the nurse when a set volume of fluid has been infused or indicates malfunctioning of the equipment.*

**7. Monitor the infusion.**

- Check the volume of fluid infused at least every hour, and compare it with the time tape on

▶

▶ **Procedure 38–2 Using an Infusion Controller or Pump** *CONTINUED*

the IV container. *This confirms the actual volume of fluid infused.*

- If the volume infused does not coincide with the time tape or the alarm sounds, check that:

  **a.** The time tape is accurate.

  **b.** The rate/volume settings are accurate.

  **c.** The drip chamber is correctly filled.

  **d.** The IV tubing clamp is fully open.

  **e.** The container still has solution.

  **f.** The drop sensor is correctly placed.

  **g.** The IV container is correctly placed.

  **h.** The tubing is not pinched or kinked.

**Infusion Pump**

**8. Attach the pump to the IV pole.**

- Attach the pump at eye level on the IV pole. *Because the pump does not depend on gravity pressure, it can be placed at any level. Eye level is convenient for checking its functioning.*

- Plug the machine into the electric outlet, unless battery power is used.

**9. Set up the infusion.**

- Check the manufacturer's directions before using an IV filter or before infusing blood. *Infusion pump pressures may damage filters or cause rate inaccuracies. Certain models may also cause hemolysis of red blood cells.*

- Open the IV container, maintaining the sterility of the port, and spike the container with the administration set.

- Place the IV container on the IV pole above the pump.

- Fill the drip chamber, and rotate it as described in step 2 above.

- Prime the tubing, and close the clamp. Most volumetric chamber pumps, i.e., pumps calibrated to infuse a specific volume of fluid at a specific rate (ml/hour), have a cassette that must also be primed. Manufacturers give instructions for doing this. Often the cassette must be inverted or tilted to be filled with fluid. Some volumetric pumps use special tubing that is gravity-primed.

**10. Attach the IV drop sensor, and insert the IV tubing into the pump.**

- Position the drop sensor, if required, on the drip chamber. See step 3.

- Load the machine according to the manufacturer's instructions.

- Ensure the correct pressure is set.

**11. Initiate the infusion.**

- See step 4.

**12. Set dials for the required drops per minute or milliliters per hour.**

- Close the door to the pump, and ensure that the IV tubing clamps are open.

- Press the power button to the "on" position, and press the start button.

**13. Set the alarm, and monitor the infusion.**

- See steps 6 and 7.

- If the tubing does not contain a regular cassette, slightly change the sections of tubing placed inside the infusion clamp. *This prevents tubing collapse from continual squeezing by the pump.*

**14. Document relevant information.**

- Record the date and time of starting the infusion, the type and amount of fluid being infused, the rate at which it is being infused, the infusion device used, the status of the IV insertion site, and any adverse responses of the client.

| **EVALUATION FOCUS** | Amount of fluid infused in designated time period; status of IV insertion site, especially the presence of infiltration. |
|---|---|

**SAMPLE RECORDING**

| Date | Time | Notes |
|---|---|---|
| 02/12/95 | 0900 | 1000 ml IV D$_5$W started at 125 ml/hour using controller. Venipuncture site clean and dry with no signs of infiltration or infection. Rodney Stewart, SN |

**38-3**

# Using an Implantable Venous Access Device (IVAD)

| | |
|---|---|
| **PURPOSES** | • To administer intravenous infusions, or medications<br>• To administer blood and blood products<br>• To obtain blood samples for laboratory analysis |
| **ASSESSMENT FOCUS** | Client's understanding and response to the system; type of therapy prescribed. |

## EQUIPMENT

- Priming solution of bacteriostatic saline
- IV solution container and administration set
  *or*
- Blood or blood product with transfusion set
  *or*

- Blood specimen tubes and syringe and needle
- Sterile gloves
- 5 ml syringes of normal saline flush and heparinized saline (100 $\mu$/ml of heparin)
- 2% lidocaine with subcutaneous syringe and needle (optional)

- Povidone-iodine and alcohol solution and swabs
- #22-gauge Huber needle
- Adhesive or nonallergenic tape
- Occlusive dressing materials
- Povidone or antibiotic ointment

## INTERVENTION

### 1. Assemble the equipment.

- Attach the IV tubing to the infusion or transfusion container.

- Prime the infusion tubing with saline.

- Prepare syringes of normal saline and heparinized saline. Currently, saline is used to flush the device either before and after medications or just periodically (once per day or per shift— check agency policy) followed by heparanized saline each time. *Heparinized saline helps prevent clotting.*

### 2. Position the client appropriately, and locate the implant port.

- Position the client in either a supine or sitting position.

- Locate the IVAD device, and grasp it between two fingers of your nondominant hand to stabilize it. Palpate and locate the septum, the rubber disc at the center of the port where the needle will be inserted.

### 3. Prepare the site.

- Wash hands, and put on sterile gloves.

- *Optional:* Insert 2 percent lidocaine subcutaneously in the injection site. *This anesthetizes the area for injection.* It may be ordered during the first few weeks after the implant surgery, when the area is tender and swollen and more pain from the needle puncture is felt.

- Prepare the skin in accordance with agency policy and let the area dry after applying such solutions as povidone-iodine and alcohol.

### 4. Insert the Huber needle.

- Grasp the device, and again palpate the septum for injection.

- Insert the needle at a 90° angle to the septum, and push it firmly through the skin and septum until it contacts the base of the IVAD chamber.

- Avoid tilting or moving the needle when the septum is punc-

**S** tured. *Needle movement can damage the septum and cause fluid leakage.*

### 5. Secure the needle, and ensure proper placement of the IVAD catheter.

- Aspirate blood when the needle contacts the base of the septum.

- Support the Huber needle with 2×2 dressings and Steristrips.

- Infuse the saline flush and priming solution. There should be no sign of subcutaneous infiltration after infusion of the saline fluid and priming solution.

### 6. After use, flush the system with heparinized saline.

- When flushing, maintain a positive pressure, and clamp the tubing as soon as the flush is finished. *These actions avoid reflux of the heparinized saline.*

### 7. Attach an IV-lock ("hep-lock" or saline-lock) to the Huber needle.

- A Huber needle with an IV-lock

▶

▶ **Procedure 38–3  Using an Implantable Venous Access Device** *CONTINUED*

can remain in place for one week before it needs to be changed. *The IV-lock allows for infusion of medications or fluid without continuous puncturing of the skin covering the IVAD.*

**8. Prevent manipulation or dislodgement of the needle.**

- Apply occlusive transparent dressings to the needle site.

- Apply povidone or antibiotic ointment to the site before dressings are applied as agency protocol dictates.

**9. Document all relevant information.**

- Record the procedure performed and all nursing assessments.

---

**VARIATION:** Obtaining a Blood Specimen

To obtain a blood specimen:

- Withdraw 10 ml of blood and discard it. *This initial specimen may be diluted with saline and heparin from previous flushes.*

- Draw up the required amount of blood and transfer it to the appropriate containers (see Procedure 38–5).

- *Slowly* instill 20 ml of normal saline over a 5-minute period (Holder and Alexander 1990, p. 45). *This thoroughly flushes the catheter and avoids excess pressure.*

- Inject 5 ml of heparin (100 $\mu$/ml) to prevent clotting.

---

**EVALUATION FOCUS**

> Infusion or transfusion rate; appearance of IVAD site; clinical signs indicating venous thrombosis (pain in the neck, arm, and/or shoulder on the side of the insertion site; neck and/or supraclavicular swelling); infection (redness and swelling at the site); and dislodgement of the needle or catheter (shortness of breath, chest pain, coolness in the chest).

**SAMPLE RECORDING**

| Date | Time | Notes |
|------|------|-------|
| 7/7/95 | 800 | IVAD accessed per protocol. 1000 cc 10% dextrose started at 100ml/hr via IV pump. IV site clean and dry with no signs of infiltration or infection. ———————————————————— Noah Andrews, RN |

## Obtaining a Capillary Blood Specimen and Measuring Blood Glucose

Before obtaining a capillary blood specimen, determine the frequency and type of testing, the client's understanding of the procedure, and the client's response to previous testing.

**PURPOSES**
- To determine or monitor blood glucose levels of clients at risk for hyperglycemia or hypoglycemia
- To promote blood glucose regulation by the client
- To evaluate the effectiveness of insulin administration

**ASSESSMENT FOCUS**

Client's learning needs.

### EQUIPMENT
- Blood glucose meter
- Blood glucose reagent strip compatible with the meter
- Paper towel
- Warm cloth or other warming
- device (optional)
- Antiseptic swab
- Disposable gloves
- Sterile lancet or #19 or #21-gauge needle
- Cotton ball to wipe the glucose reagent strip (dry wipe method)

### INTERVENTION

**1. Prepare the equipment.**

- Obtain a reagent strip from the container.

- Insert the strip into the meter according to the manufacturer's instructions, and make any required adjustments. *Some meters require calibration or the adjustment of the timer.*

- Remove the reagent strip from the meter, and place it on a clean, dry paper towel. *Moisture can change the strip, thereby altering the test results.*

**2. Select and prepare the vascular puncture site.**

- Choose a vascular puncture site, e.g., the side of an adult's finger or the heel, finger, or earlobe of an infant or child. Avoid sites beside bone.

- If either the heel or the finger is used, wrap it first in a warm cloth for 30 to 60 seconds (optional), *or* hold a finger in a dependent

position and massage it toward the site. If the earlobe is used, rub it gently with a small piece of gauze. *These actions increase the blood flow to the area, ensure an adequate specimen, and reduce the need for a repeat puncture.*

- Clean the site with the antiseptic swab, and permit it to dry.

**3. Obtain the blood specimen.**

- Don gloves.

- Place the injector, if used, against the site, and release the needle, thus permitting it to pierce the skin. Make sure the lancet is perpendicular to the site. *The lancet is designed to pierce the skin at a specific depth when it is in a perpendicular position relative to the skin.*

  *or*

  Prick the site with a lancet or needle, using a darting motion.

- Wipe away the first drop of blood

with a cotton ball. *The first blood usually contains a greater proportion of serous fluid, which can alter test results.*

- Gently squeeze the site until a large drop of blood forms.

- Hold the reagent strip under the puncture site until enough blood covers the indicator squares. The pad will absorb the blood, and a chemical reaction will occur. Do not smear the blood. *This will cause an inaccurate reading.*

- Ask the client to apply pressure to the skin puncture site with a cotton ball. *Pressure will assist hemostasis.*

**4. Expose the blood to the test strip for the period and in the manner specified by the manufacturer.**

- As soon as the blood is placed on the test strip:

  **a.** Follow the manufacturer's recommentations on the

▶

▶ **Procedure 38–4 Obtaining a Capillary Blood Specimen** *CONTINUED*

glucose meter, and monitor the time as indicated by the manufacturer, e.g., 60 seconds. *The blood must remain in contact with the test pad for a prescribed time for accurate results.*

**b.** If indicated, lay the glucose strip on a paper towel or on the side of the timer. *The strip should be kept flat so that blood will not pool on only one part of the pad.*

**5. Measure and document the blood glucose.**

• Place the strip into the meter according to the manufacturer's instructions. Some strips require that the strip be wiped, blotted, or washed (after a designated amount of time) prior to the strip being inserted in the meter. Other strips do not require blotting or wiping. Refer to the specific manufacturer's recommendations for the specific procedure.

• After the designated time most glucose meters will display the glucose reading automatically. *Correct timing ensures accurate results.*

• Turn off the meter, and discard the test strip and cotton balls.

• Document the method of testing and results on the client's record.

• Record the results.

• Report the results to the health care provider if indicated.

| EVALUATION FOCUS | Comparison of glucose meter reading with normal blood glucose levels; status of puncture site; motivation of client to perform the test independently. |
|---|---|

**SAMPLE RECORDING**

| Date | Time | Notes |
|---|---|---|
| 12/04/95 | 0700 | Skin puncture performed on right index finger for blood glucose. Results 82 by glucometer. ———————————————— Selena Daznard, RN |

# 38-5 Obtaining a Venous Blood Specimen from an Adult by Venipuncture

Before obtaining a venous blood specimen determine specific conditions to be met before obtaining the blood; previous disease, injury, or therapy that places client at risk for a venipuncture, e.g., bleeding disorder, anticoagulant therapy; presence of IV infusion that can alter test results; client's ability to cooperate with procedure.

**PURPOSES**

- To assess specific elements or constituents of venous blood (e.g., red or white blood cell count, differential white blood cell count, glucose, electrolytes, drugs, bacteria)
- To determine an individual's blood type
- To monitor a client's response to specific therapies

**ASSESSMENT FOCUS**

Condition of veins and surrounding skin for selected site.

## EQUIPMENT

- Correct test tubes for the tests (Vacuum specimen tubes are required for the vacucontainer method)
- Disposable gloves
- Topical antiseptic swab
- Tourniquet
- Sterile 1-inch needles, usually #19 or #21 gauge for adults

*or*
- Vacucontainer and sterile double-ended needles that screw into the adaptor
- Sterile syringe of appropriate size for the amount of blood required (sizes 5 to 10 ml are frequently used)

- 2 × 2 gauze pad
- Dry sterile sponges
- Band-Aid
- Completed labels for each container
- Completed requisition

## INTERVENTION

**1. Verify the physician's orders for the tests to be obtained, and obtain the correct test tubes specific for the test ordered.**

**2. Identify the client appropriately.**

- Check the client's wristband, and compare the name with the name on the requisition and chart.

**3. Don gloves, and perform venipuncture.**

- See Procedure 38–1 in *Fundamentals of Nursing*.

**4. Obtain the specimen.**

### Using Sterile Syringe and Needle

- When the needle is in the vein, gently pull back on the syringe plunger until the appropriate amount of blood is obtained (usually about 5 ml).

- Remove the tourniquet when sufficient blood is obtained, and remove the needle from the vein. Withdraw the needle in line with the vein while placing a 2 × 2 gauze pad over the site without applying pressure. *Removing the tourniquet and applying the gauze pad minimizes bleeding at the site when the needle is withdrawn. Careful removal of the needle reduces vein trauma and client discomfort.*

- Cover the venipuncture site with a sterile gauze, and ask the client to hold it firmly in place for 2 to 3 minutes, if able. *This facilitates clotting and minimizes bleeding from the site.*

- Transfer the specimens to the tubes:

  **a.** Remove the top from the laboratory test tube. Avoid touching the inside of the tube or spilling the contents. *This maintains asepsis of the test tube and contents.*

  **b.** Remove the needle from the blood-filled syringe, and gently insert the blood down one side of the tube. *Careful ejection of the blood sample is essential to prevent damage to the erythrocytes.*

  **c.** Replace the test tube lid or stopper.
  *or*
  Insert the needle directly through the stopper of the blood tube, and allow the vacuum to fill the tube with blood (Figure 38–1). Some nurses change the needle to a sterile #18-gauge needle to

▶

▶ **Procedure 38–5 Obtaining a Venous Blood Specimen** *CONTINUED*

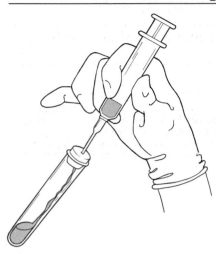

**FIGURE 38–1** Inserting a blood specimen directly through the stopper of the blood tube.

facilitate transfer of the blood by this method.

- For all blood tubes containing additives, gently rotate or invert the test tube several times. *This mixes the blood with the tube contents. Shaking is contraindicated because it can cause the erythrocytes to rupture.*

**Using a Vacucontainer System**

- Do not advance the venipuncture needle of a vacucontainer into the vein after the venipuncture.

- As soon as the venipuncture needle is positioned in the vein, hold the plastic adapter securely, and press the vacuum tube firmly into the short needle until it pierces the top of the tube. Blood will then spurt rapidly into the tube.

- Fill the vacucontainer with blood, release it, and set it aside.

- Insert another vacucontainer if more blood is required.

- Release the tourniquet, and remove the needle from the vein as described above.

- Cover the venipuncture site with a sterile gauze as above.

**5. Ensure client comfort and safety.**

- Assess the client's venipuncture site for oozing. This is especially important for clients who have prolonged blood coagulation times.

- If clots have not begun to form at the site, continue to apply pressure until bleeding has stopped.

- When bleeding is minimized, apply a Band-Aid over the site.

**6. Label the test tubes appropriately, and send them to the laboratory.**

- Attach labels to all test tubes. Ensure that the information on each label and the laboratory requisition is completely correct. *Inappropriate identification of specimens can lead to errors of diagnosis or therapy for the client.*

- Arrange for the specimen to be taken to the laboratory or stored appropriately, e.g., in a refrigerator. Blood obtained for culture should be transported immediately and should not be refrigerated. See Variation, next.

**7. Document and report relevant information.**

- Record the date and time blood is withdrawn, the test(s) to be performed, description of the venipuncture site after specimen collection.

- Report "stat" or any abnormal test results to the physician.

---

**VARIATION:** Collecting a Blood Specimen For Culture

In addition to blood withdrawal equipment, two sets of paired culture media bottles (Figure 38–2), a povidone-iodine or alcohol swab, and additional needles are required for this specimen collection.

- Prepare the venipuncture site

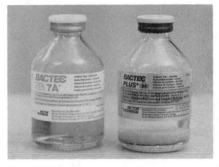

**FIGURE 38–2** Culture bottle set for blood cultures.

with povidone-iodine. Use alcohol if the client is allergic to iodine.

- Collect 5 ml of blood from a vein that does *not* have an IV running into it. *A specimen drawn through an intravenous infusion site will alter the test results.*

- Remove the venipuncture needle, and replace it with a sterile needle. *The needle used to puncture the skin may contaminate the specimen and affect culture results.*

- Swab the top(s) of the blood culture blood bottle(s). Insert the needle through the tops, and carefully inject 2½ to 5 ml of blood into one or both bottles, according to agency protocol.

- Use a new sterile needle when puncturing each bottle top. *This will avoid transmitting microorganisms to the blood from the bottle top.*

- Collect the second specimen after 15 minutes or according to agency protocol. Prepare the skin again with povidone-iodine or alcohol solution.

- Place this second sample in a set of paired culture bottles as above and according to the practice at your agency.

- Remove gloves.

- Label the bottles, and transport the specimen to the laboratory *immediately.*

▶ **Procedure 38–5** *CONTINUED*

**EVALUATION FOCUS**

Appearance of the venipuncture site after venipuncture; results of the laboratory tests.

**SAMPLE RECORDING**

| Date | Time | Notes |
|------|------|-------|
| 12/22/95 | 0700 | Venipuncture performed in antecubital vein. Specimen for complete blood count and electrolytes sent to laboratory. Venipuncture site has minimal bleeding. No evidence of hematoma.————————— George Sawyers, RN |

# 38-6 Assisting with the Insertion of a Central Venous Catheter

**PURPOSE**

- To administer nutritional fluids and medications that cannot be given by a peripheral route or when peripheral routes cannot be obtained

**ASSESSMENT FOCUS**

Baseline vital signs; actual and desired mobility status of the client, which may affect the approach used (supraclavicular or infraclavicular); exit sites for skin integrity and signs of infection; status of antecubital veins if PIC is to be inserted; client's ability to hold breath, maintain the required position, and not move when requested; agency protocol regarding care of central lines and sites.

## EQUIPMENT

### For insertion

- □ Sterile gloves for the physician and the nurse (2 pairs for the nurse)
- □ Skin preparation set, if the area needs to be shaved, or soap, water, a washcloth, and a towel
- □ Povidone-iodine sponges and ointment, or, if the client is allergic to iodine, 70% alcohol with sterile gauze squares and a combination of antifungal and antimicrobial ointment
- □ Masks for the nurse and the physician (in some agencies the client is also required to wear a mask)
- □ Bath blanket (if subclavian or jugular insertion is used)

- □ Sterile or clean gown for the physician (check agency policy)
- □ Subclavian insertion tray
- □ Cut-down tray
- □ Sterile 3-ml syringe with a 1-in #25 gauge needle
- □ Skin anesthetic (e.g., lidocaine 1 or 2% without epinephrine)
- □ Radiopaque subclavian catheter of suitable size and length
- □ Sterile 4 × 4 gauze squares
- □ Moistureproof sterile dressing material
- □ Adhesive tape

### For establishing the infusion

- □ Small IV solution container of normal saline or 5% dextrose in water

- □ Sterile TPN tubing or IV administration set with drip chamber and tubing (microdrip tubing is used when less than 100 ml/hour is administered; macrodrip tubing is used when more than 100 ml/hour is given)
- □ Extension tubing (30 in)
- □ *Optional:* A 0.22-micron cellulose membrane air-eliminating filter
- □ Tape to secure the tubing connections if Luer-Lok connections are not available
- □ IV pole
- □ Soft-tipped clamp without teeth to clamp tubing if problems arise

## INTERVENTION

### 1. Prepare the client.

- Describe the procedure, and explain the purpose of the catheter and the procedures involved in care and maintenance of the line.

- Before commencing, ensure that the client has given an informed consent.

- Instruct the client on how to perform Valsalva's maneuver (forced expiration against a closed glottis), i.e., to take a breath, close the mouth, breathe

out, and bear down. Encourage the client to practice this maneuver before the procedure, unless contraindicated by the client's condition.

- If the client is unable to perform Valsalva's maneuver

  **a.** Ask the client to hold the breath at the end of a deep inspiration or during the expiratory phase of the respiratory cycle and/or

  **b.** Have an assistant compress

the client's abdomen with both hands.

### 2. Prepare the IV infusion equipment for attachment to the catheter.

- Connect in sequence:

  **a.** The infusion tubing spike into the port of the normal saline or 5% dextrose in water solution container, using surgical aseptic technique.

  **b.** The filter.

▶ **Procedure 38–6** *CONTINUED*

c. The extension tubing. Place the filter between the infusion tubing and the extension tubing to avoid subsequently disrupting the dressing.

- Tape the tubing connections. **S** *This will prevent inadvertent separation, which can lead to air embolism, leakage, and contamination.* For easy reopening, double-tabbed tapes are available.

- Start the flow of solution, and prime the tubing to remove air. **S** *This dislodges air bubbles and prevents air embolism.*

- Stop the flow of solution, place the tubing protector cap on the end of the tubing, and hang the tubing on the IV pole. *The protector cap maintains the sterility of the open-ended tubing.*

**3. Position the client appropriately.**

- Assist the client to a Trendelenburg position (approximately a 15° to 30° angle). If the client cannot tolerate this position, use a supine position and modified Trendelenburg position with only the feet elevated 45° to 60°. *In Trendelenburg's position, the veins will dilate, and the risk of an air embolism is reduced because slight positive pressure is induced in the central veins.*

- For *subclavian insertion*, place a rolled bath blanket under the client's back between the shoulders. *In this position, venous distention is increased.*
  *or*
  For *jugular insertion:*

  a. Place a rolled bath blanket under the opposite shoulder. *The blanket will extend the neck, making anatomic structures more visible for selecting the site.*

b. Turn the client's head to the opposite side. *This position makes the site more visible and reduces the chance of contamination from microorganisms in the client's respiratory tract.*

*or*

For a *peripheral vein insertion* in the brachiocephalic vein or the superior vena cava, place the client supine with the dominant arm at a 90° angle to the trunk. *This arm position provides the straightest, most direct route to the central venous system. The dominant arm is often used because movement accelerates blood flow and decreases the risk of dependent edema.*

**4. Clean and shave the insertion area.**

- Open skin preparation equipment and don gloves.

- Wash and dry the insertion site with soap and water. *Washing will remove dirt and reduce the number of microorganisms present.*

- Shave the client's neck and upper thorax *if ordered.*

- Discard the gloves.

- Don a mask and sterile gloves.

- Clean the site with povidone-iodine sponges for 2 minutes or, if using 70% alcohol, for 10 minutes or according to agency protocol. Use a circular motion, working outward. *This reduces the number of microorganisms. Working outward prevents reintroducing microorganisms to the site.*

**5. Support and monitor the client.**

- Explain to the client what is going on, and provide support.

- Maintain the client in position.

- Monitor the client for signs of respiratory distress, complaints **S** of chest pain, tachycardia, pallor, and cyanosis. *These observations facilitate early detection of pneumothorax and air embolism. An improperly placed catheter may cause pneumothorax, resulting in chest pain and labored breathing.*

**6. Attach the primed IV tubing to the catheter.**

- While the physician removes the stylet from the catheter, quickly **S** attach the IV tubing to the catheter, and simultaneously ask the client to perform Valsalva's maneuver as practiced. *Valsalva's maneuver increases intrathoracic pressure, creating more pressure on the large veins entering the heart and reducing the return of blood to the heart. It therefore reduces the risk of air entering the large heart vein via the opened catheter and the risk of subsequent air embolism.*

**7. After the infusion is attached, apply a temporary dressing to the site.**

- Put on the second pair of sterile gloves.

- Apply povidone-iodine ointment to the site if agency protocol dictates. Many agencies no longer use ointment, believing it causes skin maceration.

- Apply a 4 × 4 sterile gauze dressing or a transparent occlusive dressing according to agency protocol.

**8. After X-ray examination or fluoroscopy confirms the position of the catheter, secure the dressing with tape.**

- See Procedure 38–8.

▶

▶ **Procedure 38–6 Assisting with the Insertion of a Central Venous Catheter** *CONTINUED*

- Tape the IV tubing to the catheter. *Taping prevents inadvertent separation of parts, leakage, and potential infection.*

- Label the dressing with the date and time of insertion and the length of the catheter, if it is not indicated on the catheter.

**9. Establish the appropriate infusion.**

- See Procedure 38–7.

**10. Document all relevant information.**

- Document the time of insertion, the size and length of the catheter, the site of insertion, the name of the physician, the time of the X-ray examination and the results, the kind of infusion, the rate of flow, and all nursing assessments and interventions.

**EVALUATION FOCUS**

| Clinical signs of sepsis and air embolism and pneumothorax. |
|---|

**SAMPLE RECORDING**

| Date | Time | Notes |
|---|---|---|
| 12/12/95 | 1900 | 18-cm subclavian catheter inserted by Dr. R. Sullivan. 1,000 ml D5W started at 36 ml/hr. Placement confirmed by fluoroscopy at 1850 hr. Vital signs stable. Slight pallor. ——————————— Naomi Treasure, NS |

# 38-7 Maintaining and Monitoring a CVC System

Before monitoring a CVC system, determine agency policy about central line care, the type of catheter (single- or multiple-lumen) used, and the type and sequence of solutions to be infused.

**PURPOSES**
- To maintain the prescribed infusion flow rate
- To maintain patency of the central venous system
- To prevent complications associated with central venous lines

**ASSESSMENT FOCUS**
Appearance of catheter site; rate of flow; any adverse response of the client.

## EQUIPMENT

- Tape
- Items for tubing change and dressing change (see Procedure 38–8).
- #21 gauge 1-in needles
- Luer-Lok adapters
- Soft-tipped clamp without teeth
- Alcohol or povidone-iodine wipes
- 10-ml syringe
- Sterile normal saline
- 3-ml syringe
- Heparin flush solution (e.g., 100 units heparin per 1 ml of saline)

## INTERVENTION

**1. Label each lumen of multilumen catheters.**

- Mark each lumen or port of the tubing with a description of its purpose (e.g., the distal lumen for CVP monitoring and infusing blood; the middle lumen for TPN; and the proximal lumen for other IV solutions or for blood samples.
*or*
Use a color code established by the agency to label the proximal, middle, and distal lumens. *Labeling prevents mixing of incompatible medications or infusions and reserves each lumen for specific therapies.*

**2. Monitor tubing connections.**

- Ensure that all tubing connections are taped or secured according to agency protocol.
- Check the connections every 2 hours.
- Tape cap ends if agency protocol indicates.

**3. Change tubing according to agency policy.**

- See Procedure 38–8.
- Some agencies advocate changing TPN tubing every 24 hours and tubing for other infusions every 48 to 72 hours.

**4. Change the catheter site dressing according to agency policy.**

- See Procedure 38–8.
- Most agencies recommend that the dressing be changed every 48 to 72 hours.

**5. Administer all infusions as ordered.**

- Use a controller or pump for all fluids (see Procedure 38–2).
- Prime all tubing to remove air.
- Maintain the fluid flow at the prescribed rate.
- *Optional:* If a *nonviscous* or *intermittent* solution is used, attach a #21 gauge short needle to the infusion tubing, and insert it through a clean Luer-Lok adapter cap. Tape this connection.
- If a *viscous* solution is to be infused, remove the Luer-Lok adapter, and apply the infusion tubing directly to the port or lumen.
- Whenever the line is interrupted for any reason, instruct the client to perform Valsalva's maneuver. If the client is unable to perform Valsalva's maneuver, place the client in a supine position, and clamp the lumen of the catheter with a soft-tipped clamp. Place a strip of tape (about 3 in from the end) over the catheter before applying the clamp. *The clamp is placed over the taped area to prevent damage to the tubing. A clamp without teeth prevents piercing.*

**6. Cap lumens without continuous infusions, and flush them regularly.**

▶ **Procedure 38–7 Maintaining and Monitoring a CVC System** *CONTINUED*

- Cap ports not in use with an intermittent infusion cap to seal **S** the end of a catheter.

- Clean the adapter caps with alcohol or povidone-iodine swab before penetration.

- Flush noninfusing tubings with 1 or 2 ml of heparin flush solution every 8 hours or according to agency protocol. *Flushing prevents obstruction of the catheter by a blood clot.*

- Always aspirate for blood before flushing tubings (or infusing **S** medications). *This validates that the catheter is appropriately placed in the vein.*

- Use a #25 gauge 5/8-in needle to penetrate the adapter cap when flushing the catheter. *A small gauge needle minimizes the possibility of leakage through the adapter plug, and a short needle minimizes the possibility of damaging the catheter.*

**7. Administer medications as ordered.**

- If a capped port is used for medications, first flush the line with 5 or 10 ml of normal saline according to agency protocol. *Many medications are incompatible with heparin.*

- After the medication is instilled through the port, inject normal saline first and then the heparin flush solution according to agency protocol. *The saline solution flushes the line of the medication. The heparin maintains the patency of the catheter by preventing blood clotting.*

**8. Monitor the client for complications.**

- At least every 4 hours, assess the client's vital signs, skin color, mental alertness, appearance of the catheter site, and presence of adverse symptoms.

- If air embolism is suspected, give the client 100% oxygen by mask, place the person in a left Trendelenburg position (Durant maneuver), and notify the physi-

cian. *Lowering the head increases intrathoracic pressure, decreasing the flow of air into the vein during inhalation. A left side-lying position helps prevent the air from moving to the pulmonary artery.*

- If sepsis is suspected, replace a TPN, blood, or other infusion with 5% or 10% dextrose solution, change the IV tubing and dressing, save the remaining solution for lab analysis, record the lot number of the solution and any additives, and notify the physician immediately. When changing the dressing, take a culture of the catheter site as ordered by the physician or according to agency protocol.

**9. Document all relevant information.**

- Record the date and time of any infusion started; type of solution, drip rate, and number of milliliters infusing per hour; dressing or tubing changes; appearance of insertion site; and all other nursing assessments.

| | |
|---|---|
| **EVALUATION FOCUS** | Rate of infusion flow; appearance of catheter site; any adverse response of the client. |

**SAMPLE RECORDING**

| Date | Time | Notes |
|---|---|---|
| 12/02/95 | 1410 | Bag #6 of hyperalimentation infusion started and running at 80 ml per hour per infusion pump. Catheter insertion site clean without inflammation or tenderness. ——————————————————— Carolyn Churchill, RN |

# 38-8 Changing a CVC Tubing and Dressing

| | |
|---|---|
| **PURPOSES** | • To prevent excessive growth of microorganisms and infection<br>• To inspect the catheter insertion site<br>• To maintain the flow of required fluids |
| **ASSESSMENT FOCUS** | Allergy to tape or iodine; infusion rate and amount absorbed; patency of IV system; presence of infiltration at catheter site. |

## EQUIPMENT

**For tubing change**
- New solution container and administration set (tubing)
- Sterile gloves
- Mask (especially if the client is immunocompromised)
- Sterile 2 × 2 gauze squares
- Antiseptic
- Tape

**For dressing change**
- Central catheter dressing set
  *or*

- Two face masks (one for the nurse and one for the client)
- 70% isopropyl alcohol
- Gloves (2 pairs)
- 4 × 4 gauze sponges
- Antiseptic swabs (e.g., 10% acetone and 1% iodine tincture or povidone-iodine solutions or, if client is allergic to iodine, 70% alcohol)

- Povidone-iodine ointment or, if client is allergic to iodine, a combination of antimicrobial and antifungal agents (optional)
- Precut sterile drain gauze or 2 × 2 gauze and sterile scissors
- Tincture of benzoin
- Elastoplast tape or transparent occlusive dressing such as Op-Site
- Nonallergenic 2.5-cm (1-in) tape

## INTERVENTION

### Tubing Change

**1. Prepare the client.**

- Assist the client to the supine position. *This lowers the negative pressure in the vena cava, thus decreasing the risk of air embolism when the catheter is opened.*

**2. Prepare the equipment.**

- Prepare the solution container, attach the new IV tubing, and prime the tubing as you would for a conventional IV. See Procedure 38–3 in *Fundamentals of Nursing.*

- Remove the tape securing the tubing to the dressing and the catheter hub connection.

- Don sterile gloves and mask.

- Place the sterile gauze underneath the connection site of the catheter and tubing. Clean the junction of the catheter and tubing with the antiseptic, if re-

quired by agency protocol. *This prevents the transfer of microorganisms from the client's skin to the open CVC catheter tip when it is detached; it also decreases the number of microorganisms at the catheter-tubing junction.*

**3. Change the tubing.**

- Ask the client to perform Valsalva's maneuver (that is, to take a deep breath and bear down) and to turn the head away while you detach the IV tubing by rotating it out of the hub. *Performance of Valsalva's maneuver reduces the risk of air embolism, and turning the head to the side reduces the chances of contaminating the equipment.*
  *or*
  Use the soft-tipped clamp to close the line.

- Quickly attach the new primed IV tubing to the TPN catheter, ensuring a tight seal. *The tubing must be attached quickly while the*

*client is performing Valsalva's maneuver.*

- Release the soft-tipped clamp, if used.

- Open the clamp on the new tubing, and adjust the flow to the rate ordered.

- Secure the tubing to the catheter with tape if a Luer-Lok connection is not present. *This prevents accidental separation of the tubes and contamination of the system.*

- Loop and tape the tubing over the dressing. *This prevents tension on the catheter and inadvertent separation of the tubing and the catheter.*

**4. Label the tubing, and document the tubing change.**

- Mark the date and time of the tubing change on the new IV tubing or drip chamber.

- Document the tubing change and all assessments.

▶

▶ **Procedure 38–8 Changing a CVC Tubing and Dressing** *CONTINUED*

**Dressing Change**

**5. Prepare the client.**

- Assist the client to a supine or a semi-Fowler's position.

- Don a mask, and have the client don a mask (if tolerated or as agency protocol indicates), and/or ask the client to turn the head away from the insertion site. *This helps protect the insertion site from the nurse's and client's nasal and oral microorganisms. Turning the client's head also makes the site more accessible.*

**6. Prepare the equipment.**

- Wash hands before handling sterile supplies and, if agency policy indicates, apply alcohol, and allow the hands to air dry.

- Open the sterile supplies.

**7. Change the dressing.**

- Remove the soiled dressing by pulling the tape slowly and gently from the skin. *This prevents catheter displacement and skin irritation.*

- Inspect the skin for signs of irritation or infection. Inspect the catheter for signs of leakage or other problems. If infection is suspected, take a swab of the drainage for culture, label it, send it to the laboratory, and notify the physician.

- Don sterile gloves.

- Clean the catheter insertion site with sterile gauze sponges soaked in a solvent such as 10% acetone. Clean in a circular motion, moving from the insertion site outward to the edge of the adhesive border. Take care not to jostle or get acetone on the catheter. Take a new sponge for each wipe. Repeat until the sponge is unstained after use. *Acetone defats the skin, destroys bacterial cell walls, and removes old adhesive tape, which could irritate the skin. Cleaning from the insertion*

*site outward and discarding the sponges after each wipe avoids introducing contaminants from the uncleaned area to the site. Jostling the catheter can cause discomfort to the client and could dislodge the catheter. Acetone is kept off the catheter because it could damage the catheter.*

- Using the method described above, clean the insertion site with povidone-iodine solution. If using 70% alcohol as a substitute for iodine, clean the area for 5 minutes. *The iodine solution is an antiseptic with antimicrobial properties that last a long time, even after drying.* Some agencies require cleansing with alcohol before applying povidone-iodine solution, and some require cleansing with alcohol afterward to remove the povidone-iodine solution, which can burn some people's skin.

- Optional. Apply the povidone-iodine ointment to the insertion site and to the catheter hub. Check agency policy.

- Apply a precut sterile drain gauze around the catheter (Figure 38–3). (If precut gauze is not available, cut a 2 × 2 sterile gauze square, using the sterile scissors.) Apply sufficient sterile gauze dressings to cover the catheter and skin. *This protects*

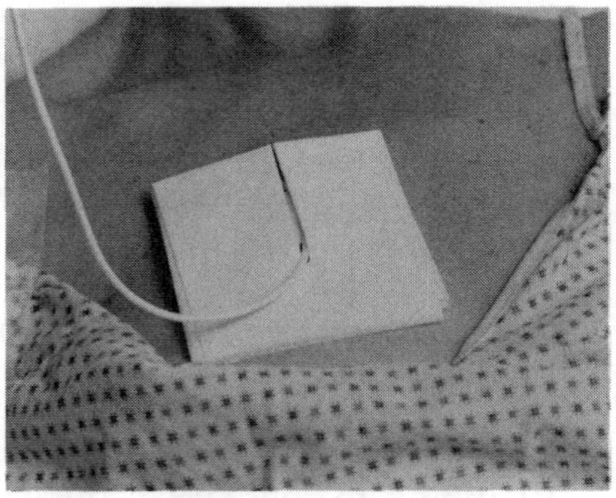

**FIGURE 38–3** A precut sterile gauze placed around a central venous catheter over the insertion site.

*the catheter and skin surrounding the insertion site from airborne contaminants.*
*or*
If using Elastoplast dressing, apply tincture of benzoin to the skin surrounding the dressing gauzes, and allow it to air dry about 1 minute. *This protects the skin when adhesive tape or Elastoplast is applied and promotes adhesion of the cover dressing. Appropriate drying time is essential to prevent skin breakdown when the dressing is removed.*

- Remove your gloves.

**8. Secure the dressing and the tubing.**

- Ask the client to abduct the arm and turn the head away from the dressing site. Tape the dressing securely to the skin with transparent occlusive dressing or Elastoplast. Make sure that the adhesive covering is occlusive. *Arm abduction and head rotation ensure that the client's range of motion is not limited by the dressing and decreases the potential for skin abrasion caused by movement of the adhesive.*

- Loop and tape the IV tubing (not the filter) over the occlusive dressing. *Looping prevents tension on the catheter and its inadvertent detachment if the tubing is pulled.*

- Label the dressing with the date, time, and your initials.

- See Procedure 38–3 in *Fundamentals of Nursing.*

**9. Document the tubing and the dressing change, including all nursing assessments.**

▶ **Procedure 38–8** *CONTINUED*

<table>
<tr><td>EVALUATION FOCUS</td><td>Appearance of catheter insertion site; presence of drainage, patency of tubing, infusion rate.</td></tr>
</table>

**SAMPLE RECORDING**

| Date | Time | Notes |
|------|------|-------|
| 12/12/95 | 1805 | CVC container and tubing changed. D5W infusing via IVAC pump at 60 ml/hr. Dressing changed at right subclavian triple-lumen catheter site using aseptic technique. No redness, edema or drainage. Povidone-iodine ointment applied. ———————————————————— Evylin Loo, RN |

# 38-9 Removing a Central Venous Catheter

**ASSESSMENT FOCUS**

Exit site of CV catheter for skin integrity and signs of infection; baseline vital signs.

## EQUIPMENT

- Sterile suture removal set
- Sterile drape
- Alcohol sponges
- Povidone-iodine ointment and 4 × 4 sterile gauze squares, or
- Vaseline gauze
- Mask for the nurse; one for the client if an infection is suspected
- Sterile gloves
- Sterile moistureproof dressing materials

## INTERVENTION

### 1. Prepare the equipment.

- Open a sterile suture removal set, and establish a sterile field.
- Open the sterile packages, i.e., sterile gauze squares and alcohol sponges.
- Place some povidone-iodine ointment on one of the sterile gauze squares if this ointment is to be used. Check agency protocol.
- Don a mask, and put one on the client if necessary.
- Close the clamp on the infusion.

### 2. Position the client appropriately.

- Place the client in a supine or slight Trendelenburg position. *These positions distend the central veins with blood, increase intrathoracic pressure, and limit air entry into the central vein.*
- Loosen and remove the dressing.
- Don sterile gloves.
- Remove any sutures that secure the catheter.

### 3. Remove the catheter.

- Ask the client to perform Valsalva's maneuver during removal. *This maneuver also raises intrathoracic pressure and prevents air entry into the central vein.*
- Grasp the catheter hub or needle, and carefully withdraw it, maintaining the direction of the vein.
- Inspect the catheter to make sure it is intact. If it is not, immediately place the client in a left lateral Trendelenburg position and notify the nurse in charge or physician immediately. *A piece of the catheter in a vein could cause an embolus.*

### 4. Immediately after catheter removal, apply pressure with an air-occlusive dressing over the subclavian site.

- Use an air-occlusive dressing, such as Vaseline gauze or Telfa covered with antibiotic ointment or plain sterile gauze (check agency policy). *Manual pressure and the occlusive dressing force the tissues together and seal off an air entry path.*
- When bleeding is controlled, replace the gauze dressing with an air-occlusive dressing while the client again performs Valsalva's maneuver.
- Completely cover the insertion site with povidone-iodine ointment, if used, sterile gauze pads, and moistureproof tape. *Nonporous tape helps to ensure impermeability to air.*
  or
  If agency protocol indicates, use a sterile transparent air-occlusive dressing. *A transparent dressing allows direct observation of the puncture site for signs of infection and bleeding.*
- Leave the air-occlusive dressing in place for 24 to 72 hours or the length of time agency protocol recommends. *The longer the duration of the catheter, the more time required for the subclavian tunnel to seal.*

### 5. Ensure client safety.

- Ask the client to remain flat and supine for a short time after the subclavian catheter is removed. *This position helps to maintain a positive intrathoracic pressure and allows the tissue tract to begin sealing.*
- Observe the client for signs of air embolism.
- If an air embolism is suspected, immediately place the client in a left lateral Trendelenburg position, and administer 100% oxygen by face mask. *The left lateral Trendelenburg position increases intrathoracic pressure, preventing air entry, and oxygen by mask provides oxygen to poorly perfused tissues.*

### 6. Document all pertinent information.

- Document the time of removal; the size, length, and condition of the catheter; and all nursing assessments and interventions.

▶ **Procedure 38–9** *CONTINUED*

<table>
<tr><td align="right">**EVALUATION**<br>**FOCUS**</td><td>Appearance of exit site for catheter; comparison of vital signs to baseline data; presence of signs of air embolism.</td></tr>
</table>

**SAMPLE RECORDING**

| Date | Time | Notes |
| --- | --- | --- |
| 01/06/95 | 1100 | 18-cm subclavian catheter removed intact. Transparent air occlusive dressing applied. BP 150/90, P 62 and regular, R 15. —— Rosanna Rodrigues, NS |

# 38-10 Measuring Central Venous Pressure

**PURPOSES**
- To assess hydration status
- To monitor fluid replacement and determine specific fluid requirements
- To evaluate blood volume, e.g., to monitor the degree of hemorrhage in a postoperative client

**ASSESSMENT FOCUS**

> Patency of CVC line; presence of infection or air embolism; central venous pressure.

## EQUIPMENT

- Intravenous tubing
- Manometer set, including stopcock
- A leveling device, if available
- Nonallergenic tape or an indelible marker
- Masks
- Sterile gloves

## INTERVENTION

### 1. Prepare the client.

- Place the client in a supine position without a pillow unless this position is contraindicated. If the client feels breathless, elevate the head of the bed slightly; note the exact position, because it must be used for all subsequent CVP readings, and the manometer level must be adjusted accordingly. *The client must always be in the same position to ensure reliable comparative CVP readings.*

- Locate the level of the client's right atrium at the 4th intercostal space on the midaxillary line.

- Mark this site with indelible pen or piece of nonallergenic tape.

### 2. Prepare the equipment.

- Prepare the IV tubing and infusion, prime the tubing, and then close the clamp on the tubing.

- If you are using a separate manometer and stopcock, attach the manometer to the stopcock. The manometer is attached to the vertical arm of the stopcock.

- If you are using a one-piece manometer and stopcock, attach these to the IV pole.

- Attach the IV tubing to the left side of the three-way stopcock.

### 3. Flush the manometer and stopcock.

- Do *not* attach the stopcock to the client's catheter until it is flushed free of air. *Air in the line will interfere with the CVP reading and could cause an air embolism.*

- Turn the stopcock to the IV-container-to-manometer position (Figure 38–4, *A*).

- Open the IV tubing clamp and fill the manometer with the IV solution to a level of about 18 to 20 cm.

- Close the IV tubing clamp.

- Turn the stopcock to the IV-container-to-client position (Figure 38–4, *C*), and flush the stopcock.

- Close the IV tubing clamp.

### 4. Attach the manometer to the central catheter.

- Place sterile 4 × 4 gauze under the catheter hub.

- Ask the client to perform Valsalva's maneuver (take a deep breath and bear down) and to

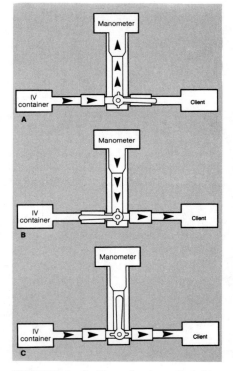

**FIGURE 38–4** Positions of a stopcock; *A*, IV container to manometer; *B*, Manometer to client; *C*, IV container to client.

turn the head away while you quickly attach the manometer tubing to the catheter. *Performing Valsalva's maneuver reduces risk of air embolism, and turning*

▶ **Procedure 38–10** *CONTINUED*

*the head reduces the chance of contaminating the equipment.*

- Turn the stopcock so that the IV runs into the client. (Figure 38–4, *C*) and open the IV clamp.

**5. Measure the central venous pressure.**

- Check that the level of the client's right atrium (zero reference point) is aligned with the zero point on the manometer scale. To align them, use the leveling rod on the manometer or a yardstick with a level attached (Figure 38–5). When the rod is horizontal (i.e., aligned with the client's right atrium), a bubble appears between two lines in the viewing window of the leveling

device. If an adjustment is required, first raise or lower the bed, and second readjust the manometer on the IV pole. *To ensure an accurate reading, the zero mark of the manometer must correspond with the level of the client's right atrium, and the manometer must be vertical.*

- Adjust the stopcock to the manometer-to-client setting (Figure 38–4, *B*).

- Observe the fall in fluid level in the manometer tube. Note also the slight fluctuations in the fluid level with the client's inspiration and expiration. If the fluid level does not fluctuate, ask the client to cough. *The fluid level falls with*

*inspiration because of a decrease in intrathoracic pressure. It rises with expiration because of an increase in intrathoracic pressure. No fluctuation may indicate that the CVP catheter is lodged against the vein wall. Coughing can change the catheter position.*

- Lightly tap the manometer tube with your index finger when the fluid level stabilizes. *This dislodges air bubbles that can distort the reading.*

- Take a reading at the end of an expiration or according to agency protocol. Inspect the column at eye level, and take the CVP reading from the base of the meniscus. If the manometer tube contains a small floating ball, take the reading from its midline.

- Refill the manometer, and take another reading of the CVP. *A repeat measurement ensures accuracy.*

- Readjust the stopcock to the IV-container-to-client position (see Figure 38–4, *C*) and adjust the infusion to the ordered rate of flow.

**6. Return the client to a comfortable position.**

**7. Document CVP.**

- Include the date and time of the CVP reading, the condition and rate of infusion flow, and all assessments.

- Report the changes in CVP as ordered. In many instances a change of 5 cm or more is reported immediately.

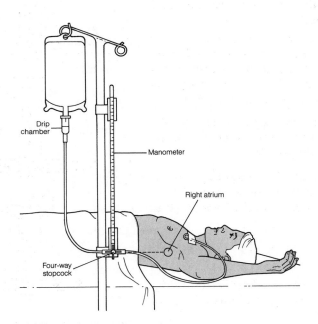

**FIGURE 38–5** The zero point on the manometer scale must be at the level of the client's right atrium.

Labels in figure: Drip chamber; Manometer; Right atrium; Four-way stopcock

| EVALUATION FOCUS | Central venous pressure; degree of fluctuation of pressure. |
| --- | --- |

**SAMPLE RECORDING**

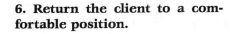

| Date | Time | Notes |
| --- | --- | --- |
| 06/06/95 | 1500 | CVP 9. Skin warm and moist. Central line dressing dry. IV infusing at 40 ml/hr. ——————————————————— Roberta Smith, SN |

# 39

# Oxygenation

## PROCEDURES

# 39-1  Collecting a Sputum Specimen

Before collecting a sputum specimen, identify the purpose for which it is to be obtained. This often determines the number of specimens to obtain and the time of day to obtain them.

**PURPOSES**
- To identify a specific microorganism and its drug sensitivities or the presence of cancerous cells
- To assess the effectiveness of therapy

**ASSESSMENT FOCUS**

Client's ability to cough and expectorate secretions; type of assistance required to produce the specimen (e.g., the need to splint an abdominal incision, the need to be placed in postural drainage position beforehand, or the need to perform deep-breathing exercises beforehand); skin color and rate, depth, and pattern of respirations as baseline data.

## EQUIPMENT

- Container with a cover
- Disposable gloves (if assisting the client)
- Disinfectant and swabs, or
- liquid soap and water
- Paper towels
- Completed label
- Completed laboratory requisition
- Mouthwash

## INTERVENTION

**1. Give the client the following information and instructions:**

- The purpose of the test and how to provide the sputum specimen.

- Not to touch the inside of the sputum container.

- To expectorate the sputum directly into the sputum container.

- To keep the outside of the container free of sputum, if possible.

- How to hold a pillow firmly against an abdominal incision if the client finds it painful to cough.

- The amount of sputum required. Usually 1 to 2 tsp (5 to 10 ml) of sputum is sufficient for analysis.

**2. Provide necessary assistance to collect the specimen.**

- Assist the client to a standing or a sitting position (e.g., high- or semi-Fowler's position or on the edge of a bed or in a chair). *These positions allow maximum lung ventilation and expansion.*

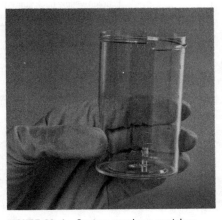

**FIGURE 39–1**  Sputum specimen container.

- Ask the client to hold the sputum cup on the outside, or, for a client who is not able to do so, don gloves and hold the cup (Figure 39–1).

- Ask the client to breathe deeply and then cough up secretions. *A deep inhalation provides sufficient air to force secretions out of the airways and into the pharynx.*

- Hold the sputum cup so that the client can expectorate into it, making sure that the sputum does not come in contact with the outside of the container. *Containing the sputum within the cup restricts the spread of microorganisms to others.*

- Assist the client to repeat coughing until a sufficient amount of sputum has been collected.

- Cover the container with the lid immediately after the sputum is in the container. *Covering the container prevents the inadvertent spread of microorganisms to others.*

- If spillage occurs on the outside of the container, clean the outer surface with a disinfectant. Some agencies recommend washing the outside of all containers with liquid soap and water and then drying with a paper towel.

- Remove and discard the gloves.

**3. Ensure client comfort.**

- Assist the client to rinse the mouth with a mouthwash as needed.

▶

▶ **Procedure 39–1  Collecting a Sputum Specimen** *CONTINUED*

- Assist the client to a position of comfort that allows maximum lung expansion as required.

**4. Label and transport the specimen to the laboratory.**

- Ensure that the specimen label and the laboratory requisition carry the correct information. Attach them securely to the specimen. *Inaccurate identification and/or information on the specimen container can lead to errors of diagnosis or therapy.*

- Arrange for the specimen to be sent to the laboratory immediately or refrigerated. *Bacterial cultures must be started immediately, before any contaminating organisms can grow, multiply, and produce false results.*

**5. Document all relevant information.**

- Document the collection of the sputum specimen on the client's chart. Include the amount, color, consistency, and odor of the sputum, any measures needed to obtain the specimen (e.g., postural drainage), the general amount of sputum produced, and any discomfort experienced by the client.

| EVALUATION FOCUS | Amount, color, and consistency (thick, tenacious, watery) of sputum; presence of hemoptysis; respiration rate and any abnormalities or difficulty breathing after the specimen collection; color of the client's skin and mucous membranes, especially any cyanosis, which can indicate impaired blood oxygenation. |
|---|---|

**SAMPLE RECORDING**

| Date | Time | Notes |
|---|---|---|
| 06/21/95 | 0600 | Sputum specimen sent to laboratory. Produced approximately 2 tbsp of green-yellow thick sputum. States has "sharp, knifelike pain" in right anterior lower chest when coughing. ———————— Sheila D. Wry, NS |

# Obtaining Nose and Throat Specimens

Before collecting a nose or throat specimen, determine (a) whether the client is suspected of having a contagious disease, e.g., diptheria, which requires special precautions; and (b) whether a specimen is required from the nasal cavity as well as from the pharynx and/or the tonsils.

**PURPOSE**

- To identify the presence of specific organisms and their drug sensitivities.

**ASSESSMENT FOCUS**

Appearance of nasal mucosa and throat (note in particular areas of inflammation and purulent drainage); complaints of soreness or tenderness; clinical signs of infection (e.g., fever, chills, fatigue).

## EQUIPMENT
- Gloves (optional)
- Two sterile swabs in sterile culture tubes
- Penlight
- Tongue blade (optional)
- Otoscope with a nasal speculum
- Container for the used nasal speculum
- Completed labels for each specimen container
- Completed laboratory requisition

## INTERVENTION

### 1. Prepare the client and the equipment.

- Assist the client to a sitting position. *This is the most comfortable position for many people and the one in which the pharynx is most readily visible.*

- Don gloves if the client's mucosa will be touched.

- Remove the cap from one culture tube. Lay the cap on a firm surface, inner side upward. *This prevents the inside of the cap from coming into contact with microorganisms on the surface.*

- Remove one sterile applicator, and hold it carefully by the stick end, keeping the remainder sterile. *The swab end is kept from touching any objects that could contaminate it.*

### 2. Collect the specimen.

### For a Throat Specimen

- Ask the client to open the mouth, extend the tongue, and say "ah." *When the tongue is extended, the*

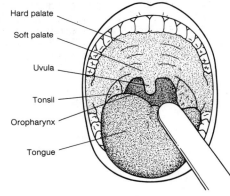

**FIGURE 39–2**  Diagram of the mouth.

*pharynx is exposed. Saying "ah" relaxes the throat muscles and helps minimize contraction of the constriction muscle of the pharynx (the gag reflex).*

- If the posterior pharynx cannot be seen, adjust the light, and depress the tongue with a tongue blade. Depress the tongue firmly without touching the throat (Figure 39–2). *Touching the throat stimulates the gag reflex.*

- Insert a swab into the mouth, taking care not to touch any part

of the mouth or tongue. *The swab should not pick up microorganisms in the mouth.*

- Quickly run the swab along the tonsils, making sure to contact any areas on the pharynx that are particularly erythematous (reddened) or that contain exudate. *By moving the swab quickly, you can avoid initiating the gag reflex or causing discomfort. Erythematous areas and areas with exudate will likely have the most microorganisms.*

- Remove the swab without touching the mouth or lips. *This prevents the swab from transmitting microorganisms to the mouth.*

- Insert the swab into the sterile tube containing transport medium without allowing it to touch the outside of the container. Make sure the swab is placed in the correctly labeled tube. *Touching the outside of the tube could transmit microorganisms to it and then to others.*

- Place the top securely on the tube, taking care not to touch the

▶

▶ **Procedure 39–2 Obtaining Nose and Throat Specimens** *CONTINUED*

inside of the cap. *Touching the inside of the cap could transmit additional microorganisms into the tube.*

- Repeat the above steps with the second swab.

- Discard the tongue blade in the waste container.

- Discard gloves.

**For a Nasal Specimen**

- Gently insert the lighted nasal speculum up one nostril.

- Insert the sterile swab carefully through the speculum, without touching the edges. *This prevents the swab from picking up microorganisms from the speculum.*

- Wipe along the reddened areas or the areas with the most exudate.

- Remove the swab without touching the speculum, and place it in a sterile tube.

- Repeat the above steps for the other nostril.

**3. Label and transport the specimens to the laboratory.**

- See Procedure 39–1, step 4.

**4. Document all relevant information.**

- Record the collection of the nose and/or throat specimens on the client's chart. Include the assessments of the nasal mucosa and pharynx, and any discomfort the client experienced.

| EVALUATION FOCUS | Appearance of nasal mucosa and throat; color of any drainage; any complaints of the client. |
|---|---|

**SAMPLE RECORDING**

| Date | Time | Notes |
|---|---|---|
| 06/22/95 | 0800 | Throat specimen for culture and sensitivity sent to lab. Throat is inflamed with patches of yellow discharge on tonsillar pillars. Unable to swallow fluids without soreness. ———————————————— Glenda Irvine, RN |

# 39-3 Assisting a Client to Use a Sustained Maximal Inspiration (SMI) Device

Before assisting a client to use an SMI device, determine the prescribed inspiratory volume level.

**PURPOSES**
- To improve pulmonary ventilation
- To counteract the effects of anesthesia and/or hypoventilation
- To loosen respiratory secretions
- To facilitate respiratory gaseous exchange
- To expand collapsed alveoli

**ASSESSMENT FOCUS**

Vital signs; breathing pattern (rhythm, ease or effort of breathing, volume); chest movements (retractions, flail chest); character of secretions and cough; breath sounds; presence of pallor or cyanosis; presence of clinical signs of hypoxia or anoxia (e.g., restlessness, increased heart rate, anxiety, rapid or deep respirations); location of a surgical incision that could impede lung expansion.

## EQUIPMENT

- ☐ Flow-oriented or volume-oriented SMI
- ☐ Mouthpiece or breathing tube
- ☐ Sterile water
- ☐ Label for mouthpiece
- ☐ Nose clip (optional)

## INTERVENTION

### 1. Prepare the client.

- Explain the procedure.
- Assist the client to an upright sitting position in bed or in a chair. If the person is unable to assume a sitting position for a flow spirometer, have the person assume any position. *A sitting position facilitates maximum ventilation of the lungs.*

### For a Flow-Oriented SMI

### 2. Set the spirometer.

- If the spirometer has an inspiratory volume-level pointer, set the pointer at the prescribed level. The physician's or respiratory therapist's order should indicate the level.

### 3. Instruct the client to use the spirometer as follows:

- Hold the spirometer in the upright position. *A tilted spirometer requires less effort to raise the balls or discs.*
- Exhale normally.
- Seal the lips tightly around the mouthpiece; take in a slow deep breath to elevate the balls: and then hold the breath for 2 seconds initially, increasing to 6 seconds (optimum), to keep the balls elevated if possible. Instruct the client to avoid brisk low-volume breaths that snap the balls to the top of the chamber. The client may use a noseclip if the person has difficulty breathing only through the mouth. *A slow, deep breath ensures maximal ventilation. Greater lung expansion is achieved with a very slow inspiration than with a brisk shallow breath, even though a slow inspiration may not elevate or keep the balls elevated while the client holds the breath* (Luce, Tyler, and Pierson 1984). *Sustained eleva-tion of the balls ensures adequate alveolar ventilation.*

- Remove the mouthpiece, and exhale normally.
- Cough productively, if possible and not contraindicated, after using the spirometer. *Deep ventilation may loosen secretions, and coughing can facilitate their removal.*
- Relax, and take several normal breaths before using the spirometer again.
- Repeat the procedure several times and then four or five times hourly. *Practice increases inspiratory volume, maintains alveolar ventilation, and prevents atelectasis.*

### For a Volume-Oriented SMI

### 4. Set the spirometer.

- Set the spirometer to the predetermined volume. Check the

▶

▶ **Procedure 39–3 Assisting a Client to Use an SMI Device** CONTINUED

physician's or respiratory therapist's order.

- Since some SMIs are battery-operated, ensure that the spirometer is functioning. Place the device on the client's bedside table.

### 5. Instruct the client to use the spirometer as follows:

- Exhale normally.

- Seal the lips tightly around the mouthpiece, and take in a slow, deep breath until the piston is elevated to the predetermined level. The piston level may be visible to the client, or lights or the word "Hold" may be illuminated to identify the volume obtained.

- Hold the breath for 6 seconds to ensure maximal alveolar ventilation.

- Remove the mouthpiece, and exhale normally.

- Cough productively, if possible and not contraindicated, after using the spirometer. *Deep ventilation may loosen secretions, and coughing can facilitate their removal.*

- Relax, and take several normal breaths before using the spirometer again.

- Repeat this procedure several times and then four or five times hourly. *Practice increases inspiratory volume, maintains alveolar ventilation, and prevents atelectasis.*

### For All Devices

### 6. Clean and put away the equipment.

- Clean the mouthpiece with sterile water, and shake it dry. Label the mouthpiece and a disposable SMI with the client's name, and store them in the bedside unit. *Only the mouthpiece of a volume SMI is stored with the client because volume SMIs are used by many clients.* Disposable mouthpieces are changed every 24 hours.

### 7. Document all relevant information.

- Record the procedure, including type of spirometer, number of breaths taken, volume or flow levels achieved, and results of auscultation.

- For a flow SMI, calculate the volume achieved by multiplying the setting by the length of time the client kept the balls elevated. For example, if the setting was 500 ml and the balls were kept suspended for 2 seconds, the volume is 500 × 2, or 1000 ml.

- For a volume SMI, take the volume directly from the spirometer, e.g., 1500 ml.

| EVALUTION FOCUS | Sounds heard on auscultation of the lungs to compare with those heard before procedure. |
|---|---|

**SAMPLE RECORDING**

| Date | Time | Notes |
|---|---|---|
| 07/06/95 | 1100 | Instructed in use of Triflo II spirometer. 5 breaths taken at volume of 1,000 ml (500 ml × 2 sec). Bilateral breath sounds normal on auscultation before and after spirometry. ————————————————— Nicholas Coscos, SN |

# 39-4 Administering Percussion, Vibration, and Postural Drainage (PVD) to Adults

Before administering PVD to an adult client, determine (a) the lung segments affected; (b) the ordered sequence of percussion, vibration, and postural drainage and the length of time specified; (c) whether the bronchodilator or moisturizing nebulization therapy is ordered prior to the postural drainage (secretions are easier to raise after the bronchi are dilated and secretions are thinned); and (d) preexisting or potential respiratory conditions.

**PURPOSES**
- To assist the removal of accumulated secretions
- To prevent the accumulation of secretions in clients at risk, e.g., the unconscious and those receiving mechanical ventilation

**ASSESSMENT FOCUS**

Lung sounds by auscultation; whether the cough is productive or nonproductive; color, amount, and character of expectoration; rate, depth, and pattern of respirations; vital signs.

## EQUIPMENT

- Bed that can be placed in Trendelenburg's position
- Pillows
- Gown or pajamas
- Towel
- Sputum container
- Tissues
- Mouthwash
- Specimen label and requisition, if a specimen of sputum is required
- Suction, as needed

## INTERVENTION

### 1. Prepare the client.

- Provide visual and auditory privacy. *Coughing and expectorating secretions can embarrass the client and disturb others.*

- Explain which positions the client will need to assume, and explain about percussion and vibration techniques.

### 2. Assist the client to the appropriate position for the postural drainage.

- Use pillows to support the client comfortably in the required positions.

### 3. Percuss the affected area.

- Ensure that the area to be percussed is covered, e.g., by a gown or towel. *Percussing the skin directly can cause discomfort.*

- Ask the client to breathe slowly and deeply. *Slow deep breathing promotes relaxation.*

- Cup your hands, i.e., hold your fingers and thumb together, and flex them slightly to form a cup, as you would to scoop up water. *Cupped hands trap the air against the chest. The trapped air sets up vibrations through the chest wall to the secretions, helping to loosen them.*

- Relax your wrists, and flex your elbows. *Relaxed wrists and flexed elbows help obtain a rapid, hollow, popping action.*

- With both hands cupped, alternately flex and extend the wrists rapidly to slap the chest (Figure 39–3). *The hands must remain cupped so that the air cushions the impact and injury to the client can be avoided.*

- Percuss each affected lung segment for 1 to 2 minutes. The per-

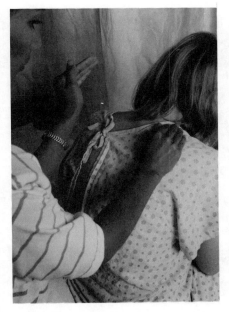

**FIGURE 39–3** Percussing the upper posterior chest.

cussing action should produce a hollow, popping sound when done correctly.

► **Procedure 39–4 Administering PVD to Adults** *CONTINUED*

### 4. Vibrate the affected area.

- Place your flattened hands, one over the other (or side by side) against the affected chest area (Figure 39–4).

- Ask the client to inhale deeply through the mouth and exhale slowly through pursed lips or the nose.

- During the exhalation, straighten your elbows, and lean slightly against the client's chest while tensing your arm and shoulder muscles in isometric contractions. *Isometric contractions will transmit fine vibrations through the client's chest wall.*

- Vibrate during five exhalations over one affected lung segment.

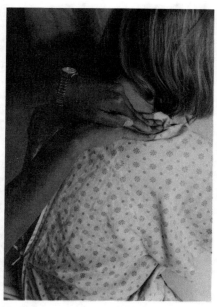

**FIGURE 39–4** Vibrating the upper posterior chest.

- Encourage the client to cough and expectorate secretions into the sputum container. Offer the client tissues and mouthwash as required.

- Auscultate the client's lungs, and compare the findings to the baseline data.

### 5. Label and transport the specimen, if obtained.

- Ensure that the specimen label and requisition carry the correct information.

- Arrange for the specimen to be sent to the laboratory immediately, or refrigerated.

### 6. Document the percussion, vibration, and postural drainage and assessments.

---

**EVALUATION FOCUS**

Amount, appearance, and character of secretions; tolerance of therapy (note signs of intolerance such as pallor, diaphoresis, dyspnea, or fatigue); change in breath sounds and rate, depth, and pattern of respirations.

**SAMPLE RECORDING**

| Date | Time | Notes |
|------|------|-------|
| 06/06/95 | 0600 | PVD for right anterior basal segment performed for 5 min. Large amount thick grey sputum produced. Specimen sent to lab. No pain or dyspnea. Inspiratory crackles unchanged. ——————— Robert Loo, RN |

# PVD for Infants and Children

Percussion, vibration, and postural drainage for infants and children is similar to that of the adult. It is usually performed three to four times daily and is more effective following bronchodilation and/or nebulization therapy. The length and duration of therapy depend on the child's condition and tolerance. To minimize the chance of vomiting, PVD is performed before meals (or 1 to 1½ hours after meals) and at bedtime. In a hospital setting, an older child can be positioned over the elevated knee rest of the hospital bed. Smaller children and infants can be positioned with pillows or over the nurse's lap.

Various methods may be employed to stimulate deep breathing, e.g., blowing feathers, blowing up balloons, using whistle toys, or using blow bottles designed to move colored liquid from one container to another. Because many children have difficulty coughing when in a dependent position, they should be allowed to sit up while they cough. The nurse can also reinforce the child's efforts by encircling the chest with the hands and compressing the sides of the lower chest during the cough.

For an infant whose chest is too small for conventional hand percussion, a small face mask or a bulb syringe cut in half can be used. Cut the syringe, leaving the nozzle with one half, and tape the cut edge to cushion it. Hold the bulb by the nozzle for percussion (Figure 39–5). To make a vibrator for an infant, remove the brush from a portable electric toothbrush and tape padding over the vibrating end.

Procedure 39–5 explains how to provide PVD to infants and children.

---

## 39-5 Administering Percussion, Vibration, and Postural Drainage (PVD) to Infants and Children

Before administering PVD to an infant or child, determine (a) the lung segments affected; (b) the ordered sequence of percussion, vibration, and postural drainage and the length of time specified; (c) whether the bronchodilator or moisturizing nebulization therapy is ordered prior to the postural drainage (secretions are easier to raise after the bronchi are dilated and secretions are thinned); and (d) preexisting or potential respiratory conditions.

**PURPOSES**
- To assist the removal of accumulated secretions
- To prevent the accumulation of secretions

**ASSESSMENT FOCUS**

Lung sounds; whether the cough is productive or nonproductive; color, amount, and character of expectorations; rate, depth, and pattern of respirations; vital signs.

---

### EQUIPMENT

- ▢ Pillows
- ▢ Gown or shirt and diapers
- ▢ Towel
- ▢ Face mask or other percussion device for small infant

- ▢ Sputum container
- ▢ Tissues
- ▢ Mouthwash, if the child is old enough to use it

- ▢ Suction apparatus as required
- ▢ Specimen label and requisition, if a specimen of sputum is required

---

### INTERVENTION

**1. Prepare the infant or child.**

- Provide an explanation that is suitable to the child's age.

- Assist the child to the appropri-ate position for postural drain-age.

- Use pillows to support the client comfortably in the required po-sitions.

**2. Perform PVD as ordered.**

- Percuss the affected area, using a percussion device if appropriate (Figure 39–5) or three fingertips flexed and held together.

▶

▶ **Procedure 39–5 Administering PVD to Infants and Children** *CONTINUED*

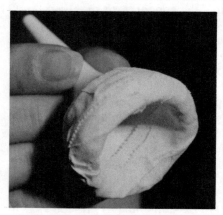

**FIGURE 39–5** A bulb syringe modified for chest percussion.

- Vibrate the affected area as appropriate, using a vibrator appropriate to the child's age. See Procedure 39–4, step 4.

- Instruct the child to sit up, and encourage deep breathing and coughing to remove loosened secretions.
  *or*
  Suction airway.

- Repeat percussion, vibration, deep breathing, and coughing for each lobe requiring drainage.

**7. Document the PVD and all assessments.**

- See Sample Recording in Procedure 39–4.

| EVALUATION FOCUS | Changed breath sounds; cough; amount, color, and character of expectorated secrections; rate, depth, and pattern of respirations; dyspnea; tolerance of treatment. |
|---|---|

# Infant Bulb Suctioning

A bulb syringe is frequently used to suction the oral and nasal cavities of infants and children, particularly when secretions are not severe enough to require deeper suctioning. This technique may be used for a newborn who has amniotic fluid in the air passages or an infant with increased mucus that is causing labored breathing. The technique requires medical aseptic practice rather than surgical asepsis, since only the mouth or nose is entered, not the pharynx. The bulb syringe should be sterile initially, but it can be rinsed and used for subsequent suctions without resterilizing. The same syringe can be used for the nose and mouth. See Procedure 39–6.

## 39-6  Bulb Suctioning an Infant

**PURPOSES**
- To establish and maintain a patent airway
- To prevent or relieve labored respirations

**ASSESSMENT FOCUS**

Rate and depth of respirations; presence or absence of breath sounds and chest movements: color and pulse rate; color, consistency, and amount of secretions.

## EQUIPMENT

- ☐ Large towel or blanket
- ☐ Clean towel or bib
- ☐ Bulb syringe
- ☐ Kidney basin or other receptacle
- ☐ Disposable gloves as needed

## INTERVENTION

**1. Position the infant appropriately for the procedure.**

Ⓢ • Bundle the infant in a large towel or blanket to restrain the arms, or cradle the child in your arm, tucking the infant's near arm behind your back and holding the other arm securely with your hand (Figure 39–6).

- Put the bib or towel under the infant's chin.

**2. Suction the oral and nasal cavities.**

Ⓢ • Compress the bulb of the syringe with your thumb before inserting the syringe (Figure 39–7). *Compressing the bulb while the tip is in the mouth or nose can force secretions deeper into the respiratory tract.*

- Keeping the bulb compressed, insert the tip of the syringe into the infant's nose or mouth.

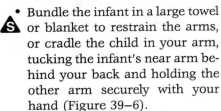

**FIGURE 39–6**  Restraining the arms of an infant for bulb suctioning. The infant's right arm is tucked behind the nurse's back.

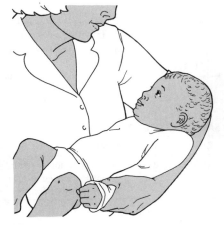

- Release the bulb compression gradually, and slowly move it outward to aspirate the secretions.

- Remove the syringe, hold the tip over the waste receptacle, and compress the bulb again. *Com-*

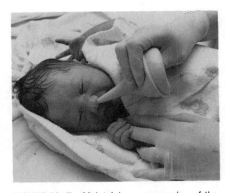

**FIGURE 39–7**  Maintaining compression of the bulb of the syringe during insertion into the nose. *Source:* S. B. Olds, M. L. London, and P. W. Ladewig, *Maternal-newborn nursing: A family-centered approach,* 4th ed. (Redwood City, Calif.: Addison-Wesley Nursing, 1992), p. 899.

*pressing the bulb expels the contents into the waste receptacle.*

- Repeat the above until the infant's nares and mouth are clear of secretions and the breathing sounds are clear.

▶

**Procedure 39–6 Bulb Suctioning an Infant** *CONTINUED*

**3. Ensure infant comfort and safety.**

- Cuddle and soothe the infant as necessary, and place the infant in a side-lying position after suctioning. *In a back-lying position, the infant is more likely to aspirate secretions.*

**4. Ensure availability of the equipment for the next suction.**

- Rinse the syringe and the waste receptacle.

- Place the syringe in a clean folded towel at the cribside for use as needed.

**5. Document all relevant information.**

- Report to the nurse in charge any problems or untoward responses of the infant.

- Record the procedure and relevant observations in the appropriate records.

**VARIATION:** The DeLee Suction Device (Mucus Trap)

The DeLee mucus trap is a negative-pressure mouth suction device used for infants (Figure 39–8). To use the device, carefully insert the catheter to 12 cm (3 to 5 in) into the infant's nose or mouth without applying suction, and connect the other end to low suction. Apply suction as the tube is removed. Continue to reinsert the tube and provide suction as long as fluid is aspirated. Avoid excessive suctioning. *This can cause vagal stimulation and subsequent bradycardia.*

The DeLee device is commonly used in the delivery room to clear the neonate's nose, mouth, and pharynx of mucus and amniotic fluid and to initiate breathing. Suctioning of the mouth is often needed as soon as the neonate's head presents. The mouth is suctioned before the nose. *Nasal stimulation can precipitate the sneezing reflex and cause the infant to inhale and*

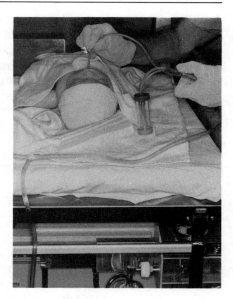

**FIGURE 39–8** Suctioning a neonate using the DeLee suction device. *Source:* S. B. Olds, M. L. London, and P. W. Ladewig, *Maternal-newborn nursing: A family-centered approach*, 4th ed. (Redwood City, Calif.: Addison-Wesley Nursing, 1992), p. 678.

*aspirate any secretions in the mouth.* Suctioning is often repeated after the neonate's first cry.

| | |
|---|---|
| **EVALUATION FOCUS** | Response to suctioning in terms of respiratory rate, rhythm, and depth; pulse rate and rhythm; skin color; and appearance of secretions suctioned. |

**SAMPLE RECORDING**

| Date | Time | Notes |
|------|------|-------|
| 11/02/95 | 0730 | Admitted to nursery from delivery room. Color pink, P 142, R 30. Clear mucuous drainage removed from mouth and nose with bulb syringe. Placed in side-lying position. ———————————————— Kay Kergstra, RN |

# Humidity Tent and Incubator

A variety of humidity/oxygen tents are available for children beyond early infancy until they are old enough to cooperate and use a nasal cannula. Each unit generally comes with the manufacturer's instructions for use. However, all have common elements. The tent consists of a rectangular, clear, plastic canopy with outlets that connect to an oxygen or compressed air source and to a humidifier that moisturizes the air or oxygen (Figure 39–9). Because the enclosed tent becomes very warm, some type of cooling mechanism such as an ice chamber or a refrigeration unit is provided to maintain the desired temperature. Administering oxygen by humidity tent is discussed in Procedure 39–7.

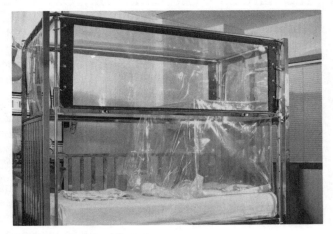

**FIGURE 39–9** A humidity tent.

---

## **39-7** Administering Oxygen by Humidity Tent

Before administering oxygen by humidity tent, determine (a) whether the damper valve is to be kept open, kept partially open, or intermittently closed and opened; and (b) whether aerosol medications are to be administered. Check the physician's orders.

**PURPOSES**
- To facilitate breathing by humidifying respiratory membranes and loosening secretions
- To increase blood oxygenation levels if oxygen is required
- To cool the body and reduce body temperature to normal range

**ASSESSMENT FOCUS**

> See Procedure 39–3 in *Fundamentals of Nursing.*

---

**EQUIPMENT**
- Gown or cotton blanket
- Humidity tent
- Ice
- Sterile distilled water
- Oxygen source or compressed air
- Additional gowns and bath blankets
- Small pillow or rolled towel

---

**INTERVENTION**

1. **Verify the physician's orders.**

2. **Prepare the child.**
- Provide an explanation appropriate to the age of the child, and offer emotional support.
- Cover the child with a gown or a cotton blanket. Some agencies provide gowns with hoods, or a small towel may be wrapped around the head. *The child needs protection from chilling and from*

*the dampness and condensation in the tent.*

3. **Prepare the humidity tent.**
- Close the zippers on each side of the tent.
- Fanfold the front part of the canopy into the bedclothes or into an overlying drawsheet, and ensure that all sides of the canopy are tucked well under the mattress (Figure 39–9, earlier).

- If cool mist is ordered, fill the trough with ice to the depth indicated by a line on the trough.
- Ensure that the drainage tube for the trough is in place.
- Fill the water jar with sterile distilled water. *The water moisturizes the air or the oxygen.*
- Connect the tent to the wall oxygen or compressed air.

▶

► **Procedure 39–7 Administering Oxygen by Humidity Tent** *CONTINUED*

- Flood the tent with oxygen by setting the flow meter at 15 liters per minute for about 5 minutes. Then, adjust the flow meter according to orders, e.g., 10 to 15 liters per minute. *Flooding the tent quickly increases the oxygen to the desired level.*

- Open the damper valve for about 5 minutes to increase humidity. The valve controls mist output and may be left open or partially open.

**4. Place the child in the tent, and assess the child's respiratory status.**

- Assess vital signs, skin color, breathing, and chest movements.

**5. Provide required care for the child.**

- Change the bedding and clothing as they become damp.

- Place a small pillow or rolled towel at the head of the tent. *This padding prevents bumping of the child's head and helps absorb excess moisture.*

- When administering care, be sure to maintain the humidity of the air and oxygen therapy. The canopy can be moved up around the infant's head and neck and secured under a pillow while care is being provided.

**6. Monitor the functioning of the humidity tent.**

- Monitor air or oxygen flows frequently to maintain required concentrations, and ensure that all connections are airtight.

- Minimize opening of the tent to avoid lowering the prescribed oxygen concentration. Plan care accordingly.

- Monitor the concentration of oxygen inside the tent according to agency protocol.

- Maintain the temperature of the tent at 20° to 21° C (68° to 70° F).

**7. Document relevant data.**

- Record the initiation of therapy, all assessments, and the data from oxygen analyzer.

| EVALUATION FOCUS | Vital signs; cough; skin color; lung sounds; signs of hypoxia, hypercarbia; blood gas levels. |
| --- | --- |

**SAMPLE RECORDING**

| Date | Time | Notes |
| --- | --- | --- |
| 5/5/95 | 0600 | Placed in humidity tent. T 98.6, P 108, R 32, Slightly cyanotic. $O_2$ set at 8 L/min., mist continuous. ———————————————— Nina Sims, SN |
| | 0630 | P 96, R 24, no cyanosis, Resting ———————————————— Nina Sims, SN |

# 39-8  Inserting and Maintaining a Pharyngeal Airway

**PURPOSES**

- To prevent obstruction of the airway by the tongue of an unconscious client (oropharyngeal tube)
- To maintain a patent air passage for clients who have or may become obstructed

**ASSESSMENT FOCUS**

> Level of consciousness and presence or absence of gag reflex; clinical signs indicating need for airway (e.g., upper airway "gurgling," labored respiration, increased respiratory and pulse rates).

## EQUIPMENT

- Disposable gloves
- Tongue blade (for oropharyngeal tube)
- Water-soluble lubricant or cool water
- Sterile oropharyngeal airway of the appropriate size (length should extend from the teeth to the end of the jawline)

  *or*

- Nasopharyngeal airway of the appropriate size (diameter should be slightly narrower than the client's naris)
- Soft tissues or washcloth
- Topical anesthetic, if ordered (for nasopharyngeal tube)
- Tape
- Suction equipment

## INTERVENTION

### 1. Insert the airway.

#### Oropharyngeal Airway

- Place the client in a supine position with the neck hyperextended or with a pillow placed under the shoulders. *This position prevents the tongue from falling back to block the pharynx.* Note: This position may be contraindicated for clients with head, neck, or back injuries.

- Don disposable gloves, open the client's mouth, and place a tongue depressor on the anterior half of the tongue. *This flattens the tongue and facilitates airway insertion.*

- Remove dentures, if present.

- Lubricate the airway with a water-soluble lubricant or with cool water.

- Turn the airway upside down, with the curved end upward or sideways, and advance it along the roof of the mouth.

- When the airway passes the uvula (or is at the posterior half of the tongue), rotate the airway until the curve of the airway follows the natural curve of the tongue.

- Remove excess lubricant from the client's lips with a soft tissue or washcloth.

#### Nasopharyngeal Airway

- Assess the patency of each naris. Ask the client, if conscious, to breathe through one naris while occluding the other.

- Ask the client, if conscious, to blow the nose to clear it of excess secretions.

- Lubricate the entire tube with a topical anesthetic (if ordered). *This prevents irritation of the nasopharyngeal mucosa and undue discomfort.*

- Hold the airway by the wide end, and insert the narrow end into the naris, applying gentle inward and downward pressure when advancing the airway. Follow the natural course of the nasal passage.

- Advance the airway until the external horn fits against the outer naris.

- If resistance is felt, try the other naris.

- Remove excess lubricant from the nares, as required.

### 2. Tape the airway in position, if required.
*Stabilizing the airway maintains the airway's position and prevents injury to the oropharyngeal or nasopharyngeal mucosa.* Smith and Johnson (1990) recommend the following method:

- Prepare two long strips of tape—one 35 cm (14 in), and the other 60 cm (24 in). This should be performed before donning the gloves.

▶

▶ **Procedure 39–8  Inserting and Maintaining a Pharyngeal Airway** *CONTINUED*

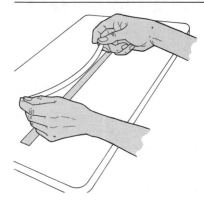

**FIGURE 39–10**  Attaching the shorter tape over the center of the longer tape.

- Lay the longer strip down, sticky side up.

- Place the shorter strip, sticky side down, over the center (Figure 39–10).

- Split each end of the longer tape (Figure 39–11).

- Place the nonsticky tape under the client's neck.

- For an *oral airway*, press half of the split tape across the upper airway flange and the other across the lower flange (Figure 39–12).
  *or*
  For a *nasal airway*, press half of the split tape across the upper lip and the other half around the tube without occluding the nares. Repeat for the other side.

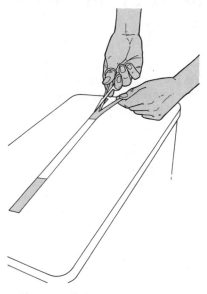

**FIGURE 39–11**  Splitting one end of the longer tape.

**3. Ensure the client's comfort and safety.**

**Oropharyngeal Tube**

- Maintain the client in a lateral or semiprone position so that any blood, vomitus, and mucus will drain out of the mouth and not be aspirated.

- Suction secretions as required.

- Provide mouth care as required to maintain moisture and tissue integrity.

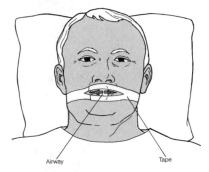

**FIGURE 39–12**  An oral airway taped in place.

- Remove the airway once the client has regained consciousness and has the swallow, gag, and cough reflexes.

**Nasopharyngeal Tube**

- Remove the tube, clean it in warm, soapy water, and insert it in the other nostril at least every 8 hours, or as ordered by the physician, to prevent irritation of the mucosa.

- Provide nasal hygiene every 4 hours or more often if needed.

**4. Document all relevant information.**

- Record the time the airway was inserted, type of airway inserted, client response to insertion, and character of any secretions suctioned.

| | |
|---|---|
| **EVALUATION FOCUS** | Client response to insertion (e.g., comparison of respiratory rate and depth and pulse rate to baseline data); integrity of oral or nasal mucous membrane and lips; character of secretions suctioned. |

**SAMPLE RECORDING**

| Date | Time | Notes |
|---|---|---|
| 4/6/95 | 0930 | Responding to painful stimuli only. Gurgling during aspiration. R 14, P 88. Oral airway inserted. Clear secretions suctioned from mouth. Turned to L lateral position. Mouth care given. Skin on lips and oral mucous membrane intact. ————————————————— Mary Beth Holly, RN |

# 39-9   Deflating and Inflating a Cuffed Tracheostomy Tube

**PURPOSES**
- To prevent aspiration of oropharyngeal secretions while the client is comatose or is eating or receiving oral medications
- To prevent tracheal edema, ulceration, and necrosis

**ASSESSMENT FOCUS**

> Size of cuff; maximum cuff inflation pressure recommended by the manufacturer; physician's orders and agency policy about the prescribed schedule for deflation and inflation; client respiratory rate and character; breath sounds.

## EQUIPMENT

- Equipment needed for suctioning the oropharyngeal cavity
- 5- or 10-ml syringe
- Manual resuscitator (Ambu bag)
- Stethoscope
- Soft-tipped hemostat
- Manometer specifically designed to measure cuff
- pressure, or blood pressure manometer
- Sterile three-way stopcock (optional)

## INTERVENTION

**1. Position the client appropriately.**

- Assist the client to a semi-Fowler's position unless contraindicated.
- Place clients receiving positive pressure ventilation in a supine position. *This position enables secretions above the cuff site to move up into the mouth.*

**2. Deflate the cuff.**

- First suction the oropharyngeal cavity. See Procedure 39–2 in *Fundamentals of Nursing*. *Suctioning prevents pooled oral secretions from descending into the trachea after the cuff is deflated. The secretions could cause irritation and infection.*

- Discard the catheter. *This catheter is discarded to avoid introducing microorganisms into the lower airway when it is suctioned later.*

- If a soft-tipped hemostat is clamping the cuff inflation tube, unclamp it. Some tubes have

one-way valves that replace the hemostat.

- Attach the 5- or 10-ml syringe to the distal end of the inflation tube, making sure the seal is tight.

- While the client inhales, *slowly* withdraw the amount of air from the cuff indicated by the manufacturer (e.g., about 5 ml), or as orders indicate, while providing a positive pressure breath with a manual resuscitator (an Ambu bag). *Removal of air on inhalation under positive pressure allows secretions to ascend from the bronchi. Slow deflation allows positive lung pressure to move secretions upward from the bronchi.*

- Keep the syringe attached to the tubing. *The syringe is left attached for reinflation of the cuff.*

- If the cough reflex is stimulated during cuff-deflation, suction the lower airway with a sterile catheter. *Cuff deflation can stimulate the cough reflex, which may produce additional secretions.*

- Assess the client's respirations, and suction the client as needed. If the client experiences breathing difficulties, reinflate the cuff immediately.

**3. Reinflate the cuff to the minimal occluding volume (MOV) using the minimal air leak technique (MLT).**

- Use a stethoscope over the client's neck adjacent to the trachea while inflating the cuff (Figure 39–13). *The stethoscope helps you gauge the proper cuff inflation point.*

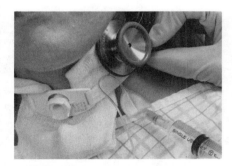

**FIGURE 39–13** Inflating a cuff while auscultating breath sounds over the neck beside the trachea.

►

▶ **Procedure 39–9  Deflating and Inflating a Cuffed Tracheostomy Tube** *CONTINUED*

- Inflate the cuff on inhalation, and inject the least amount of air needed (usually 2 to 5 ml) to achieve a tracheal seal. *This prevents tracheal damage.*

- Continue to inflate the cuff until you cannot hear an air leak, i.e., a harsh, squeaking, or gurgling sound.

- Stop cuff inflation when there is no audible air leak on auscultation. The cuff is sufficiently inflated when

  a. You cannot hear the client's voice.

  b. You cannot feel any air movements from the client's mouth, nose, or tracheostomy site.

  c. You hear no leak from the positive pressure ventilation when auscultating the neck adjacent to the trachea during inspiration.

- Establish a minimum air leak by listening to the client's neck with your stethoscope and aspirating a small amount of air (e.g., 0.1 to 0.3 ml) until a slight leak (i.e., a slight hissing sound) is detected. *This creates a minimal air leak, which indicates that the cuff is inflated at the lowest pressure possible to create an adequate seal. An air leak that is audible without a stethoscope is greater than a minimal leak.*

- Note the exact amount of air used to inflate the cuff to achieve a minimal air leak. *This prevents overinflation in subsequent cuff inflations and detects tracheal problems if more air is consistently needed.*

- If the tube does not have a one-way valve, clamp the inflation tube with a soft-tipped hemostat, or apply a one-way valve.

- Remove the syringe.

**4. Measure the cuff pressure.**

- Make sure the client is in the same position for each pressure cuff reading. *A change in position can alter the pressure needed to make an adequate seal.*

- Attach the cuff's pilot port to the cuff pressure manometer tubing.

- Read the dial on the manometer. The pressure should not exceed 15 to 20 mm Hg or 25 cm $H_2O$. Check physician's orders. *Excessive cuff pressure causes tracheal edema, ulceration, and necrosis. Underinflation may cause inadequate ventilation and may allow aspiration of blood, food, or secretions.*

- If the pressure is appropriate, clamp the inflation tube with a soft-tipped hemostat, provided that tube does not have a one-way valve.

- Remove the syringe.

- See also the variation below.

**5. Ensure client comfort and safety.**

- Check cuff pressure every 8 to 12 hours or as recommended by agency protocol. Note whether the minimal occlusive volume increases or decreases.

- Suspect an air leak if

  a. Air injection fails to inflate the cuff or increase cuff pressure.

  b. You are not able to inject the amount of air withdrawn.

  c. The client can speak.

  d. You can hear harsh gurgling breath sounds without a stethoscope.

- Make sure the client is comfortable and that the call signal and  communication aids are within easy reach.

**6. Document all relevant information.**

- Document the time of the deflation and/or inflation, the amount of air withdrawn and/or injected, and your assessments.

---

**VARIATION:** Using a Stopcock to Measure Cuff Pressure

- Attach the ends of the stopcock to the manometer tubing, the syringe, and the pilot port of the cuff (Figure 39–14).

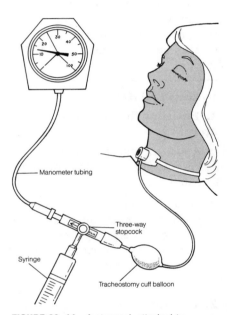

**FIGURE 39–14** A stopcock attached to manometer tubing, a syringe, and the pilot port of the cuff.

- Make sure the stopcock dial to the pilot balloon port is in the "off" position when you connect the setup to the pilot balloon port. *This prevents air leakage during equipment attachment.*

- Ensure a tight seal at all connections. *A tight seal prevents an air leak that could alter cuff pressure.*

- Turn the stopcock dial to the "off" position to the syringe. *This*

▶ **Procedure 39–9** *CONTINUED*

*establishes the connection between the cuff and the manometer.*

- Note the pressure reading on the manometer as the client exhales.

- If the amount of air needs to be adjusted, inflate or deflate the cuff by first turning the stopcock dial to the "off" position to the manometer. *This establishes a connection between the syringe and the cuff.*

- Turn the stopcock dial to the "off" position to the pilot balloon, and disconnect the apparatus.

| | |
|---|---|
| **EVALUATION FOCUS** | Respiratory rate and depth; pulse rate; tracheal breath sounds; skin and nail bed color. |

**SAMPLE RECORDING**

| Date | Time | Notes |
|------|------|-------|
| 7/21/95 | 1700 | Oropharyngeal cavity suctioned and tracheal cuff deflated. 3.7 ml air withdrawn from cuff. No coughing after deflation. R 16, regular, and nonlabored, P 84. ———————————————————— Sally S. Lee, RN |
| | 1800 | Tracheal cuff inflated to 15 mm Hg. R 14, regular, and eupneic. Lung sounds clear bilaterally. Skin color and nailbeds pink. ———————————————————— Sally S. Lee, RN |

# Plugging a Tracheostomy Tube

**39-10**

| PURPOSE | • To establish ventilation through the natural airway |
|---|---|

**ASSESSMENT FOCUS**
> Pulse and respirations before plugging the tube; excessive secretions in the respiratory tract (may contraindicate plugging of the tube).

## EQUIPMENT

- Suction apparatus
- Sterile suction catheters
- Sterile 10-ml syringe
- Sterile gloves
- Sterile tracheostomy plug

## INTERVENTION

### 1. Position the client.

- Assist the client to a semi-Fowler's position if not contraindicated. *This position enhances lung expansion and may decrease fears about not being able to breathe.*

### 2. Suction the airways.

- Suction the client's nasopharynx if there are any secretions present.

- Change suction catheters, and suction the tracheostomy. If there are excessive secretions, report this finding to the nurse in charge or physician to determine whether to proceed with the procedure.

### 3. Deflate the tracheal cuff if ordered.

- See Procedure 39–9.

- Suction the tracheostomy tube again if secretions are present.

### 4. Insert the tracheostomy plug.

- Using sterile gloves, fit the tracheostomy plug into either the inner or the outer cannula, depending on whether the tracheostomy tube has a double or single cannula.

- Monitor the client closely for 10 minutes for signs of respiratory distress, e.g., noisy and/or rapid respirations and use of accessory muscles for breathing. At the first signs of distress, remove the tracheostomy plug, and suction the tracheostomy if necessary.

- Clean the inner cannula, if it was removed, so that it is ready to be reinserted.

- Observe the client frequently while the tube is plugged.

### 5. Remove the plug at the designated time.

- After removing the plug, suction the tracheostomy if indicated, and replace the inner cannula if removed.

- Reinflate the cuff if ordered.

### 6. Document all relevant information.

- Document the amount, color, and consistency of the secretions, the times the plug was inserted and removed, and your assessments.

**EVALUATION FOCUS**
> Respiratory status while the tube is plugged (i.e., breath sounds, respiratory rate, and the use of accessory muscles for breathing).

**SAMPLE RECORDING**

| Date | Time | Notes |
|---|---|---|
| 7/11/95 | 1500 | P 82 regular, R 14 and effortless. Tracheostomy tube plugged after suctioning nasopharynx and tracheostomy tube. Cuff deflated—2.5 ml air withdrawn. |
| | 1515 | Breathing effortless while plug in place, pulse rate and respiratory rate unchanged. Plug removed. ———————————————— Briona R. King, SN |

# 39-11 Assisting with the Insertion of a Chest Tube

Prior to assisting with the insertion of a chest tube, verify that an informed consent has been obtained and that the client has been prepared for the procedure.

**PURPOSES**
- To remove air, fluid, and/or blood from the pleural space
- To allow full re-expansion of the lungs
- May be used to permit the administration of sclerosing agents in the treatment of malignant effusions

**ASSESSMENT FOCUS**

Respiratory rate, rhythm, and quality; vital signs, bilateral breath sounds; chest expansion and respiratory excursion; chest movements; presence/absence of retractions; dressing site; presence/absence of drainage and subcutaneous emphysema; level of comfort; client's emotional status.

## EQUIPMENT

- Sterile chest tube tray, which includes
  - Drapes
  - 10-ml syringe
  - Sponges
  - 1-in #22 gauge needle
  - ⅝-in #25 gauge needle
  - Scalpel
  - #11 blade
  - Forceps
- Two rubber-tipped clamps for each tube inserted
- Several 4 × 4 gauze squares
- Split drain gauzes
- Chest tube with a trocar
- Suture materials (e.g., 2-0 silk with a needle)
- Pleural drainage system with sterile drainage tubing and connectors
- Y-connector, if two tubes will be inserted
- Sterile gloves for the physician and the nurse
- Vial of local anesthetic (e.g., 1% lidocaine) if required
- Alcohol sponges to clean the top of the vial
- Antiseptic (e.g., povidone-iodine)
- Tape (nonallergenic is preferable)
- Sterile petrolatum gauze (optional)

## INTERVENTION

### 1. Prepare the client.

- Explain placement and rationale for chest tube(s) to client and family.

- Assist the client to a lateral position with the area to receive the tube facing upward. Determine from the physician whether to have the bed in the supine position or semi-Fowler's position. *A supine position is generally preferred for tube insertion into the second or third intercostal space, a semi-Fowler's position for the sixth to eighth intercostal spaces.*

### 2. Prepare the equipment.

- Open the chest tube tray and the sterile gloves on the overbed table.

- Pour antiseptic solution onto the sponges.

- After cleansing rubber stopper of local anesthetic with an alcohol swab, invert vial and hold it for physician to aspirate the medication.

- Be sure to maintain sterile technique.

### 3. Provide emotional support and monitor the client as required.

### 4. Provide an airtight dressing.

After tube insertion

- Don sterile gloves. Wrap a piece of sterile petrolatum gauze around the chest tube. Place drain gauzes around the insertion site (one from the top and one from the bottom). Place several 4 × 4 gauze squares over these. *The gauze makes an airtight seal at the insertion site.*

- Remove your gloves and tape the dressings, covering them completely.

### 5. Secure the chest tube appropriately.

- Tape the chest tube to the client's skin away from the insertion site. *Taping prevents accidental dislocation of the tube.*

▶

# ▶ Procedure 39-11 Assisting with the Insertion of a Chest Tube CONTINUED

- Tape the connections of the chest tube to the drainage tube and to the drainage system. *Taping prevents inadvertent separation.*

- Coil the drainage tubing, and secure it to the bed linen, ensuring enough slack for the person to turn and move. *This prevents kinking of the tubing and impairment of the drainage system.*

## 6. When all drainage connections are completed, ask the client to

- Take a deep breath and hold it for a few seconds.

- Slowly exhale. *These actions facilitate drainage from the pleural space and lung re-expansion.*

## 7. Ensure client safety.

- Place rubber-tipped chest tube clamps at the bedside. *These are used to clamp the chest tube and prevent pneumothorax if the tube becomes disconnected from the drainage system or the system breaks or cracks.*

- Assess the client regularly for signs of pneumothorax and subcutaneous emphysema. *Subcutaneous emphysema can result from a poor seal at the chest tube insertion site. It is manifested by a "crackling" sound that is heard when the area around the insertion site is palpated.*

- Assess the client's vital signs every 15 minutes for the first hour following tube insertion and then as ordered, e.g., every hour for 2 hours, then every 4 hours or as often as the client's condition indicates.

- Auscultate the lungs at least every 4 hours for breath sounds and the adequacy of ventilation in the affected lung.

- Check for intermittent bubbling in the water of the water-seal bottle or chamber. *Intermittent bubbling normally occurs when the system removes air from the pleural space, especially when the client takes a deep breath or coughs. Absence of bubbling usually indicates that the pleural space has healed and is sealed, but it may also indicate obstructed tubing. Continuous bubbling or a sudden change from the established pattern can indicate a break in the system, i.e., an air leak, and should be reported immediately.*

- Check for gentle bubbling in the suction-control chamber or bottle. *Gentle bubbling indicates proper suction pressure.*

- Inspect the drainage in the collection container at least every 30 minutes during the first 2 hours after chest tube insertion and then every 2 hours. Report bright red bleeding or drainage over 100 cc per hour to the physician.

## 8. Document relevant information.

- Document the date and time of chest tube insertion and the name of the physician.

- Include the insertion site, drainage system used, presence of bubbling, characteristics of the drainage, vital signs, breath sounds by auscultation, and any other assessment findings.

## 9. Prepare the client for a portable chest x-ray to check for re-expansion of the lung.

---

| EVALUATION FOCUS | Respiratory rate, rhythm, and quality; vital signs; breath sounds; dressing and character, quality, and amount of any drainage; patency of drainage system and character, quality and amount of drainage; presence/absence of subcutaneous emphysema. |
|---|---|

### SAMPLE RECORDING

| Date | Time | Notes |
|---|---|---|
| 12/6/95 | 2200 | Sudden sharp pain in L chest, diaphoretic, pale, and dyspneic. ——————————————— Karen P. Smith, RN |
| 12/6/95 | 2300 | BP 100/70, TPR 98.6, 105, 24. Diminished breath sounds in L lung and absence of chest movement. Two chest tubes inserted by Dr. Jung in L 2nd and 8th ICS. Connected by Y-connector and attached to Pleur-evac. Drainage system patent. Fluid level in water-seal chamber fluctuating with respiration. Drainage 25 cc clear amber. —————————————— Karen P. Smith, RN |
| 12/6/95 | 2305 | BP 110/70, TPR 98.6, 100, 20. Breath sounds present in L lung. ——————————————— Karen P. Smith, RN |

# 39-12 Monitoring a Client with Chest Drainage

**PURPOSES**

- To maintain patency of the chest drainage system and facilitate lung reexpansion
- To prevent complications associated with chest drainage (e.g., infection)

**ASSESSMENT FOCUS**

See Intervention, step 1.

## EQUIPMENT

### To Remedy Tube Problems

- Sterile gloves
- Two rubber-tipped Kelly clamps
- Sterile petrolatum gauze
- Sterile drainage system
- Antiseptic swabs
- Sterile 4 × 4 gauzes
- Air-occlusive tape

### To Milk Tubing

- Lubricating gel, soap, hand lotion, or alcohol sponge

### To Obtain a Specimen

- Povidone-iodine swab
- Sterile #18 or #20 gauge needle
- 3- or 5-ml syringe

- Needle protector
- Label for the syringe
- Laboratory requisition

## INTERVENTION

### 1. Assess the client.

- Assess vital signs every 4 hours, or more often, as indicated.

- Determine ease of respirations, breath sounds, respiratory rate and depth, and chest movements.

- Monitor the client for signs of pneumothorax.

- Inspect the dressing for excessive and abnormal drainage, such as bleeding or foul-smelling discharge. Palpate around the dressing site, and listen for a crackling sound indicative of subcutaneous emphysema. *Subcutaneous emphysema can result from a poor seal at the chest tube insertion site. It is manifested by a "crackling" sound that is heard when the area around the insertion site is palpated.*

- Assess level of discomfort. *Analgesics often need to be administered before the client moves or does deep-breathing and coughing exercises.*

### ⚠ 2. Implement all necessary safety precautions.

- Keep two 15- to 18-cm (6- to 7-in) rubber-tipped Kelly clamps within reach at the bedside, to clamp the chest tube in an emergency, e.g., if leakage occurs in the tubing.

- Keep one sterile petrolatum gauze within reach at the bedside to use with an air-occlusive material if the chest tube becomes dislodged.

- Keep an extra drainage system unit available in the client's room. In most agencies, the physician is responsible for changing the drainage system except in emergency situations, such as malfunction or breakage. In these situations:

  a. Clamp the chest tube close to the insertion site with two rubber-tipped clamps placed in opposite directions (Figure 39–15).

  b. Reestablish a water-sealed drainage system.

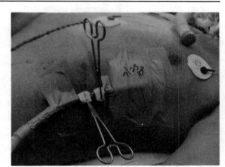

**FIGURE 39–15** Clamping a chest tube.

  c. Remove the clamps, and notify the physician.

- Keep the drainage system below chest level and upright at all times, unless the chest tubes are clamped. *Keeping the unit below chest level prevents backflow of fluid from the drainage chamber into the pleural space. Keeping the unit upright maintains the glass tube below the water level, forming the water seal.*

### 3. Maintain the patency of the drainage system.

- Check that all connections are secured with tape to ensure that the system is airtight.

▶

## ▶ **Procedure 39–12 Monitoring Chest Drainage** *CONTINUED*

- Inspect the drainage tubing for kinks or loops dangling below the entry level of the drainage system.

- Coil the drainage tubing and secure it to the bed linen, ensuring enough slack for the client to turn and move (Figure 39–16). *This prevents kinking of the tubing and impairment of the drainage system.*

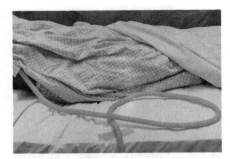

**FIGURE 39–16** Coiled drainage tubing secured to the bed linen.

- Inspect the air vent in the system periodically to make sure it is not occluded. A vent must be present to allow air to escape. *Obstruction of the air vent causes an increased pressure in the system that could result in pneumothorax.*

- Milk or strip the chest tubing **as ordered and only in accordance with agency protocol.** *Too vigorous milking can create excessive negative pressure that can harm the pleural membranes and/or surrounding tissues.* Always verify the physician's orders before milking the tube; milking of only short segments of the tube may be specified (e.g., 10 to 20 cm, or 4 to 8 in). To milk a chest tube, follow these steps:

  a. Lubricate about 10 to 20 cm (4 to 8 in) of the drainage tubing with lubricating gel, soap, or hand lotion, or hold an alcohol sponge between your fingers and the tube. *Lubrication reduces friction*

*and facilitates the milking process.*

  b. With one hand, securely stabilize and pinch the tube at the insertion site.

  c. Compress the tube with the thumb and forefinger of your other hand and milk it by sliding them down the tube, moving away from the insertion site. *Milking the tubing dislodges obstructions, such as blood clots. Milking from the insertion site downward prevents movement of the obstructive material into the pleural space.*

  d. If the entire tube is to be milked, reposition your hands farther along the tubing, and repeat steps **a** through **c** in progressive overlapping steps, until you reach the end of the tubing.

**4. Assess any fluid level fluctuations and bubbling in the drainage system.**

- In gravity drainage systems, check for fluctuation (tidaling) of the fluid level in the water-seal glass tube of a bottle system or the water-seal chamber of a commercial system as the client breathes. Normally, fluctuations of 5 to 10 cm (2 to 4 in) occur until the lung has reexpanded. In suction drainage systems, the fluid line remains constant. *Fluctuations reflect the pressure changes in the pleural space during inhalation and exhalation. The fluid level rises when the client inhales and falls when the client exhales. The absence of fluctuations may indicate tubing obstruction from a kink, dependent loop, blood clot, or outside pressure (e.g., because the client is lying on the tubing), or may indicate that full lung reexpansion has occurred.*

- To check for fluctuation in suction systems, temporarily turn off the suction. Then observe the fluctuation.

- Check for intermittent bubbling in the water of the water-seal bottle or chamber. *Intermittent bubbling normally occurs when the system removes air from the pleural space, especially when the client takes a deep breath or coughs. Absence of bubbling indicates that the pleural space has healed and is sealed. Continuous bubbling or a sudden change from an established pattern can indicate a break in the system, i.e., an air leak, and should be reported immediately.*

- Check for gentle bubbling in the suction-control bottle or chamber. *Gentle bubbling indicates proper suction pressure.*

**5. Assess the drainage.**

- Inspect the drainage in the collection container at least every 30 minutes during the first 2 hours after chest tube insertion and every 2 hours thereafter.

- Every 8 hours, mark the time,

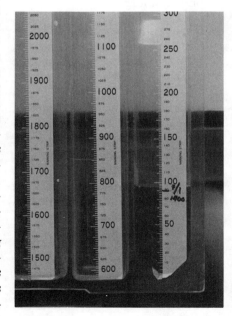

**FIGURE 39–17** Marking the date, time, and drainage level.

► **Procedure 39–12** *CONTINUED*

date, and drainage level on a piece of adhesive tape affixed to the container, or mark it directly on a disposable container (Figure 39–17).

• Note any sudden change in the amount or color of the drainage.

• If drainage exceeds 100 ml per hour or if a color change indicates hemorrhage, notify the physician immediately.

**6. Watch for dislodgement of the tubes, and remedy the problem promptly.**

• If the chest tube becomes disconnected from the drainage system

  **a.** Have the client exhale fully.

  **b.** Clamp the chest tube close to the insertion site with two rubber-tipped clamps placed in opposite directions. *Clamping the tube prevents external air from entering the pleural space. Two clamps ensure complete closure of the tube.*

  **c.** Quickly clean the ends of the tubing with an antiseptic, reconnect them, and tape them securely.

  **d.** Unclamp the tube as soon as possible. *Having the client exhale and clamping the tube for no longer than necessary prevents an air or fluid buildup in the pleural space, which can cause further lung collapse.*

  **e.** Assess the client closely for respiratory distress (dyspnea, pallor, diaphoresis, blood-tinged sputum, or chest pain).

  **f.** Check vital signs every 10 minutes or as the client's condition indicates.

• If the chest tube becomes dislodged from the insertion site

  **a.** Remove the dressing, and immmediately apply pressure with the petrolatum gauze, your hand, or a towel.

  **b.** Cover the site with sterile 4 × 4 gauze squares.

  **c.** Tape the dressings with air-occlusive tape.

  **d.** Notify the physician immediately.

  **e.** Assess the client for respiratory distress every 10 to 15 minutes or as client condition indicates.

• If the drainage system is accidentally tipped over

  **a.** Immediately return it to the upright position.

  **b.** Ask the client to take several deep breaths. *Deep breaths help force air out of the pleural cavity that might have entered when the water seal was not intact.*

  **c.** Notify the nurse in charge and the physician.

  **d.** Assess the client for respiratory distress.

**7. If continuous bubbling persists in the water-seal collection chamber, indicating an air leak, determine its source.** *Continuous bubbling in the water-seal collection chamber normally occurs for only a few minutes after a chest tube is attached to drainage, because fluid and air initially rush out from the intrapleural space under high pressure.*

• To detect an air leak, follow the next steps sequentially (Quinn 1986 and Palau 1986):

  **a.** Check the tubing connection sites. Tighten and retape any connection that seems loose. *The tubing connection sites are the most likely places for leaks to occur. Bub-*

*bling will stop if these are the sources of the leak.*

  **b.** If bubbling continues, clamp the chest tube near the insertion site, and see whether the bubbling stops while the client takes several deep breaths. *Clamping the chest tube near the insertion site will help determine whether the leak is proximal or distal to the clamp. Chest tube clamping must be done only for a few seconds at a time. Clamping for long periods can aggravate an existing pneumothorax or lead to a recurrent pneumothorax.*

  **c.** If bubbling stops, proceed with the next step. The source of the air leak is above the clamp, i.e., between the clamp and the client. It may be either at the insertion site or inside the client.

  **d.** If bubbling continues, the source of the air leak is below the clamp, i.e., in the drainage system below the clamp. See next step below.

• To determine whether the air leak is at the insertion site or inside the client:

  **a.** Unclamp the tube and palpate gently around the insertion site. If the bubbling stops, the leak is at the insertion site. To remedy this situation, apply a petrolatum gauze and a 4 × 4 gauze around the insertion site, and secure these dressings with adhesive tape.

  **b.** If the leak is not at the insertion site, it is inside the client and may indicate a dislodged tube or a new pneumothorax, a new disruption of the pleural space.

►

▶ **Procedure 39–12 Monitoring Chest Drainage** *CONTINUED*

In this instance, leave the tube unclamped, notify the physician, and monitor the client for signs of respiratory distress.

- To locate an air leak below the chest tube clamp

  **a.** Move the clamp a few inches farther down and keep moving it downward a few inches at a time. Each time the clamp is moved, check the water-seal collection chamber for bubbling. The bubbling will stop as soon as the clamp is placed between the air leak and the water-seal drainage.

  **b.** Seal the leak when you locate it by applying tape to that portion of the drainage tube.

  **c.** If bubbling continues after the entire length of the tube is clamped, the air leak is in the drainage device. To remedy this situation, replace the drainage system according to agency protocol.

**8. Take a specimen of the chest drainage as required.**

- Specimens of chest drainage may be taken from a disposable chest drainage system because these systems are equipped with self-sealing ports. If a specimen is required

  **a.** Use a povidone-iodine swab to wipe the self-sealing diaphragm on the back of the drainage collection chamber. Allow it to dry.

  **b.** Attach a sterile #18 or #20 gauge needle to a 3- or 5-ml

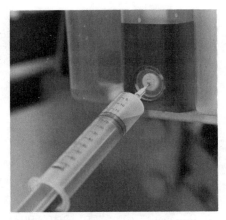

**FIGURE 39–18** Obtaining a specimen through a self-sealing port.

syringe, and insert the needle into the diaphragm (Figure 39–18).

  **c.** Aspirate the specimen (discard the needle in the appropriate container), label the syringe, and send it to the laboratory with the appropriate requisition form.

**9. Ensure essential client care.**

- Encourage deep-breathing and coughing exercises every 2 hours if indicated (this may be contraindicated in clients with a lobectomy). Have the client sit upright to perform the exercises, and splint the tube insertion site with a pillow or with a hand to minimize discomfort. *Deep breathing and coughing help remove accumulations from the pleural space, facilitate drainage, and help the lung to reexpand.*

- While the client takes deep breaths, palpate the chest for thoracic expansion. Place your hands together at the base of the sternum so that your thumbs meet. As the client inhales, your thumbs should separate at least

2.5 to 5 cm (1 to 2 in). Note whether chest expansion is symmetric.

- Reposition the client every 2 hours. When the client is lying on the affected side, place rolled towels beside the tubing. *Frequent position changes promote drainage, prevent complications, and provide comfort. Rolled towels prevent occlusion of the chest tube by the client's weight.*

- Assist the client with range-of-motion exercises of the affected shoulder three times per day to maintain joint mobility.

- When transporting and ambulating the client:

  **a.** Attach rubber-tipped forceps to the client's gown for emergency use.

  **b.** Keep the water-seal unit below chest level and upright.

  **c.** If it is necessary to clamp the tube, remove the clamp as soon as possible or in accordance with the client's condition.

  **d.** Disconnect the drainage system from the suction apparatus before moving the client, and make sure the air vent is open.

**10. Document all relevant information.**

- Record patency of chest tubes; type, amount, and color of drainage; presence of fluctuations, appearance of insertion site; laboratory specimens, if any were taken; respiratory assessments; client's vital signs and level of comfort; and all other nursing care provided to the client.

▶ **Procedure 39–12** *CONTINUED*

**EVALUATION FOCUS**

Amount and appearance of drainage; rate, depth, and pattern of respirations; breath sounds, pulse, blood pressure, and body temperature; complaints of discomfort; status of chest tube insertion site; amount and appearance of insertion site drainage.

**SAMPLE RECORDING**

| Date | Time | Notes |
|------|------|-------|
| 8/6/95 | 0800 | Respirations 12 and effortless. Breath sounds auscultated in all lung lobes. Chest expansion is symmetric. T 37.6, P 78, BP 126/78. 25 ml of serosanguineous chest drainage in last hour. Fluid level in water-seal chamber fluctuating with respiration. Dressing dry and intact. Chest tubes intact. ——————————————————————— Holly Wilson, RN |

## ‹39-13› Assisting with the Removal of a Chest Tube

**PURPOSE**
- To remove a chest tube when the lung is re-expanded

**ASSESSMENT FOCUS**

Respiratory rate, rhythm, and quality; vital signs, bilateral breath sounds; chest expansion and respiratory excursion; chest movements; presence/absence of retractions; dressing site; presence/absence of drainage and subcutaneous emphysema; level of comfort; client's emotional status.

---

### EQUIPMENT

- Nonsterile gloves to remove the dressing
- Sterile gloves to remove the tube
- Sterile suture removal set, with forceps and suture scissors

- Sterile petrolatum gauze
- Several 4 × 4 gauze squares
- Air-occlusive tape, 2 or 3 in wide (nonallergenic is preferred)
- Scissors

- Absorbent linen-saver pad
- Moistureproof bag
- Sterile swabs or applicators in sterile containers to obtain a specimen (optional)

---

### INTERVENTION

**1. Prepare the client.**

- Administer an analgesic, if ordered, 30 minutes before the tube is removed.

- Ensure that the chest tube is securely clamped. *Clamping prevents air from entering the pleural space.*

- Assist the client to a semi-Fowler's position or to a lateral position on the unaffected side.

- Put the absorbent pad under the client beneath the chest tube. *The pad protects the bed linen from drainage and provides a place for the chest tube after removal.*

- Instruct the client to perform the Valsalva maneuver (exhale fully and bear down) when the physician removes the chest tube.

**2. Prepare sterile field and sterile air-tight gauze.**

- Open the sterile packages, and prepare a sterile field.

- Wearing sterile gloves, place the sterile petrolatum gauze on a 4 × 4 gauze square. *This will quickly provide an airtight dress-*

*ing over the insertion site after the tube is removed.*

**3. Remove the soiled dressing.**

- Wearing gloves, be careful not to dislodge the tube when removing underlying gauzes.

- Discard soiled dressings in the moisture-resistant bag.

**4. Prepare strips of air-occlusive tape.**

- While the physician is removing the tube, remove gloves and prepare three 15-cm (6-in) strips of air-occlusive tape.

- After the petrolatum gauze dressing is applied over the insertion site immediately after tube removal, completely cover it with the air-occlusive tape. *This makes the dressing as airtight as possible.*

**5. Provide emotional support and monitor the client's response to removal of the chest tube.**

**6. Assess the client.**

- Monitor the vital signs, and assess the quality of the respirations as the client's condition in-

dicates, e.g., every 15 minutes for the first hour following tube removal and then less often or as condition indicates.

- Auscultate the client's lungs every hour for the first 4 hours to assess breath sounds and the adequacy of ventilation in the affected lung.

- Assess the client regularly for signs of pneumothorax, subcutaneous emphysema, and infection.

**7. Document relevant information.**

- Document the date and time of chest tube insertion or removal and the name of the physician.

- Include the amount, color, and consistency of drainage, and vital signs.

**8. Prepare the client for a chest x-ray, which is usually done 1 to 2 hours after removal of chest tube to assess lung expansion.**

▶ **Procedure 39–13** *CONTINUED*

| | |
|---|---|
| **EVALUATION FOCUS** | Respiratory rate, rhythm, and quality; vital signs; breath sounds; dressing and character, quality, and amount of any drainage; presence/absence of subcutaneous emphysema. |

**SAMPLE RECORDING**

| Date | Time | Notes |
|---|---|---|
| 12/12/95 | 1000 | Chest tubes removed by Dr. Jung. 100 mL clear pink drainage. BP 120/70, TPR 98.6, 76, 16. ———————————————— Susan March, RN |

# Clearing an Obstructed Airway

There are several possible causes of airway obstruction and, as a result, several different ways of clearing an obstructed airway. Causes include

- Aspirated food, mucus plug, or foreign bodies, such as partial dentures or small toys. Food is the most common cause of choking, particularly meat that has been ineffectively chewed.

- Unconsciousness or seizures, which cause the tongue to fall back and block the airway.

- Severe trauma to the nose, mouth, or neck that produces blood clots that obstruct the airway, especially in unconscious victims.

- Acute edema of the trachea, from smoke inhalation, facial and neck burns, or anaphylaxis. In these instances, a tracheostomy is often indicated.

Foreign bodies may cause either partial or complete airway obstruction. When an airway is partially obstructed, the victim may have either good air exchange or poor air exchange. If sufficient air is obtained, even though there is frequent wheezing between coughs, do *not* interfere with the victim's attempts to expel the foreign object. Stay with the individual and call the emergency medical service (EMS). Partial obstructions with inadequate air exchange are dealt with in the same manner as complete obstructions.

The victim with complete airway obstruction is unable to speak, breathe, or cough and may clutch at the neck. *Subdiaphragmatic abdominal thrusts* (also known as the Heimlich maneuver) are recommended to relieve the obstruction for persons over 1 year of age. By elevating the diaphragm, this maneuver forces air from the lungs to create an artificial cough to expel the obstruction. It may be necessary to perform this maneuver numerous times to clear the airway. Abdominal thrusts can be performed when the victim is conscious and standing or sitting. For infants under 1 year of age, a combination of back blows and chest thrusts is recommended. Chest thrusts are used with clients who are pregnant or markedly obese.

Any individual who receives intervention to treat an obstructed airway should seek immediate follow-up medical evaluation, even if the person remains conscious and the airway is cleared with abdominal thrusts.

---

 **39-14**

# Clearing an Obstructed Airway

**PURPOSE**
- To clear an obstructed airway in order to permit adequate ventilation

**ASSESSMENT FOCUS**

| Patency of airway (inability to speak, breathe, or cough); hand(s) at throat (universal sign of choking); rate, rhythm, and quality of respirations, quality of cough; skin color; level of consciousness. |
| --- |

---

## EQUIPMENT
- ☐ Mouth shield, if indicated
- ☐ Nonsterile gloves, if indicated

---

### INTERVENTION

**Abdominal Thrusts to a Standing or Sitting Victim**

To perform abdominal thrusts to a conscious victim who is standing or sitting:

**1. Identify yourself as a trained rescuer.**

- Stand behind the victim, and wrap your arms around the victim's waist.

- Direct a bystander to contact EMS.

**2. Give abdominal thrusts.**

- Make a fist with one hand, tuck the thumb inside the first, and place the flexed thumb just above the victim's navel and below the xiphoid process. *(A protruding thumb could inflict injury.)*

- With the other hand, grasp the fist (see Figure 39–19), and press it into the victim's abdomen with a firm, quick upward thrust (see Figure 39–20). Avoid tightening the arms around the rib cage, and thrust in the direction of the chin. Deliver quick upward thrusts.

- Deliver successive thrusts as separate and complete movements until the victim's airway clears or the victim becomes unconscious.

▶ **Procedure 39–14** *CONTINUED*

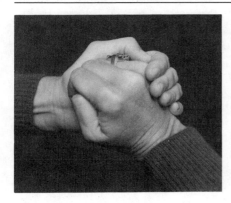

FIGURE 39–19 The hand and fist position used to deliver abdominal thrusts to a conscious victim.

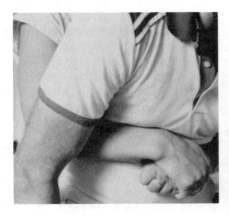

FIGURE 39–20 The position to provide abdominal thrusts to a conscious victim.

### Abdominal Thrusts to an Unconscious Victim Lying on the Ground

To implement abdominal thrusts to an unconscious victim who is lying on the ground

**1. Direct a bystander to contact EMS.**

**2. Airway management**

• Tilt the victim's head back, lift the chin, and pinch the nose shut.

• Give two slow breaths.

• If unable to ventilate, re-tilt the head and repeat breaths.

**3. Give abdominal thrusts**

• Straddle one or both of the victim's legs.

• Place the heel of one hand slightly above the victim's navel and well below the xiphoid process.

• Place the other hand directly on top of the first. Make sure that the shoulders are over the victim's abdomen and the elbows are straight.

• Point the fingers of both hands toward the victim's head and give five quick inward and upward abdominal thrusts. See Figure 39–21. Be sure the thrust is midline of the abdomen and not to the left or right.

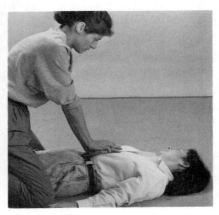

FIGURE 39–21 The position to provide abdominal thrusts to an unconscious victim.

**4. Foreign object check**

• Using your fingers and thumb, lift the victim's lower jaw and tongue. Slide one finger down inside the victim's cheek and attempt to hook the object out, being careful not to push it down. In children, try hooking out the object only if you can see it.

• Repeat abdominal thrusts, airway maneuvers, and foreign object checks until the airway clears or the victim breathes.

### Chest Thrusts to a Conscious Standing or Sitting Victim

Chest thrusts are to be administered only to women in advanced stages of pregnancy and markedly obese persons who cannot receive abdominal thrusts. To administer chest thrusts:

**1. Identify yourself as a trained rescuer.**

• Stand behind the victim with your arms under the victim's armpits and encircling the victim's chest.

• Direct a bystander to contact EMS.

• Place the thumb side of the fist on the middle of the breast bone, not on the xiphoid process.

**2. Deliver thrusts.**

• Grab the fist with the other hand and deliver a quick backward thrust.

• Repeat thrusts until the obstruction is relieved or the victim becomes unconscious.

### Chest Thrusts to an Unconscious Victim Lying Flat

Chest thrusts to unconscious victims lying on the ground are administered only to women in advanced stages of pregnancy or markedly obese persons. To administer this maneuver:

**1. Airway management**

• Tilt the victim's head back, lift the chin, and pinch the nose shut. Put on mouth shield.

• Give two slow breaths.

• If unable to ventilate, re-tilt the head and repeat breaths.

**2. Deliver thrusts**

• Position the victim supine and kneel close to the side of the victim's trunk.

• Position the hands as for cardiac compression with the heel of the hand on the lower half of the sternum. (See Procedure 39–16, step 4.)

▶

▶ **Procedure 39–14 Clearing an Obstructed Airway** *CONTINUED*

**3. Foreign object check**

- Using your fingers and thumb, lift the victim's lower jaw and tongue. Slide one finger down inside the victim's cheek and attempt to hook the object out, being careful not to push it down.

**4. Repeat chest thrusts, airway maneuvers, and foreign object checks until the airway clears or the person breathes.**

**Back Blows and Chest Thrusts for Infants**

To administer a combination of back blows and chest thrusts to infants:

**1. Deliver back blows and chest thrusts.**

- Straddle the infant over your forearm with his or her head lower than the trunk.
- Support the infant's head by firmly holding the jaw in the hand.
- Rest your forearm on your thigh.
- With the heel of the free hand, deliver five sharp blows to the back over the spine between the shoulder blades. See Figure 39–22.

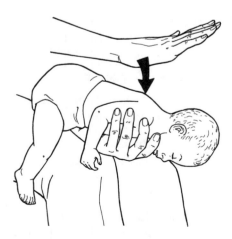

**FIGURE 39–22** The correct position to administer back blows to an infant.

- Turn the infant as a unit to the supine position:

  **a.** Place the free hand on the infant's back.

  **b.** While continuing to support the jaw, neck, and chest with the other hand, turn and place the infant on the thigh with the baby's head lower than the trunk.

- Using two fingers, administer five chest thrusts over the sternum in the same location as external chest compression for cardiac massage, i.e., one finger width below the nipple line. See Procedure 39–16.

- In the conscious infant, continue chest thrusts and back blows until the airway is cleared or the infant becomes unconscious.

- If the infant is unconscious, assess the airway and give two breaths. If unable to ventilate, re-tilt the infant's head and try to give two breaths. If the air does not go in, then give back blows and chest thrusts (see above). Following the chest thrusts, lift the jaw and tongue and check for foreign object. If an object is noted, sweep it out with finger. Repeat this sequence of foreign object checks, breaths, back blows, and chest thrusts until the airway clears or the infant begins to breathe.

**Finger Sweep**

If foreign material is visible in the mouth it must be expediently removed. The finger sweep maneuver should be used only on unconscious persons and with extreme caution in infants and children since the foreign material can be pushed back into the airway, causing increased obstruction. To remove visible foreign material from the mouth:

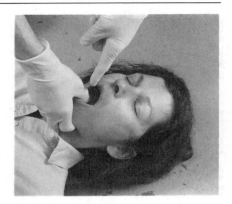

**FIGURE 39–23** The finger sweep maneuver.

- Don nonsterile gloves.

- Open the person's mouth by grasping the tongue and lower jaw between the thumb and fingers, and lifting the jaw upward. (See Figure 39–23.) This pulls the tongue away from the back of the throat.

- To remove solid material insert the index finger of your free hand along the inside of the person's cheek and deep into the throat. With your finger hooked, use a sweeping motion to try to dislodge and lift out the foreign object. If these measures fail, try more abdominal thrusts in adults and children. In infants, give back blows and chest thrusts.

- After removing the foreign object, clear out liquid material, such as mucus, blood, or emesis, with a scooping motion, using two fingers wrapped with a gauze pad, tissue, or piece of cloth.

- After the digital maneuver, assess air exchange. If it is ineffective, proceed with Procedures 39–15 and 39–16, as indicated.

**Document relevant information:**

- Document the date and time of the procedure, including the precipitating events and the client's response to the intervention.

▶ **Procedure 39–14** *CONTINUED*

- Describe the type of the procedure, the duration of breathlessness, and the type and size of any foreign object.

- Note vital signs, any complications, and type of follow-up care.

EVALUATION FOCUS

Patency of airway; rate, rhythm, and quality of respirations; level of consciousness; bilateral breath sounds; complications (injuries).

**SAMPLE RECORDING**

| Date | Time | Notes |
|---|---|---|
| 6/17/95 | 1800 | Found choking in bed during evening meal, conscious with both hands on neck. Five abdominal thrusts given with quick return of 1″ by 1″ piece of meat. Alert, able to speak following thrusts. R 20, even and unlabored. Breath sounds clear to auscultation. Dr. Hood in to examine. ——————————— —————————————————————— Matthew B. Corwin, RN |

<39-15> ## Administering Oral ᴊcitation

**PURPOSES**
- To provide ventilation during a respiratory or cardiac arrest
- To provide oxygen to the brain, heart, and vital organs during a respiratory or cardiac arrest

**ASSESSMENT FOCUS**

Patency of airway; rate, rhythm, quality of respirations; level of consciousness; skin color; presence/absence of carotid pulse.

### EQUIPMENT

- Pocket face mask with one-way valve or mouth shields or hand-compressible breathing bag with mask with one-way valve (see Figure 39–24).
- Disposable gloves

### INTERVENTION

**1. Position the client appropriately.**

- If the victim is lying on one side or face down, turn the client as a unit supporting head and neck, onto the back, and kneel beside the head.

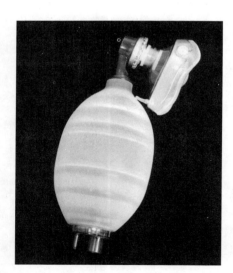

**FIGURE 39–24** An Ambu bag with a face mask.

**2. Open the airway.**

- Use the head-tilt, chin-lift maneuver or the jaw-thrust maneuver. A modified jaw thrust is used for victims with suspected neck injury. In unconscious victims, the tongue lacks sufficient muscle tone, falls to the back of the throat, and obstructs the pharynx. *Because the tongue is attached to the lower jaw, moving the lower jaw forward and tilting the head backward lifts the tongue away from the pharynx and opens the airway.* See Figure 39–25.

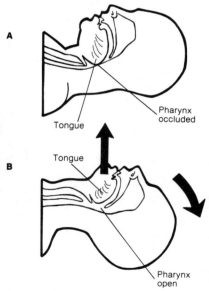

**FIGURE 39–25** The position of an unconscious person's tongue: *A*, pharynx occluded; *B*, pharynx open.

**Head-tilt, chin-lift maneuver:**

- Place one hand palm downward on the forehead.

- Place the fingers of the other hand under the bony part of the lower jaw near the chin. The teeth should then be almost closed. The mouth should not be closed completely.

- Simultaneously press down on the forehead with one hand, and lift the victim's chin upward with the other. See Figure 39–26. Avoid pressing the fingers deeply into the soft tissues under the chin, since too much pressure can obstruct the airway.

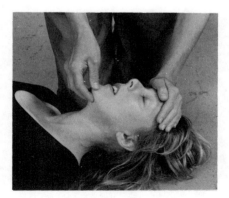

**FIGURE 39–26** The head-tilt, chin-lift maneuver.

▶ **Procedure 39-15** *CONTINUED*

- Open the victim's mouth by pressing the lower lip downward with the thumb after tilting the head.

- Remove dentures if they cannot be maintained in place. However, dentures that can be maintained in place make a mouth-to-mouth seal easier should rescue breathing be required.

**Jaw-thrust maneuver:**

- Kneel at the *top* of the victim's head.

- Grasp the angle of the mandible directly below the earlobe between your thumb and forefinger on each side of the victim's head.

- While tilting the head backward, lift the lower jaw until it juts forward and is higher than the upper jaw. See Figure 39–27.

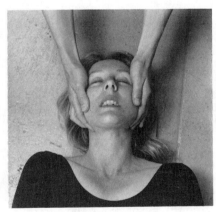

**FIGURE 39–27** The jaw-thrust maneuver.

- Rest your elbows on the surface on which the victim is lying.

- Retract the lower lip with the thumbs prior to giving artificial respiration.

- If the victim is suspected of having a spinal neck injury, *do not hyperextend the neck.* Instead, *use the modified jaw thrust for a person with a spinal injury.*

**Modified jaw-thrust maneuver:**

- Perform first two steps for jaw-thrust maneuver.

- Do not tilt the head backward while lifting the lower jaw forward.

- Support the head carefully without hyperextending it or moving it from side to side.

**3. Determine the victim's ability to breathe.**

- Place your ear and cheek close to the victim's mouth and nose.

- Look at the chest and abdomen for rising and falling movement.

- Listen for air escaping during exhalation.

- Feel for air escaping against your cheek.

**4. If no breathing is evident, provide rescue breathing if required.**

- Use one of the following methods: mouth-to-mouth, mouth-to-nose, mouth-to-mask, or hand-compressible breathing bag.

**Mouth-to-mouth method:**

- Put on a mouth shield.

- Maintain the open airway by using the head-tilt, chin-lift maneuver.

- Pinch the victim's nostrils with the index finger and thumb of the hand on the victim's forehead. *Pinching closes the nostrils and prevents resuscitation air from escaping through them.*

- Take a deep breath, and place the mouth, opened widely, around the victim's mouth. Ensure an airtight seal. See Figure 39–28.

- Give two full breaths (1½ seconds per breath). Pause and take a breath after the first ventilation. *The 1½-second time span closely matches the victim's in-*

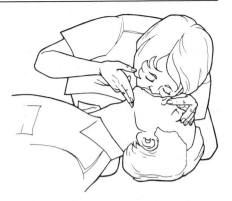

**FIGURE 39–28** Mouth-to-mouth rescue breathing.

*spiratory time, allows adequate time to provide good chest expansion, and decreases the possibility of gastric distention. Excessive air volumes and rapid inspiratory flow rates can cause pharyngeal pressures that are great enough to open the esophagus, thus allowing air to enter the stomach.*

- Ensure adequate ventilation by observing the victim's chest rise and fall and by assessing the person's breathing as outlined in step 3.

- If the initial ventilation attempt is unsuccessful, reposition the victim's head and repeat the rescue breathing as above. If the victim still cannot be ventilated, proceed to clear the airway of any foreign bodies using the finger sweep, abdominal thrusts, or chest thrusts described earlier. (See Procedure 39–14.)

**Mouth-to-nose method:**

This method can be used when there is an injury to the mouth or jaw or when the client is edentulous (toothless), making it difficult to achieve a tight seal over the mouth.

- Maintain the head tilt and chin lift.

- Close the victim's mouth by pressing the palm of your hand

▶

▶ **Procedure 39–15  Administering Oral Resuscitation** *CONTINUED*

against the victim's chin. The thumb of the same hand may be used to hold the bottom lip closed.

• Put on a mouth shield.

• Take a deep breath, and seal your lips around the victim's nose. Ensure a tight seal by making contact with the cheeks around the nose.

• Deliver two full breaths of 1½ seconds each, and pause to inhale before delivering the second breath.

• Remove your mouth from the nose, and allow the victim to exhale passively. It may be necessary to separate the victim's lips or to open the mouth for exhaling, since the nasal passages may be obstructed during exhalation.

**Mouth-to-mask method:**

• Remove the mask from its case and push out the dome.

• Connect the one-way valve to the mask port.

• Position yourself at the top of the victim's head, and open the airway using the jaw-thrust maneuver.

• Place the bottom rim of the mask between the victim's lower lip and chin. Place the rest of the mask over the face using your thumbs on each side of the mask to hold it in place. *This keeps the mouth open under the mask.*

• Perform the jaw-thrust maneuver to tilt the head backward. Use your index, middle, and ring fingers of both hands behind the angles of the jaw, and grasp the victim's temples with the palms of your hands.

• Maintain this head position while blowing intermittently into the mouthpiece.

**Hand-compressible breathing bag method:**

• Stand at the victim's head.

• Use one hand to secure the mask at the top and bottom and to hold the victim's jaw forward. Use the other hand to squeeze and release the bag. See Figure 39–29.

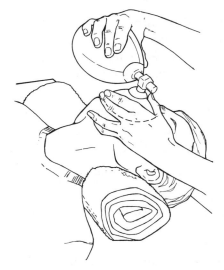

**FIGURE 39–29**  An Ambu bag in position.

• Compress the bag until sufficient elevation of the victim's chest is observed. Then release the bag.

**5. Determine whether the victim's breathing is restored.** See step 3.

**6. Determine the presence of a carotid pulse** (see Figure 39–30).

• Take about 5 to 10 seconds for this pulse check. *Adequate time is needed since the victim's pulse may be very weak and rapid, irregular, or slow.*

• To palpate the carotid artery, first locate the larynx, then slide your fingers alongside it into the groove between the larynx and the neck muscles on the same side you are. Use gentle pressure. *This avoids compressing the artery. The carotid pulse site is used because the femoral pulse is diffi-*

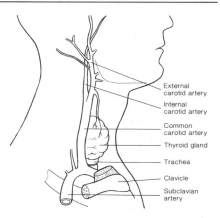

**FIGURE 39–30**  Location of the carotid artery.

*External carotid artery*
*Internal carotid artery*
*Common carotid artery*
*Thyroid gland*
*Trachea*
*Clavicle*
*Subclavian artery*

*cult to locate on a fully clothed victim and because a pulse can often be palpated there when more peripheral pulses, such as the radial, are imperceptible.*

**7. If the carotid pulse is palpable, but breathing is not restored, repeat rescue breathing.**

• Inflate at the rate of 12 breaths per minute (1 breath every 5 seconds).

• Blow forcibly enough to make the victim's chest rise.

• If chest expansion fails to occur, ensure that the head is hyperextended and the jaw lifted upward, or check again for the presence of obstructive material, fluid, or vomitus.

• After each inflation, move your mouth away from the victim's mouth by turning your head toward the victim's chest. *This movement allows the air to escape when the victim exhales. It also gives the nurse time to inhale and to watch for chest expansion.*

**8. Reassess the carotid pulse after every 12 inflations (after 1 minute).**

• If you cannot locate the pulse, the victim's heart has stopped, and cardiac compression also needs to be provided. See Pro-

▶ **Procedure 39–15** *CONTINUED*

cedure 39–16. **Accurate assessment of the victim's pulse is essential because performing external chest compressions on victims who have a pulse can lead to serious medical complications.**

**9. Document relevant information:**

- Document the date and time of resuscitation, including assessment findings prior to the respiratory arrest. Assess events during and after the respiratory arrest and the victim's responses to the intervention.

- Describe the duration of breathlessness.

- Note vital signs, any complications, and type of follow-up care.

| | |
|---|---|
| **EVALUATION FOCUS** | Patency of airway; rate, rhythm, and quality of respirations; level of consciousness; breath sounds; vital signs. |

**SAMPLE RECORDING**

| Date | Time | Notes |
|---|---|---|
| 10/3/95 | 1600 | Found breathless and unresponsive. Skin color pale and ashen. Airway opened, two breaths given mouth-to-mask. Carotid pulse 64 and regular. Mouth-to-mask ventilations given at 12 breaths/minute with carotid pulse present and full every 1 minute. Skin color pale, pink. Awake, responsive to painful stimuli. Breath sounds clear to auscultation. Dr. Walker present. ———————— Deanna Matson, RN |
| 10/3/95 | 1604 | Transferred to ICU for mechanical ventilation. ———————— Deanna Matson, RN |

# 39-16 Administering External Cardiac Compressions

**PURPOSES**
- To provide ventilation and circulation following cardiac arrest
- To provide oxygen to the brain, heart, and vital organs following cardiac arrest
- To increase pressure in the chest causing blood to circulate

**ASSESSMENT FOCUS**

Level of consciousness, patency of airway, presence/absence of breathing, pulse.

## EQUIPMENT

- A hard surface, such as a cardiac board or the floor, on which to place the victim
- A face shield or mask with a one-way valve

## INTERVENTION

**1. Survey the scene for safety hazards, presence of bystanders, and other victims.**

**2. Position the victim appropriately if not already done.**

- Place the victim supine on a firm surface. *Blood flow to the brain will be inadequate during CPR if the victim's head is positioned higher than the thorax. A hard surface facilitates compression of the heart between the sternum and the hard surface.*

- If the victim is in bed in a health care facility, place a cardiac board—preferably the full width of the bed—under the back. If necessary, place the victim on the floor.

- If the victim must be turned, turn the body as a unit while firmly supporting the head and neck so that the head does not roll, twist, or tilt backward or forward. *Turning the person as a unit prevents further injury (if present) to the neck or spine.*

- Have a bystander elevate the lower extremities (optional). *This may promote venous return and augment circulation during external cardiac compressions.*

**3. Follow procedures for assessing responsiveness, airway, breathing, and circulation (see next page).**

**4. Position the hands on the sternum.** Proper hand placement is essential for effective cardiac compression. Position the hands as follows:

- With the hand nearest the victim's legs, use your middle and index fingers to locate the lower margin of the rib cage.

- Move the fingers up the rib cage to the notch where the lower ribs meet the sternum. See Figure 39–31.

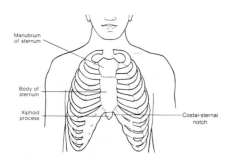

**FIGURE 39-31** The sternum and ribs.

- Place the heel of the other hand (nearest the person's head)

along the lower half of the victim's sternum, close to the index finger that is next to the middle finger in the costal-sternal notch. *Proper positioning of the hands during cardiac compression prevents injury to underlying organs and the ribs.* See Figure 39–32. ⚠ *Compression directly over the xiphoid process can lacerate the victim's liver.*

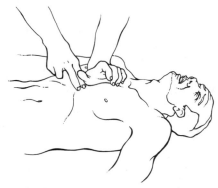

**FIGURE 39–32** Proper positioning of hands during cardiac compression.

- Then place the first hand on top of the second hand so that both hands are parallel. The fingers may be extended or interlaced. *Compression occurs only on the sternum through the heels of the hands.*

▶ **Procedure 39–16** *CONTINUED*

---

**5. Administer cardiac compression.**

- Lock your elbows into position, straighten your arms, and position your shoulders directly over your hands. See Figure 39–33.

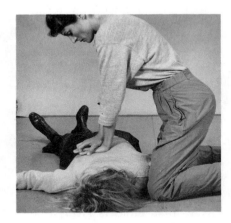

**FIGURE 39–33** Arm and hand position for external cardiac massage.

- For each compression, thrust *straight down* on the sternum. For an adult of normal size, depress the sternum 3.8 to 5.0 cm (1.5 to 2 in). *The muscle force of both arms is needed for adequate cardiac compression of an adult. The weight of your shoulders and trunk supplies power for compression. Extension of the elbows ensures an adequate and even force throughout compression.*

- Completely release the compression pressure. However, do *not* lift your hands from the chest or change their position. *Releasing the pressure allows the sternum to return to its normal position and allows the heart chambers to fill with blood. Leaving the hands on the chest prevents taking a malposition between compressions and possibly injuring the person.*

- Provide external cardiac compressions at the rate of 80 to 100 per minute. Maintain the rhythm by counting "One and, two and,"

and so on. *The specified compression rate and rhythm stimulate normal heart contractions.*

- Administer 5 or 15 external compressions, depending on the number of rescuers, and coordinate them with rescue breathing. See CPR performed by one rescuer or by two rescuers, next.

---

**VARIATION: CPR performed by one rescuer**

- Survey the scene.

- Call for help and have another person call for EMS. In many communities the emergency telephone number is 911. The person who calls the local EMS must be able to impart all of the following information:

  **a.** Location of the emergency

  **b.** Telephone number from which the call is being made

  **c.** What happened

  **d.** Number of people needing assistance

  **e.** Condition of the victim(s)

  **f.** What aid is being given

  **g.** Any other information that is requested

- If there is no bystander and the rescuer is alone, summon help and then perform CPR.

- Position the victim on the back on a flat, firm surface.

- Kneel beside the victim's chest. If the person is in bed, you may have to kneel on the bed.

**6. Assess responsiveness. If unconscious, open airway, assess breathing and circulation prior to initiating compressions.**

**Airway:**

- Open the airway with the head-

tilt, chin-lift maneuver or, if neck injury is suspected, the modified jaw thrust.

- Clear the airway, if you suspect airway obstruction from food or some other foreign object.

**Breathing:**

- Assess breathing: *Look for* chest movement; *listen for* exhalation; and *feel for* air flow against the cheek.

- Ventilate the victim, if breathing is not present. See Procedure 39–15 for detailed steps.

- Deliver two full breaths into the victim's mouth. Between the breaths, remove your mouth, turn your head to the side, and pause to take a breath.

- If unable to give two breaths, reposition the victim's head, and attempt to ventilate again.

- If still unsuccessful, follow procedures for obstructed airway (Procedure 39–14).

**Circulation:**

- Assess for the presence of the carotid pulse for 5–10 seconds.

- If pulse is present:

  **a.** Continue rescue breathing at 12 times per minute while continuing to monitor the pulse.

- If pulse is absent:

  **a.** Begin external chest compression.

  **b.** Perform chest compression: 15 external chest compressions at the rate of 80 to 100 per minute. Count, "One and, two and, three and . . ." up to 15.

  **c.** Open the airway, and give two rescue breaths.

▶

▶ **Procedure 39–16 Administering External Cardiac Compressions** *CONTINUED*

**d.** Repeat four complete cycles of 15 compressions and two ventilations.

**e.** Assess the victim's carotid pulse. If there is no pulse, continue with CPR and check for the return of the pulse every few minutes.

**VARIATION: CPR performed by two rescuers**

When help arrives, one rescuer can provide external cardiac compression, and the other can provide pulmonary resuscitation, inflating the lungs once after every five compressions, a 5:1 ratio.

- The second rescuer identifies himself or herself as a trained rescuer and verifies that EMS has been notified. If EMS has been notified, the second rescuer offers to help with CPR.

- The first rescuer completes a cycle of compressions with two breaths. The second rescuer gets into position to give compressions.

- The first rescuer assesses the carotid pulse for 5–10 seconds and if there is no pulse, gives one breath and then states, "No pulse, continue CPR."

- The second rescuer then:

  **a.** Provides compression.

  **b.** Sets the pace, counting aloud, "One and, two and, three and, four and, five and, ventilate."

- The first rescuer:

  **a.** Provides one ventilation after every five chest compressions.

  **b.** Observes each breath for effectiveness.

  **c.** Assesses the carotid pulse frequently between breaths

to assess the effectiveness of cardiac compression.

  **d.** Observes for abdominal (gastric) distention, which can result from overinflation of the lungs. If distention occurs, the rescuer reduces the force of the ventilations, but ensures sufficient ventilation to elevate the ribs.

- When the person compressing the chest becomes fatigued, positions should be changed. To initiate a change in position, the person compressing states, "Change one and, two and, three and, four and, five and"; moves to the person's head; and counts the pulse for 5 seconds.

- The person ventilating gives the breath and moves into position to provide compression.

- If there is no pulse, the original person compressing states, "No pulse—start compression," gives one full breath, and CPR is continued.

**When relieved from CPR**

- Stand by to assist. Often a person is needed to take notes, document the actions taken, and record the drugs given by the cardiac arrest team.

- Provide emotional support to the victim's family members and any others who may have witnessed the cardiac arrest. This is often a frightening experience for others because it is so sudden and so serious.

**VARIATION: CPR for children and infants**

Providing CPR for infants and children is similar to CPR for adults.

**a.** Providing CPR to children

- In children, follow steps 1–3.

- In children, to find the hand position for compressions, run your index and middle fingers up the ribs until you locate the sternal notch. With those two fingers on the lower end of the sternum, look at the location of the index finger and lift fingers off sternum and put the heel of the same hand on the sternum just above the location of the index finger. The other hand should remain on the child's forehead so as to maintain an open airway.

- Use the heel of one hand for compressions, keeping the fingers off the chest. Compression depth is 2.5 to 3.8 cm (1 to 1½ in.). Never lift the hand off the chest.

- CPR for a child is given at the following rate: 100 compressions/minute with cycles of five compressions and one breath.

**b.** Providing CPR to infants

- For infants, follow steps 1–3.

- When ventilating an infant, cover the infant's nose and mouth.

- For pulse checks, use the brachial pulse in the arm.

- To find the position for compressions, place your index finger on the sternum at the nipple line. Place your middle and ring fingers on the sternum next to your index finger, then lift your index finger.

- Compress the chest 1.25 to 2.5 cm (½ to 1 in.) straight down using the pads of two fingers. Keep your fingers in the compression position while the other hand remains on the forehead, maintaining the open airway.

- Give compressions at a rate of up to 120 compressions/minute with cycles of five compressions and one breath.

▶ **Procedure 39–16** *CONTINUED*

#### 7. Terminating CPR

A rescuer terminates CPR only when one of the following events occurs:

- Another trained individual takes over.
- The victim's heartbeat and breathing are re-established.
- Adjunctive life-support measures are initiated.
- A physician states that the victim is dead and that CPR is to be discontinued.

- The rescuer becomes exhausted, and there is no one to take over.

#### 8. Document relevant information:

- Document the date and time of the arrest and the initiation of CPR, including the events prior to the arrest.
- Note length of resuscitation.
- Record the time, dose, and route of any medications administered.

- Record any advanced cardiac life support interventions such as defibrillation or initiation of IV therapy.
- Include the victim's response to CPR.
- Record the victim's status and outcome of CPR.
- Document vital signs, rhythm strips, any complications, and type of follow-up care.

| EVALUATION FOCUS | Level of consciousness, patency of airway; rate, rhythm, and quality of respirations; pulse rate and blood pressure; breath sounds. |
|---|---|

**SAMPLE RECORDING**

| Date | Time | Notes |
|---|---|---|
| 3/23/95 | 1600 | Monitored arrest from ventricular fibrillation. Unresponsive, no respirations or carotid pulse. CPR initiated. ———— Deborah A. Nathan, RN |
| 3/23/95 | 1602 | Defibrillated with 200 joules with prompt return of sinus rhythm and multifocal premature ventricular beats. Lidocaine 75 mg IV push administered. $O_2$ at 2L/m via nasal canula. Alert and oriented, B/P 90/50, P 76, R 22. Dr. Peters in to examine. Transferred to ICU via bed. ———— Deborah A. Nathan, RN |

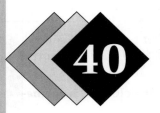

# Fecal Elimination

## PROCEDURES

# Obtaining and Testing a Specimen of Feces

Before obtaining a specimen, determine the reason for collecting the stool specimen and the correct method of obtaining and handling it (i.e., how much stool to obtain, whether a preservative needs to be added to the stool, and whether it needs to be sent immediately to the laboratory). It may be necessary to confirm this information by checking with the agency laboratory. In many situations, only a single specimen is required; in others, timed specimens are necessary, and every stool passed is collected within a designated time period.

**PURPOSE**

- To determine the presence of occult blood, parasites, bacteria, viruses, or other abnormal constituents in the stool

**ASSESSMENT FOCUS**

Client's need for assistance to defecate or use a bedpan; any abdominal discomfort before, during, or after defecation; status of perianal skin for any irritation, especially if the client defecates frequently and has liquid stools; any interventions related to the specimen collection, e.g., dietary or medication orders; presence of hemorrhoids that may bleed (particularly important for clients who are constipated, because constipated stool can aggravate existing hemorrhoids; any bleeding can affect test results); any interventions (e.g., medication) ordered to follow a defecation.

## EQUIPMENT

### Collecting a Specimen of Feces

- Clean or sterile bedpan or bedside commode (for an infant, the stool is scraped from the diaper)
- Disposable gloves
- Cardboard or plastic specimen container (labeled) with a lid

or, for stool culture, a sterile swab in a test tube, as policy dictates
- Two tongue blades
- Paper towel
- Completed laboratory requisition
- Air freshener

### Testing for Occult Blood in the Feces

- Clean bedpan or bedside commode
- Disposable gloves
- Two tongue blades
- Paper towel
- Test product

## INTERVENTION

**1. Give ambulatory clients the following information and instructions.**

- The purpose of the stool specimen and how the client can assist in collecting it.

- Defecate in a clean or sterile bedpan or bedside commode.

- Do not contaminate the specimen, if possible, by urine or menstrual discharge. Void before the specimen collection.

- Do not place toilet tissue in the bedpan after defecation, because

contents of the paper can affect the laboratory analysis.

- Notify the nurse as soon as possible after defecation, particularly for specimens that need to be sent to the laboratory immediately after collection.

**2. Assist clients who need help.**

- Assist the client to a bedside commode or a bedpan placed on a bedside chair or under the toilet seat in the bathroom.

- After the client has defecated, cover the bedpan or commode.

*Covering the bedpan reduces odor and embarrassment to the client.*

- Put on gloves to prevent hand contamination, and clean the client as required. Inspect the skin around the anus for any irritation, especially if the client defecates frequently and has liquid stools.

**3. Transfer the required amount of stool to the stool specimen container.**

- Use one or two tongue blades to transfer some or all of the stool

▶ **Procedure 40–1  Obtaining and Testing a Specimen of Feces** *CONTINUED*

to the specimen container, taking care not to contaminate the outside of the container. The amount of stool to be sent depends on the purpose for which the specimen is collected. Usually 2.5 cm (1 in) of formed stool or 15 to 30 ml of liquid stool is adequate. For some timed specimens, however, the entire stool passed may need to be sent. Visible pus, mucus, or blood should be included in the sample.
*or*
For a culture, dip a sterile swab into the specimen, preferably where purulent fecal matter is present in the feces. Place the swab in a sterile test tube using sterile technique.
*or*
For an occult blood test, see step 5 below.

- Wrap the used tongue blades in a paper towel before disposing of them in a plastic-lined waste container. *These measures help prevent the spread of microorganisms by contact with other articles.*

- Place the lid on the container as soon as the specimen is in the container. *Putting the lid on immediately prevents the spread of microorganisms.*

**4.  Ensure client comfort.**

- Empty and clean the bedpan or commode, and return it to its place.

- Remove and discard the gloves.

- Provide an air freshener for any odors unless contraindicated by the client; e.g., a spray may increase dyspnea.

**5.  Label and send the specimen to the laboratory.**

- Ensure that the specimen label and the laboratory requisition have the correct information on them and are securely attached on the specimen container. *Inappropriate identification of the specimen can lead to errors of diagnosis or therapy for the client.*

- Arrange for the specimen to be taken to the laboratory. Specimens to be cultured or tested for parasites need to be sent immediately. If this is not possible, follow the directions on the specimen container. In some instances refrigeration is indicated because bacteriologic changes take place in stool specimens left at room temperature.
*or*

**Test the stool for occult blood.**

- Select a test product.

♦ - Put on gloves.

- Follow the manufacturer's directions. For example:

  **a.** For a Guaiac test, smear a thin layer of feces on a paper towel or filter paper with a tongue blade, and drop reagents onto the smear as directed.

  **b.** For a Hematest, smear a thin layer of feces on filter paper, place a tablet in the middle of the specimen, and add two drops of water as directed.

  **c.** For a Hemoccult slide, smear a thin layer of feces over the circle inside the envelope, and drop reagent solution onto the smear.

- Note the reaction. For all tests, a blue color indicates a positive result, i.e., the presence of occult blood.

**6.  Document all relevant information.**

- Record the collection of the specimen on the client's chart and on the nursing care plan. Include in the recording the date and time of the collection and all nursing assessments. See Evaluation Focus.

- For an occult blood test, record the type of test product used and the reaction.

| EVALUATION FOCUS | Color, odor, consistency, and amount of feces; presence of abnormal constituents, e.g., blood or mucus; results of test for occult blood if obtained; discomfort during or after defecation; status of perianal skin; any bleeding from the anus after defecation. |
|---|---|

**SAMPLE RECORDING**

| Date | Time | Notes |
|---|---|---|
| 08/12/95 | 0830 | Stool specimen obtained for parasites and sent to laboratory. Stool is light brown, soft and without form. No evidence of blood or mucus. Perianal skin intact. ——————————————— Stacey McNamara, RN *or* Guaiac test performed for occult blood. Results positive. ——————— ——————————————— Stacey McNamara, RN |

## 40-2 Siphoning an Enema

In some instances, a client may be unable to expel the solution after the administration of an enema. The solution must then be siphoned off. In siphoning, the nurse uses the force of gravity to draw the fluid out of the rectum and colon. Siphoning an enema may require a physician's order.

**PURPOSE**

- To remove retained enema solution

**ASSESSMENT FOCUS**

Amount of enema solution instilled, presence of abdominal distention, abdominal pain or feeling of fullness; rate and quality of respirations.

---

## EQUIPMENT

- Bedpan
- Rectal tube
- Nonsterile gloves
- Lubricant
- Container of water at 40° C (105° F)
- Disposable large plastic volume enema container

---

## INTERVENTION

**1. Position the client appropriately.**

- Assist the client to a *right* side-lying position. *In this position, the sigmoid colon is uppermost, thus facilitating drainage of the solution from the rectum and colon by gravity.*

- Ensure that the client's hips are close to the side of the bed. *This placement prevents undue stretching and reaching by the nurse and facilitates siphoning into the container and bedpan.*

**2. Prepare the equipment.**

- Place the bedpan on a chair at the side of the bed near the client's hips. The chair must be lower than the client's hips.

- Attach the open end of the rectal tube to the partially filled enema set.

- Lubricate the rectal tube.

**3. Siphon the enema solution.**

- Fill the tube with solution, then pinch it and gently insert it into the rectum as for an enema.

- Hold the enema container about 10 cm (4 in) above the anus, release the pinched rectal tube, and quickly lower the enema container. *This action should draw the fluid from the colon and rectum, permitting it to flow through the rectal tube into the solution container.*

**4. Document all relevant information.**

- Record the amount of fluid siphoned off as well as the characteristics of the returns.

---

**EVALUATION FOCUS**

Amount of fluid returns; color, odor, and presence of any feces; abnormal constituents, e.g., blood or mucus.

**SAMPLE RECORDING**

| Date | Time | Notes |
|------|------|-------|
| 12/13/95 | 1030 | 700 ml enema fluid siphoned through anal canal. Returns tinged with mucus and dark brown hard stool. R 16 and shallow. C/O abdominal pain. ———————— Ned Zabirski, RN |

## 40-3 Removing a Fecal Impaction Digitally

 Digital removal involves breaking up the fecal mass digitally and removing it in portions. Because the bowel mucosa can be injured during this procedure, some agencies restrict and specify the personnel permitted to conduct digital disimpactions. Rectal stimulation is also contraindicated for some people because it may cause an excessive vagal response resulting in cardiac arrhythmia. After a disimpaction, the nurse can use various interventions to remove remaining feces, e.g., a cleansing enema or the insertion of a suppository.

**PURPOSES**
- To relieve pain and discomfort caused by blockage of impacted feces
- To reestablish normal defecation

**ASSESSMENT FOCUS**

Pattern of defecation; presence of an impaction confirmed by digital examination; presence of nausea, headache, abdominal pain, malaise, or abdominal distention.

---

### EQUIPMENT
- Bath blanket
- Moisture-resistant bedpan
- Bedpan and cover
- Toilet tissue
- Disposable gloves
- Lubricant
- Soap, water, and towel

---

### INTERVENTION

**1. Prepare the client.**

- Explain to the client what you plan to do and why. This procedure is distressing, tiring, and uncomfortable, so the person may desire the presence of another nurse or support person.

- Assist the client to a right lateral or Sims' position with the back toward you. *When the person lies on the right side, the sigmoid colon is uppermost; thus, gravity can aid removal of the feces.*

- Cover the client with the bath blanket.

**2. Prepare the equipment.**

- Place the disposable bedpan under the client's hips, and arrange the top bedclothing so that it falls obliquely over the hips, exposing only the buttocks.

- Place the bedpan and toilet tissue nearby on the bed or a bedside chair.

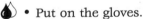 • Put on the gloves.

- Lubricate the gloved index finger. *Lubricant reduces resistance by the anal sphincter as the finger is inserted.*

**3. Remove the impaction.**

- Gently insert the index finger into the rectum, moving toward the umbilicus.

- Gently massage around the stool. *Gentle action prevents damage to the rectal mucosa. A circular motion around the rectum dislodges the stool, stimulates peristalsis, and relaxes the anal sphincter.*

- Work the finger into the hardened mass of stool to break it up. If you cannot break up the impaction with one finger, insert two fingers and try to break up the impaction scissor style.

- Work the stool down to the anus, remove it in small pieces, and place them in the bedpan.

- Carefully continue to remove as much fecal material as possible; at the same time, assess the client for signs of pallor, feelings of faintness, shortness of breath, and perspiration. Terminate the procedure if these occur. *Manual stimulation could result in excessive vagal nerve stimulation and subsequent cardiac arrhythmia.*

- Assist the client to a position on a clean bedpan, commode, or toilet. *Digital stimulation of the rectum may induce the urge to defecate.*

**4. Assist the client with hygienic measures as needed.**

- Wash the rectal area with soap and water and dry gently.

- Remove and discard the gloves.

**5. If appropriate, teach the client measures to promote normal elimination.** Alterations in diet

►

▶ **Procedure 40–3** *CONTINUED*

and fluid intake and the use of stool softeners may be necessary.

**6. Document the procedure and all assessments.**

<table>
<tr><td>EVALUATION FOCUS</td><td>Color, consistency, odor, and amount of feces; presence of abnormal constituents; passage of flatus; client comfort; vital signs; abdominal distention.</td></tr>
</table>

**SAMPLE RECORDING**

| Date | Time | Notes |
|------|------|-------|
| 09/28/95 | 1000 | Rectal examination for fecal impaction. Moderate amount dark brown feces removed digitally. Vital signs stable. Unable to defecate following procedure. — Bruce L. Ching, NS |

# 40-4  Irrigating a Colostomy

Before commencing a colostomy irrigation, determine (a) whether the stoma needs to be dilated; (b) which is the distal stoma and which is the proximal stoma, if the colostomy is not an end colostomy; and (c) why the irrigation is being performed and which stoma is to be irrigated (usually the proximal stoma is irrigated, to stimulate evacuation of the bowel; however, it may be necessary to irrigate the distal stoma in preparation for diagnostic procedures (e.g., roentgenography).

**PURPOSE**
- To distend the bowel and stimulate peristalsis and evacuation of feces

**ASSESSMENT FOCUS**

Bowel sounds; presence of abdominal distention; type of colostomy and functioning stoma; client readiness to select and use the equipment; client's mobility status to determine where the irrigation will be done.

## EQUIPMENT

- Disposable bedpad and a bedpan, if the client is to remain in bed
- Bath blanket
- Irrigation equipment
  A bag to hold the solution
  Tubing attached to the bag
  Tubing clamp or flow regulator

- #28 rubber colon catheter, calibrated in either centimeters or inches, with a stoma cone or seal
  Disposable stoma-irrigation drainage sleeve with belt to direct the fecal contents into the toilet or bedpan
- IV pole

- Moisture-resistant bag
- Clean gloves to protect the nurse's hands from contamination, and one glove to dilate the stoma if ordered by the physician
- Lubricant
- Clean colostomy appliance or dressings

## INTERVENTION

### 1. Prepare the client.

- Assist the client who must remain in bed to a side-lying position. Place a disposable bedpad on the bed in front of the client, and place the bedpan on top of the disposable pad, beneath the stoma.

- Assist an ambulatory client to sit on the toilet or on a commode in the bathroom. Ensure that the client's gown or pajamas are moved out of the way to prevent soiling, and cover the client appropriately with the bath blanket to prevent undue exposure.

- Throughout the procedure, provide explanations, and encourage the client to participate.

### 2. Prepare the equipment.

- Fill the solution bag with 500 ml of warm (body temperature) tap

water, or other solution as ordered.

- Hang the solution bag on an IV pole so that the bottom of the container is at the level of the client's shoulder, or 30 to 45 cm (12 to 18 in) above the stoma. *This height provides a pressure gradient that allows fluid to flow into the colon.*

- Attach the colon catheter securely to the tubing.

- Open the regulator clamp, and run fluid through the tubing to expel all air from it. Close the clamp until ready for the irrigation. *Air should not be introduced into the bowel because it distends the bowel and can cause cramps.*

### 3. Remove the colostomy bag and then position the irrigation drainage sleeve.

- Remove the soiled colostomy bag, and place it in the moisture-resistant bag. *Placing the colostomy bag in this container prevents the transmission of microorganisms and helps reduce odor.*

- Center the irrigation drainage sleeve over the stoma, and attach it snugly. *This prevents seepage of the fluid onto the skin.*

- Direct the lower, open end of the drainage sleeve into the bedpan or between the client's legs into the toilet.

### 4. If ordered by the physician, dilate the stoma.

- Put on gloves.

- Lubricate the tip of the little finger.

- Gently insert the finger into the stoma, using a massaging mo-

▶ **Procedure 40–4** CONTINUED

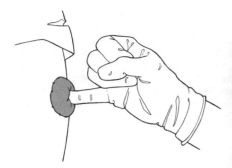

**FIGURE 40–1** Dilating a colostomy stoma.

tion (Figure 40–1). *A massaging motion relaxes the intestinal muscles.*

- Repeat the previous two steps, using progressively larger fingers, until maximum dilation is achieved. *Stoma dilation is performed to stretch and relax the stomal sphincter and to assess the direction of the proximal colon prior to an irrigation.*

**5. Insert the stoma cone or colon catheter.**

- Lubricate the tip of the stoma cone or colon catheter. *Lubricating the tip of the cone or catheter eases insertion and prevents injury to the stoma.*

- Using a rotating motion, insert the catheter or stoma cone through the opening in the top of the irrigation drainage sleeve and gently through the stoma (Figure 40–2). *A rotating motion on insertion helps to open the stoma.*

- Insert a catheter only 7 cm (3 in); insert a stoma cone just until it fits snugly. Many practitioners prefer using a cone to avoid the risk of perforating the bowel.

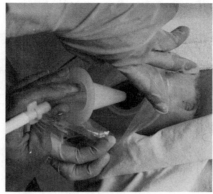

**FIGURE 40–2** The client is participating in the colostomy irrigation by directing the cone.

- If you have difficulty inserting the catheter or cone, do not apply force. *Forcing the cone or catheter may traumatize or perforate the bowel.*

**6. Irrigate the colon.**

- Open the tubing clamp, and allow the fluid to flow into the bowel. If cramping occurs, stop the flow until the cramps subside and then resume the flow. *Fluid that is too cold or administered too quickly may cause cramps.*

- If the fluid flows out as fast as you put it in, press the stoma cone or seal more firmly against the stoma to occlude it. If a stoma cone or seal is not available, press around the stoma with your fingers to close the stoma against the catheter.

- After all the fluid is instilled, remove the catheter or cone and allow the colon to empty. Although not always indicated, you may ask the client to gently massage the abdomen and sit quietly for 10 to 15 minutes until initial

emptying has occurred. *Massaging the abdomen encourages initial emptying.* In some agencies the stoma cone is left in place for 10 to 15 minutes before it is removed.

**7. Seal the drainage sleeve and allow complete emptying of the colon.**

- Clean the base of the irrigation drainage sleeve, and seal the bottom with a drainage clamp, following the manufacturer's instructions.

- Encourage an ambulatory client to move around for about 30 minutes. *Complete emptying of the colon often takes up to half an hour. Moving around promotes peristalsis.*

**8. Empty and remove the irrigation sleeve.**

**9. Ensure client comfort.**

- Clean the area around the stoma, and dry it thoroughly.

- Put a colostomy appliance on the client as needed. See Procedure 40–3 in *Fundamentals of Nursing.*

**10. Document and report relevant information.**

- Document all assessments and interventions. Include the time of the irrigation, the type and amount of fluid instilled, the returns, any problems experienced, and the client's response.

- Promptly report to the nurse in charge any problems, such as no fluid or stool returns, difficulties inserting the tube, peristomal skin redness or irritation, and stomal discoloration.

| **EVALUATION FOCUS** | Amount and consistency of fluid returns; status of stoma and peristomal skin; any difficulties encountered inserting the tube or dilating the stoma; client's response and participation. |
|---|---|

▶

▶ **Procedure 40–4  Irrigating a Colostomy** *CONTINUED*

**SAMPLE RECORDING**

| Date | Time | Notes |
|------|------|-------|
| 12/05/95 | 0900 | Colostomy irrigated with 750 ml warm tap water. Water and large amount soft brown stool expelled. Tube inserted without difficulty. Peristomal skin intact. Stoma is pink. Asked questions about irrigation, looked at stoma for first time. Observed stoma care and pouch application. ——————— ——————————————————————————— Chung-Hao Jen, NS |

# Urinary Elimination

## PROCEDURES

# 41-1  Collecting a Routine Urine Specimen from an Adult or Child Who Has Urinary Control

**PURPOSE**
- To screen the client's urine for abnormal constituents

**ASSESSMENT FOCUS**
Client's ability to provide the specimen; medications that may discolor urine or affect the test results.

## EQUIPMENT
- Nonsterile gloves as needed
- Clean bedpan, urinal, or commode for clients who are unable to void directly into the specimen container
- Wide-mouthed specimen container
- Completed laboratory requisition
- Completed specimen identification label

## INTERVENTION

**1. Give ambulatory clients the following information and instructions.**

- Explain the purpose of the urine specimen and how the client can assist.

- Explain that all specimens must be free of fecal contamination, so voiding needs to occur at a different time from defecation.

- Instruct female clients to discard the toilet tissue in the toilet or in a waste bag rather than in the bedpan, because tissue in the specimen makes laboratory analysis more difficult.

- Give the client the specimen container, and direct the client to the bathroom to void 120 ml (4 oz) into it.

**2. Assist clients who are seriously ill, physically incapacitated, or disoriented.**

- Provide required assistance in the bathroom, or help the client

to use a bedpan or urinal in bed.

- Wear gloves when assisting the client to void into a bedpan or urinal and transferring the urine from the bedpan, urinal, or commode to the specimen container.

- Empty the bedpan or urinal.

- Remove gloves if worn, and wash your hands.

**3. Ensure that the specimen is sealed and the container clean.**

- Put the lid tightly on the container. *This prevents spillage of the urine and contamination of other objects.*

- If the outside of the container has been contaminated by urine, clean it with soap and water. *This prevents the spread of microorganisms.*

**4. Label and transport the specimen to the laboratory.**

- Ensure that the specimen label

and the laboratory requisition have the correct information on them. Attach them securely to the specimen container. *Inappropriate identification of the specimen can lead to errors of diagnosis or therapy for the client.*

- Arrange for the specimen to be taken immediately to the laboratory or placed in a refrigerator. *Urine deteriorates relatively rapidly from bacterial contamination when left at room temperature; specimens should be analyzed immediately after collection.*

**5. Document all relevant information.**

- Document the collection of the specimen on the client's chart. Include the date and time of collection and the appearance and odor of the urine.

**EVALUATION FOCUS**
Color, odor, and character of the urine.

### SAMPLE RECORDING

| Date | Time | Notes |
|------|------|-------|
| 02/27/95 | 0600 | Random urine specimen collected for admission urinalysis. Urine clear, straw colored, and without odor. Specimen sent to lab.———Joyce Daynard, SN |

# 41-2   Collecting a Timed Urine Specimen

For timed urine specimens, appropriate specimen containers with or without preservative in accordance with the specific test are generally obtained from the laboratory and placed in the client's bathroom or in the utility room. Alert signs are placed in the client's unit to remind staff of the test in progress. Specimen identification labels need to indicate the date and time of each voiding in addition to the usual identification information. They may also be numbered sequentially, e.g., 1st specimen, 2nd specimen, 3rd specimen.

**PURPOSES**
- To assess the ability of the kidney to concentrate and dilute urine
- To determine disorders of glucose metabolism, e.g., diabetes mellitus
- To determine levels of specific constituents, e.g., albumin, amylase, creatinine, urobilinogen, certain hormones (e.g., estriol or corticosteroids) in the urine

**ASSESSMENT FOCUS**
Client's ability to understand instructions and to provide urine samples independently; any fluid or dietary requirements associated with the test; any medication restrictions or requirements for the test.

## EQUIPMENT

- ☐ Appropriate specimen containers with or without preservative in accordance with the specific test
- ☐ Completed specimen identification labels
- ☐ Completed laboratory requisition
- ☐ Bedpan or urinal
- ☐ Alert card on or near the bed indicating the specific times for urine collection
- ☐ Antiseptic
- ☐ Nonsterile gloves, as needed

## INTERVENTION

**1 Give the client the following information and instructions.**

- The purpose of the test and how the client can assist.

- When the specimen collection will begin and end. For example, a 24-hour urine test commonly begins at 0700 hours and ends at the same hour the next day.

- That all urine must be saved and placed in the specimen containers once the test starts.

- That the urine must be free of fecal contamination and toilet tissue.

- That each specimen must be given to the nursing staff immediately so that it can be placed in the appropriate specimen bottle.

**2. Start the collection period.**

- Ask the client to void in the toilet or bedpan or urinal. Discard this urine (check agency procedure), and document the time the test starts with this discarded specimen. Collect all subsequent urine specimens, including the one at the end of the period.

- Ask the client to ingest the required amount of liquid for certain tests or to restrict fluid intake. Follow the test directions.

- Instruct the client to void all subsequent urine into the bedpan or urinal and to notify the nursing staff when each specimen is provided. Some tests require voiding at specified times.

- Number the specimen containers sequentially, e.g., 1st specimen, 2nd specimen, 3rd specimen, if separate specimens are required.

- Place alert signs in the client's unit to remind staff of the test in progress.

**3. Collect all of the required specimens.**

- Place each specimen into the appropriately labeled container. For some tests, each specimen is not kept separately but is poured into a large bottle in the laboratory refrigerator.

- If the outside of the specimen container is contaminated with

▶

► **Procedure 41–2 Collecting a Timed Urine Specimen** CONTINUED

urine, clean it with soap and water. *Cleaning prevents the transfer of microorganisms to others.*

- Ensure that each specimen is refrigerated throughout the timed collection period. If not refrigerated, specimens are often kept on ice. *Refrigeration or other form of cooling prevents bacterial decomposition of the urine.*

- Measure the amount of each urine specimen as required.

- Ask the client to provide the last specimen 5 to 10 minutes before the end of the collection period.

- Inform the client that the test is completed.

- Remove the alert signs and the specimen equipment from the client's unit and bathroom.

**5. Document all relevant information.**

- Record the starting time of the test and completion of the specimen collection on the client's chart. Include the date and specific time. In addition, if indicated for the specific test, note the time each urine specimen was collected, the volume of each specimen, the appearance of the urine, and other relevant data such as fluid intake or restrictions.

---

**EVALUATION FOCUS**

Each urine specimen for color, odor, and clarity; results of laboratory analysis when available.

**SAMPLE RECORDING**

| Date | Time | Notes |
|------|------|-------|
| 03/21/95 | 0700 | 24 hour urine collection for quantitative albumin started after client voided. Client informed of need to save all urine and inform nursing staff after each voiding. Specimen collection bottle labeled and placed on ice in bathroom. ——————————————————————— Annette Campinola, R.N. |
| 03/22/95 | 0700 | 24 hour urine collection for albumin completed. Specimen sent to lab. Urine cloudy. ——————————————————— Thomas Timothy, R.N. |

## 41-3   Collecting a Urine Specimen from an Infant

| | |
|---|---|
| **PURPOSE** | • To screen the infant's urine for abnormal constituents |
| **ASSESSMENT FOCUS** | Skin status of infant's perineal area. |

### EQUIPMENT

- Plastic disposable urine collection bag
- Sterile cotton balls
- Soap and a basin of water
- Antiseptic solution
- Sterile water
- Diaper
- Specimen container
- Disinfectant
- Completed specimen label
- Completed laboratory form
- Nonsterile gloves, as needed

### INTERVENTION

**1. Prepare the parents and the infant.**

- If parents are present, explain why a urine specimen is being taken and the method of obtaining it.

- Before and throughout the procedure, handle the infant gently, and talk in soothing tones.

- Remove the infant's diaper and clean the perineal-genital area with soap and water and then with an antiseptic. *Cleaning is necessary to remove powder, baby oil, lotions, secretions, and fecal matter from the genitals. It also reduces the number of microorganisms on the skin and subsequent contamination of the voided urine.*

  a. For girls, separate the labia and wash, rinse, and dry the perineal area from the front to the back (clitoris to anus) on each side of the urinary meatus, and then over the meatus (Figure 41–1). Repeat this procedure, using the antiseptic solution to clean, the sterile water to rinse, and some dry cotton balls to dry.

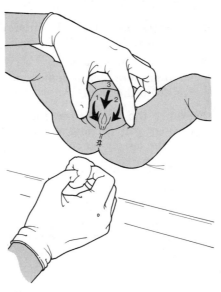

**FIGURE 41–1**   Cleaning the perineal area of a female infant.

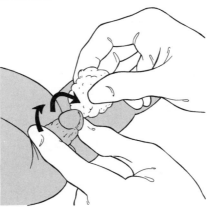

**FIGURE 41–2**   Cleaning the tip of the penis.

b. For boys, clean and disinfect both the penis and the scrotum in the manner described above. Wash the penis in a circular motion from the tip toward the scrotum, and wash the scrotum last (Figure 41–2). Retract the foreskin of an uncircumcised boy. *Freeing the skin of all moisture and secretions facilitates proper adhesion of the urine collection bag and prevents leakage of urine.*

**2. Apply the specimen bag.**

- Remove the protective paper from the bottom half of the adhesive backing of the collection bag (Figure 41–3).

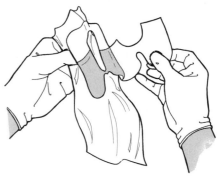

**FIGURE 41–3**   Removing the bottom half of the adhesive backing.

▶

▶ **Procedure 41–3 Collecting a Urine Specimen from an Infant** CONTINUED

- Spread the infant's legs apart as much as possible. *Spreading the legs separates and flattens the folds of the skin.*

- Place the opening of the collection bag over the urethra or the penis and scrotum. The base of the opening needs to cover the vagina or to fit well up under the scrotum (Figure 41–4).

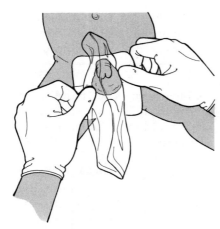

**FIGURE 41–4** Placing the opening of the collection bag over the penis and scrotum.

- Press the adhesive portion firmly against the infant's skin, starting at the perineum (the area between the anus and the genitals) and working outward. *This method prevents wrinkles, which could cause leakage of urine.*

- Remove the protective paper from the top half of the adhesive backing, and press it firmly in place, working from the top center outward.

- Apply a loose-fitting diaper. *A diaper helps keep the urine bag in place.*

- Elevate the head of the crib mattress to semi-Fowler's position. *Semi-Fowler's position aids the flow of urine by gravity into the collection portion of the urine bag.*

**3. Remove the bag, and transfer the specimen.**

- After the child has voided a desired amount, gently remove the bag from the skin.

- Empty the urine from the bag through the opening at its base into the specimen container.

- Discard the urine bag.

- Tightly apply the lid to the specimen container. *The lid will prevent spillage of urine from the container and contamination of other objects.*

- If the outside of the specimen container has been contaminated, clean it with a disinfectant. *Cleaning the outside of the container prevents the spread of microorganisms.*

**4. Ensure client comfort.**

- Apply the infant's diaper.

- Leave the infant in a comfortable and safe position held by a parent or in a crib.

**5. Transport the specimen.**

- Ensure that the specimen label and the laboratory requisition have the correct information on them. Attach them securely to the specimen. *Incorrect identification of the specimen can lead to subsequent errors of diagnosis or therapy for the infant.*

- Arrange for the specimen to be sent to the laboratory immediately or refrigerate it.

**6. Document all relevant information.**

- Record collection of the urine specimen and your assessments.

- See Sample Recording in Procedure 41–1.

**EVALUATION FOCUS**  | See Procedure 41–1.

# Changing a Urinary Diversion Ostomy Appliance

Various types of vinyl urinary stoma appliances are available. The disposable one-piece pouch may be attached either to a nonallergenic adhesive-backed faceplate, which may or may not be precut, or to a semipermeable skin barrier, which is permeable to vapor and oxygen but impermeable to liquid. The latter attachment maintains skin integrity more effectively. Reusable pouches have opaque faceplates, which may or may not be attached to the pouch. Some have belt attachments, and one type has an adaptable insert that can be adjusted to stoma size. The enterostomal therapy nurse selects the pouch that best suits the client by considering the type of ostomy, the stoma location and shape, and the peristomal skin surface, as well as the client's body size and contour, physical and mental abilities, skin allergies, financial status, and life-style.

Generally, a urinary diversion appliance adheres to the skin for 2–5 days. It is usually changed twice a week. The nurse's responsibilities include stoma and peristomal care.

## 41-4   Changing a Urinary Diversion Ostomy Appliance

**PURPOSES**
- To assess and care for the peristomal skin
- To collect urinary drainage for the assessment of the amount and type of output

**ASSESSMENT FOCUS**

> Stoma size and shape; color of stoma; presence of swelling; condition of peristomal skin; type and size of appliance currently in use; client and family learning needs; client emotional status and responses; level of comfort; behavior and attitude toward ostomy; skills learned.

---

### EQUIPMENT

If a commercially prepared stoma care kit is not available, the following supplies need to be assembled:
- Disposable gloves
- Ostomy pouch with adhesive-backed faceplate
- Ostomy pouch belt (optional)
- Graduated pitcher or receptacle for the urine
- Cleaning materials including basin filled with warm water, soap (optional), cotton balls, and towel

- Tampon
- Scissors
- Gauze pads
- Skin barrier (Skin Prep liquid or wipes or similar product, e.g., Stomahesive or ready-made wafer-type or disc-type barrier) for the peristomal skin
- Stoma measuring guide
- Pen or pencil

- Adhesive solvent in the form of presaturated sponges or liquid (optional)
- Adhesive cement (optional) for reusable pouches if double-faced adhesive disc is not used
- Electric or safety razor
- Waterproof bag for the soiled appliance

---

### INTERVENTION

**1. Determine the need for appliance change.**

- Assess the appliance in use for leakage of urine. *Urine can irritate the peristomal skin.*

- Ask the client about any discomfort at or around the stoma. *Complaints of burning may indicate urine leakage and skin breakdown beneath the faceplate.*

▶

▶ ## Procedure 41–4 Changing a Urinary Diversion Ostomy Appliance CONTINUED

- Drain the pouch into a graduated cylinder when it is one-third to one-half full and prior to removing the pouch.

- With any evidence of leakage or discomfort at or around the stoma, change the appliance.

**2. Communicate acceptance and support of the client throughout the procedure.** *This procedure may evoke negative emotional and psychologic responses.*

**3. Select an appropriate time.**

- The best time is early in the morning prior to taking fluids. *Urine output is lower at this time.* Avoid mealtimes or visiting hours. *The ostomy may embarrass the client or affect appetite.*

- Avoid times immediately after the administration of diuretics which will increase urine output. *It is best to change the pouch when urine output is at its lowest flow rate.*

**4. Prepare the client and support persons.**

- Explain the procedure to the client and support persons. Changing an ostomy appliance should not result in discomfort, but it may be distressful to the client. *Providing information to support persons will assist them in providing support.*

- Change the appliance competently and quickly. Do not convey negative feelings.

- Provide privacy, preferably in the bathroom, where clients can deal with the ostomy as they would at home.

- Assist the client into a comfortable sitting or lying position in bed or, preferably, a sitting or standing position in the bathroom. *Lying or standing positions may facilitate pouch application by avoiding skin wrinkles.*

- Don gloves, and unfasten the belt if one is being worn.

**5. Shave the peristomal skin of well-established ostomies as needed.**

- Use an electric or safety razor on a regular basis to remove excessive hair. *Hair follicles can become irritated or infected by repeated pulling out hairs during removal of the appliance and skin barrier.*

**6. Remove the emptied ostomy appliance.**

- Assess the volume and character of output.

- Peel the bag off slowly while holding the client's skin taut. *Holding the skin taut minimizes client discomfort and prevents abrasion of the skin.*

- If the appliance is disposable, discard it in a moisture-proof bag.

**7. Clean and dry the peristomal skin and stoma.**

- Using cotton balls, carefully wash the peristomal skin with warm water and mild soap if needed. Thoroughly rinse the soap from the skin. *Washing the area will remove any urine on the skin. Soap left on the skin can prevent proper adherence of the appliance and may be irritating.*

- Pat dry the skin with a towel or cotton balls. Excessive rubbing may abrade the skin.

- Place a rolled gauze or tampon to wick urine from stoma. *The capillary action of the gauze or tampon will keep urine away from skin while changing appliance.*

**8. Assess the stoma and peristomal skin.**

- Inspect the color, size, and shape of the stoma. Note any frank bleeding.

- Inspect the peristomal skin for any redness, ulcerations, or irritation. Transient redness *after the removal of adhesive is normal.*

**Applying the Skin Barrier (Peristomal Seal)**

**9. If using Skin Prep liquid or wipes or other similar product:**

- Cover the stoma with a gauze pad to avoid getting the Skin Prep on the stoma.

- Either wipe the Skin Prep evenly around the peristomal skin, or use an applicator to apply a thin layer of the liquid plastic coating to the area.

- Allow the Skin Prep to dry until it no longer feels tacky.

**10. If using a wafer- or disc-type barrier, read the manufacturer's directions as well as the steps below.** (Note that the karaya ring seal, although effective in protecting the skin, is less effective with urinary ostomies than with bowel ostomies because urine tends to melt the karaya.)

- Use the stoma measuring guide to measure the size of the stoma.

- Trace a circle on the backing of the skin barrier the same size as the stomal opening.

- Make a template of the stoma pattern. *A template aids other nurses and the client with future appliance changes.*

- Cut out the traced stoma pattern to make an opening in the skin barrier.

- Remove the backing on one side of the skin barrier to expose the sticky adhesive.

- Attach the skin barrier to the faceplate of the ostomy appliance when it is prepared. *Assembling the skin barrier and the appliance before application enhances the speed of application,*

▶ **Procedure 41–4** *CONTINUED*

*an important consideration for constantly draining urostomies.*

**11. Preparing the clean appliance**

**To prepare a disposable pouch with adhesive square:**

- If the appliance does not have the precut opening, trace a circle no more than 2–3 mm (⅛ in.) larger than the stoma size on the appliance's adhesive square. *The opening is made slightly larger than the stoma to prevent rubbing, cutting, or trauma to the stoma.*

- Cut out the traced circle in the adhesive. Take care not to cut any portion of the pouch.

- Peel off the backing from the adhesive seal, and attach the seal to a disc-type skin barrier or, if a liquid product was used, to the client's peristomal skin.

**To prepare a reusable pouch with faceplate attached:**

- Depending on the type of appliance, apply either adhesive cement or a double-faced adhesive disc to the faceplate. Follow the manufacturer's directions.

**To prepare a reusable pouch with detachable faceplate:**

- Remove the protective paper strip from one side of the double-faced adhesive disc.

- Apply the sticky side of the disc to the back of the faceplate.

- Remove the remaining protective paper strip from the other side of the adhesive disc.

- Attach the faceplate to a disc-type skin barrier or, if a liquid product was used, to the client's peristomal skin.

**12. Applying the clean appliance**

**For a disposable pouch:**

- Remove the gauze pad or tampon

over the stoma before applying the pouch.

- Gently press the adhesive backing onto the skin and smooth out any wrinkles, working from the stoma outward. *Wrinkles allow seepage of urine, which can irritate the skin and soil clothing.*

- Remove the air from the pouch. *Removing the air helps the pouch lie flat against the abdomen.*

- Attach the spout of the pouch to a urinary drainage system or cap the spout. Temporary disposable pouches are often attached to drainage systems.

**For a reusable pouch with faceplate attached:**

- Insert a coiled paper guidestrip into the faceplate opening. The strip should protrude slightly from the opening and expand to fit it. *The guidestrip helps in centering the appliance over the stoma and prevents pressure or irritation to the stoma by the appliance.*

- Using the guidestrip, center the faceplate over the stoma.

- Firmly press the adhesive seal to the peristomal skin. The guidestrip will fall into the pouch; commercially prepared guidestrips will dissolve in the pouch.

- Place a deodorant in the bag (optional).

- Close the spout of the pouch with the designated cap.

- Optional: Attach the pouch belt and fasten it around the client's waist. Wash a soiled belt with warm water and mild soap, rinse, and dry if needed.

**For a reusable pouch with detachable faceplate:**

- Press and hold the faceplate against the client's skin for a few minutes to enhance the seal.

- Press the adhesive around the circumference of the adhesive disc.

- Tape the faceplate to the client's abdomen using four or eight 7.5-cm (3-in.) strips of tape. Place the strips around the faceplate in a "picture-framing" manner, one strip down each side, one across the top, and one across the bottom. The additional four strips can be placed diagonally over the other tapes to enhance the seal.

- Stretch the opening on the back of the pouch, and position it over the base of the faceplate. Ease it over the faceplate flange.

- Place the lock ring between the pouch and the faceplate flange to secure the pouch against the faceplate.

- Close the spout of the pouch with the appropriate cap.

- Optional: Attach the pouch belt and fast it around the client's waste.

**13. Document relevant information.**

- Document the date and time of appliance change.

- Record the color and size of stoma; amount, color, and character of urine output, condition of peristomal skin; client response; type and size of appliance.

- Document client's behavior and attitudes toward ostomy and skills learned.

**14. Adjust the client's teaching plan and nursing care plan as needed. Include on the teaching plan the equipment and procedure used.** *Learning to care for the ostomy is facilitated if procedures implemented by nurses are consistent.* The client will also need to learn self-care and ways to reduce odor. Use of deodorant tablets in the ap-

▶

▶ **Procedure 41–4 Changing a Urinary Diversion Ostomy Appliance** *CONTINUED*

pliance, soaking a reusable pouch in dilute vinegar solution, a diet that makes the urine more acid, and drinking plenty of fluids all help to control odor. *A high fluid intake di-lutes the urine, making it less odorous. Ascorbic acid and cranberry juice increase the acidity of urine, which in turn inhibits bacterial action and odor. Information about os-tomy clubs and other community services available should also be included.*

|  |  |
|---|---|
| **EVALUATION FOCUS** | Stoma size and shape; color of stoma; presence of swelling; condition of peristomal skin; type and size of appliance currently in use; client and family learning needs; client emotional status and responses; level of comfort; behavior and attitudes toward ostomy; skills learned. |

**SAMPLE RECORDING**

| Date | Time | Notes |
|---|---|---|
| 1/8/95 | 800 | Ureterostomy appliance changed. 200 cc clear yellow urine. Stoma pink, 6 cm. Peristomal skin intact. Denies discomfort. 1¼-inch two piece drainage system applied. Helped to clean peristomal skin and measure appliance. ———————————— Kerry Andrews, SN |

# Medications

## PROCEDURES

**Administering Dermatologic Medications**

**PURPOSES**
- To decrease itching (pruritus)
- To lubricate and soften the skin
- To cause local vasoconstriction or vasodilation
- To increase or decrease secretions from the skin
- To provide a protective coating to the skin
- To apply an antibiotic or antiseptic to treat or prevent infection
- To reduce inflammation
- To administer sustained-action transdermal medications
- To debride necrotic tissue

**ASSESSMENT FOCUS**

Discomfort; pruritus; color of affected and surrounding area (e.g., redness, rash); swelling; discharge; amount of hair on affected area (excessive hair may need to be removed before the medication is applied).

## EQUIPMENT

Use sterile supplies and techniques for all open skin lesions.
- Gloves (disposable and sterile if required)
- Ordered solution to wash area as ordered
- 2 × 2 gauze pads for cleaning
- Medication container
- Application tube (if required)
- Tongue blades (sterile if required)
- Gauze to cover area (if required)

## INTERVENTION

### 1. Verify the order.

 • Compare the medication record with the most recent order.

- Compare the label on the medication tube or jar with the medication record.

- Determine whether area is to be washed before applying medication.

### 2. Prepare the client.

- Provide privacy.

- Expose the area of the skin to be treated.

### 3. Prepare the area for the medication.

 • Wash hands and don gloves.

- Determine that the body part to be treated is clean; if not, wash it gently as directed, and pat it dry with gauze pads.

### 4. Apply the medication and dressing as ordered.

- Place a small amount of cream (e.g., emollient) on the tongue blade, and spread it evenly on the skin.
  *or*
  Pour some lotion on the gauze, and pat the skin area with it.
  *or*
  If a liniment is used, rub it into the skin with the hands using long, smooth strokes.

- Repeat the application until the area is completely covered. *For complete coverage, no skin should show through cream or ointment.*

- Apply a sterile dressing as necessary.
  *or*
- Apply a prepackaged transdermal patch as directed.

### 5. Ensure client comfort.

- Provide a clean gown or pajamas after the application if the medication will come in contact with the clothing. *Agency clothes can be washed more easily than the client's own clothes.*

- Remove and discard the gloves.

### 6. Document all assessments and interventions.

- Record the type of preparation used; the site to which it was applied; the time; and the response of the client, including data about the appearance of the site, discomfort, itching, and so on.

- Return at a time by which the preparation should have acted to assess the reaction, e.g., redness (for a rubefacient, i.e., an agent that reddens the skin), and/or relief of itching, burning, swelling, or discomfort.

▶ **Procedure 43–1** *CONTINUED*

<table>
<tr><td>**EVALUATION FOCUS**</td><td>Presence of redness or discharge; increased or decreased comfort.</td></tr>
</table>

**SAMPLE RECORDING**

| Date | Time | Notes |
|------|------|-------|
| 8/7/95 | 2100 | Thin film of 0.5% Topicort cream applied to affected areas as ordered. Area is dry and has flaky patches (2.5 cm in diameter) scattered on chest, back, and abdomen. States no itching or pain. ———— Lawrence Campbell, RN |

# ‹43-2› Administering Nasal Instillations

**PURPOSES**
- To decrease nasal congestion and improve nasal breathing
- To treat infections, inflammations, or allergies of the nasal cavity or facial sinuses

**ASSESSMENT FOCUS**

> Appearance of nasal cavities; congestion of the mucous membranes and any obstruction to breathing; facial discomfort with or without palpation (see Intervention, step 3).

## EQUIPMENT
- ☐ Disposable tissues
- ☐ Correct medication
- ☐ Dropper

## INTERVENTION

**⚠S 1. Verify the medication or irrigation order.**

- Carefully check the physician's order for the solution to be used, its strength, the number of drops, the frequency of the instillation, and the area to receive the instillation (e.g., the eustachian (auditory) tube or specific sinuses).

**2. Prepare the client.**

- If secretions are excessive, ask the client to blow the nose to clear the nasal passages.

- Inspect the discharge on the tissues for color, odor, and thickness.

**3. Assess the client.**

- Assess congestion of the mucous membranes and any obstruction to breathing. Ask the client to hold one nostril closed and blow out gently through the other nostril. Listen for the sound of any obstruction to the air. Repeat for the other nostril.

- Assess signs of distress when nares are occluded. Block each naris of an infant or young child and observe for signs of greater distress when the naris is obstructed.

- Assess facial discomfort. An infected or congested sinus can cause an aching, full feeling over the area of the sinus and facial tenderness on palpation.

- Assess any crusting, redness, bleeding, or discharge of the mucous membranes of the nostrils. Use a nasal speculum. The membrane normally appears moist, pink, and shiny.

**4. Position the client appropriately.**

- To treat the opening of the eustachian tube, have the client assume a back-lying position. *The drops will flow into the nasopharynx, where the eustachian tube opens.*

- To treat the ethmoid and sphenoid sinuses, have the client take a back-lying position with the head over the edge of the bed or a pillow under the shoulders so that the head is tipped backward. This is called the *Proetz position* (Figure 43–1).

- To treat the maxillary and frontal sinuses, have the client assume the same back-lying position, with the head turned toward the side to be treated. This is called the *Parkinson position.* (Figure

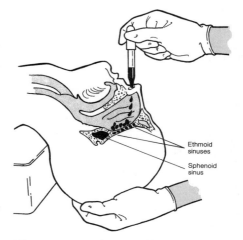

**FIGURE 43–1** The Proetz position.

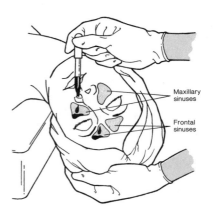

**FIGURE 43–2** The Parkinson position.

43–2). If only one side is to be treated, be sure the person is positioned so that the correct side

▶ **Procedure 43–2** *CONTINUED*

is accessible. If the client's head is over the edge of the bed, support it with your hand so that the neck muscles are not strained.

5. **Administer the medication.**

• Draw up the required amount of solution into the dropper.

• Hold the tip of the dropper just above the nostril, and direct the solution laterally toward the midline of the superior concha of the ethmoid bone as the client

breathes through the mouth. Do not touch the mucous membrane of the nares. *If the solution is directed toward the base of the nasal cavity, it will run down the eustachian tube. Touching the mucous membrane with the dropper could damage the membrane and cause the client to sneeze.*

• Repeat for the other nostril if indicated.

• Ask the client to remain in the position for 5 minutes. *The client*

*remains in the same position to help the solution come in contact with all of the nasal surface or flow into the desired area.*

• Discard any remaining solution in the dropper, and dispose of soiled supplies appropriately.

6. **Document all relevant information.**

• Document nursing assessments and interventions.

**EVALUATION FOCUS**

Relief of complaints (e.g., nasal congestion, difficulty breathing, and discomfort); amount and character of secretions; appearance of nasal mucosa; adverse reactions or side-effects of medication.

**SAMPLE RECORDING**

| Date | Time | Notes |
|------|------|-------|
| 12/6/95 | 2250 | Moderate amount clear secretions cleared from nose by blowing. Neosynephrine 2 gtts administered in both nares. No nasal or facial discomfort. Mucosa is pink. ———————————— Sharona Von Stachenberg, RN |

# 43-3 Administering an Intradermal Injection

**PURPOSES**
- To administer a medication for sensitivity and allergy testing
- To administer some types of immunizations

**ASSESSMENT FOCUS**

> Appearance of injection site; specific drug action and expected response; client's knowledge of drug action and response; agency protocol about sites to use for skin tests.

## EQUIPMENT

- Medication card or computer printout
- Vial or ampule of the correct sterile medication
- Sterile 1-ml syringe calibrated into hundredths of a milliliter and a needle ¼ to ⅝ inch
- long with #25, #26, or #27 gauge
- Acetone and 2 × 2 sterile gauze square (optional)
- Swab moistened with alcohol or other colorless antiseptic
- Nonsterile gloves (according to agency protocol)
- Band-Aid (optional)
- Epinephrine, a bronchodilator, and antihistamine on hand

## INTERVENTION

### 1. Verify the order.
- Check the physician's orders carefully for the medication, dosage, and route.

### 2. Prepare the medication from the vial or ampule.
- See Procedure 43–2 in *Fundamentals of Nursing.*

### 3. Identify and prepare the client for the injection.
- Check the client's arm band, and ask the client to tell you his or her name.
- Explain that the medication will produce a small bleb like a blister. The client will feel a slight prick as the needle enters the skin. Some medications are absorbed slowly through the capillaries into the general circulation, and the bleb gradually disappears. Other drugs remain in the area and interact with the body tissues to produce redness and induration (hardening), which will need to be interpreted at a particular time, e.g., in 24 or

48 hours. This reaction will also gradually disappear.

- Restrain a confused client or an infant or small child. *This prevents accidental injury from sudden movement.*

### 4. Select and clean the site.
- Select a site (e.g., the forearm about a hand's breadth above the wrist and three or four finger-widths below the antecubital space).
- Avoid using sites that are tender, inflamed, or swollen and those that have lesions.
- Don gloves as agency protocol indicates.
- Defat the skin if agency protocol dictates, using a gauze square or swab moistened with acetone. Start at the center and widen the circle outward.
- Using the same method, clean the site with a swab moistened with alcohol or other colorless antiseptic, according to agency protocol. Allow the area to dry thoroughly. *A colorless antiseptic*

*does not hinder the reading of the test.*

### 5. Prepare the syringe for injection.
- Remove the needle cap while waiting for the antiseptic to dry.
- Expel any air bubbles from the syringe. Small bubbles that adhere to the plunger are of no consequence. *A small amount of air will not harm the tissues.*
- Grasp the syringe in your dominant hand, holding it between thumb and four fingers, with your palm upward. Hold the needle at a 15° angle to the skin surface, with the bevel of the needle up.

### 6. Inject the fluid.
- With the nondominant hand, pull the skin at the site until it is taut, and thrust the tip of the needle firmly through the epidermis into the dermis (Figure 43–3, *A*). Do *not* aspirate.
- Inject the medication carefully so that it produces a small bleb on the skin (Figure 43–3, *B*).

▶ **Procedure 43–3** *CONTINUED*

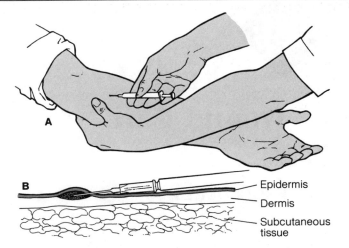

- Epidermis
- Dermis
- Subcutaneous tissue

**FIGURE 43–3** For an intradermal injection: *A*, the needle enters the skin at a 15° angle; and *B*, the medication forms a bleb under the epidermis.

- Withdraw the needle quickly while providing countertraction on the skin, and apply a Band-Aid if indicated.

- Do *not* massage the area. *Massage can disperse the medication into the tissue or out through the needle insertion site.*

- Dispose of the syringe and needle safely.

- Remove gloves, if worn.

**7. Document all relevant information.**

- Record the testing material given, the time, dosage, route, site, and nursing assessments.

**8. Assess the client.**

- Evaluate the client's response to the testing substance. *Some medications used in testing may cause allergic reactions.* An antidotal drug (e.g., epinephrine hydrochloride), may need to be given.

- Evaluate the condition of the site in 24 or 48 hours, depending on the test. Measure the area of redness and induration in millimeters at the largest diameter and document findings.

**EVALUATION FOCUS**

Client's response; size of induration and redness at the injection site. See step 8.

**SAMPLE RECORDING**

| Date | Time | Notes |
|------|------|-------|
| 02/26/95 | 1500 | Tuberculin skin test (0.1 ml) administered intradermally in inner aspect of L forearm. No adverse systemic or local response. ———— Maureen Kirkpatrick, RN |
| 02/28/95 | 1500 | Small wheal (4 mm in diameter) formed. ———— Maureen Kirkpatrick, RN |

# Wound Care

## PROCEDURES

# 44-1   Basic Bandaging

**PURPOSES**
- To provide comfort
- To prevent further injury
- To promote healing

**ASSESSMENT FOCUS**

Status of the skin area to which the bandage is to be applied; presence of an open wound; adequacy of circulation to the part; degree of pain.

## EQUIPMENT

- Clean bandage of the appropriate material and width
- Padding, such as ABD pads or gauze squares
- Tape, special metal clips, or a safety pin

## INTERVENTION

### 1. Position and prepare the client appropriately.

- Provide the client with a chair or bed, and arrange support for the area to be bandaged. For example, if a hand needs to be bandaged, ask the client to place the elbow on a table, so that the hand does not have to be held up unsupported. *Because bandaging takes a little time, holding up a body part without support can fatigue the client.*

- Make sure that the area to be bandaged is clean and dry. Wash and dry the area if necessary. *Washing and drying remove microorganisms, which flourish in dark, warm, moist areas.*

- Align the part to be bandaged with slight flexion of the joints, unless this is contraindicated. *Slight flexion places less strain on the ligaments and muscles of the joint.*

### 2. Apply the bandage.

### Circular Turns

- Hold the bandage in your dominant hand, keeping the roll uppermost, and unroll the bandage about 8 cm (3 in). *This length of unrolled bandage allows good control for placement and tension.*

- Apply the end of the bandage to the part of the body to be bandaged. Hold the end down with the thumb of the other hand (Figure 44–1).

- Encircle the body part a few times or as often as needed, making sure that each turn directly covers the previous turn. *This provides even support to the area.*

- Secure the end of the bandage with tape, metal clips, or a safety pin over an uninjured area. *Clips and pins can cause discomfort when situated over an injured area.*

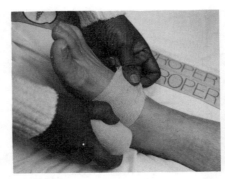

**FIGURE 44–1**   Starting a bandage with two circular turns.

### Spiral Turns

- Make two circular turns. *Two circular turns anchor the bandage.*

- Continue spiral turns at about a 30° angle, each turn overlapping the preceding one by two-thirds the width of the bandage (Figure 44–2).

- Terminate the bandage with two circular turns, and secure the end as described for circular turns.

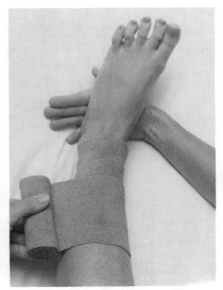

**FIGURE 44–2**   Applying spiral turns.

▶

▶ **Procedure 44–1 Basic Bandaging** *CONTINUED*

**Spiral Reverse Turns**

- Anchor the bandage with two circular turns, and bring the bandage upward at about a 30° angle.

- Place the thumb of your free hand on the upper edge of the bandage (Figure 44–3, *A*). *The thumb will hold the bandage while it is folded on itself.*

- Unroll the bandage about 15 cm (6 in), then turn your hand so that the bandage falls over itself (Figure 44–3, *B*).

- Continue the bandage around the limb, overlapping each previous turn by two-thirds the width of the bandage. Make each bandage turn at the same position on the limb so that the turns of the bandage will be aligned (Figure 44–3, *C*).

- Terminate the bandage with two circular turns, and secure the end as described for circular turns.

**Recurrent Turns**

- Anchor the bandage with two circular turns.

- Fold the bandage back on itself, and bring it centrally over the distal end to be bandaged (Figure 44–4).

- Holding it with the other hand, bring the bandage back over the end to the right of the center bandage but overlapping it by two-thirds the width of the bandage.

- Bring the bandage back on the left side, also overlapping the first turn by two-thirds the width of the bandage.

- Continue this pattern of alternating right and left until the area is covered. Overlap the preceding turn by two-thirds the bandage width each time.

- Terminate the bandage with two circular turns (Figure 44–5). Secure the end appropriately.

**Figure-Eight Turns**

- Anchor the bandage with two circular turns.

- Carry the bandage above the joint, around it, and then below it, making a figure eight (Figure 44–6).

- Continue above and below the joint, overlapping the previous turn by two-thirds the width of the bandage.

- Terminate the bandage above the joint with two circular turns, and then secure the end appropriately.

**Thumb Spica**

- Anchor the bandage with two circular turns around the wrist.

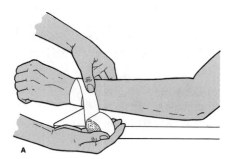

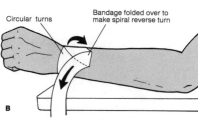

Circular turns

Bandage folded over to make spiral reverse turn

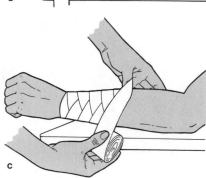

**FIGURE 44–3** Applying spiral reverse turns.

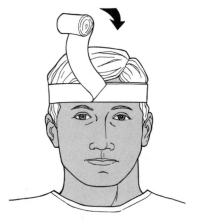

**FIGURE 44–4** Starting a recurrent bandage with two circular turns.

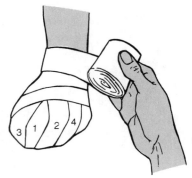

**FIGURE 44–5** Completing a recurrent bandage with two circular turns.

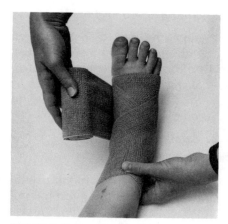

**FIGURE 44–6** Applying a figure-eight bandage.

▶ **Procedure 44–1** *CONTINUED*

- Bring the bandage down to the distal aspect of the thumb, and encircle the thumb. Leave the tip 🔺 of the thumb exposed if possible. *This allows you to check blood circulation to the thumb.*

- Bring the bandage back up and around the wrist, then back down and around the thumb, overlapping the previous turn by two-thirds the width of the bandage.

- Repeat the above two steps, working up the thumb and hand until the thumb is covered (Figure 44–7).

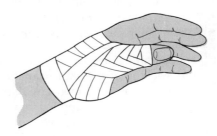

**FIGURE 44–7**  A thumb spica bandage.

- Anchor the bandage with two circular turns around the wrist, and secure the end appropriately.

**3. Document all relevant information.**

- Record the type of bandage applied, the area to which it is applied, and nursing assessments, 🔺 including skin problems or neurovascular problems.

**EVALUATION FOCUS**

Adequacy of distal circulation to bandaged part (e.g., skin color for pallor or cyanosis, skin temperature, strength of pulse, presence of numbness or tingling); client's ability to reapply the bandage when needed; client's ability to perform ADLs and assistance required.

**SAMPLE RECORDING**

| Date | Time | Notes |
|------|------|-------|
| 04/07/95 | 0700 | Elastic spiral bandage applied to right leg. Toes warm and pink. No numbness. Rt pedal pulse 60 beats per min strong. Laura R. Stenhouse, NS |

# 44-2 Applying a Stump Bandage

**PURPOSES**
- To support the return flow of venous blood
- To apply pressure and minimize bleeding and/or swelling
- To retain a surgical dressing
- To help shape a stump in preparation for a prosthesis

**ASSESSMENT FOCUS**

The amount of any drainage on the dressing; the color, temperature, and swelling of the skin near the dressing to provide baseline data for evaluating the blood circulation to and from the area after the bandage has been applied; any discomfort, e.g., "phantom" pain (pain or irritation perceived to be in the removed part of the limb).

## EQUIPMENT

- ☐ Clean bandage
- ☐ Tape, safety pins, or metal clips

## INTERVENTION

### 1. Position the client appropriately.

- Assist the client to a semi-Fowler's position in bed or to a sitting position on the edge of the bed.
- Clean the skin or stump wound, and apply a sterile dressing as needed.

### 2. Apply the bandage.

**Figure-Eight Bandage**

- Anchor the bandage with two circular turns around the hips.
- Bring the bandage down over the stump and then back up and around the hips (Figure 44–8).
- Bring the bandage down again, overlapping the previous turn, and make a figure eight around the stump and back up around the hips.
- Repeat, working the bandage up the stump (Figure 44–9).
- Anchor the bandage around the hips with two circular turns.
- Secure the bandage with adhesive tape, safety pins, or clips. *or*

- Place the end of the elastic bandage at the top of the anterior surface of the leg, and have the client hold it in place. Bring the bandage diagonally down toward the end of the stump.
- Then, applying even pressure, bring the bandage diagonally upward toward the groin area (Figure 44–10).
- Make a figure-eight turn behind the top of the leg, downward again over and under the stump, and back up to the groin area (Figure 44–11).
- Repeat these figure-eight turns at least twice.
- Anchor the bandage around the hips with two circular turns.
- Secure the bandage with tape, safety pins, or clips.

**Recurrent Bandage**

- Anchor the bandage with two circular turns around the stump.
- Cover the stump with recurrent turns.

- Anchor the recurrent bandage with two circular turns (Figure 44–12).
- Secure the bandage with tape, safety pins, or clips.

**Spiral Bandage**

- Make recurrent turns to cover the end of the stump.
- Apply spiral turns from the distal aspect of the stump toward the body (Figure 44–13).
- Anchor the bandage with two circular turns around the hips.
- Secure the bandage with tape, safety pins, or clips.

### 3. Document all relevant information.

- Record the application of the bandage, all nursing assessments, and the client's response.

▶ **Procedure 44–2** *CONTINUED*

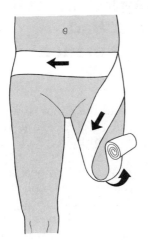

**FIGURE 44–8**  One way of beginning a figure-eight stump bandage.

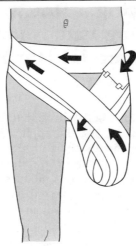

**FIGURE 44–9**  Figure-eight stump bandage applied around stump and waist.

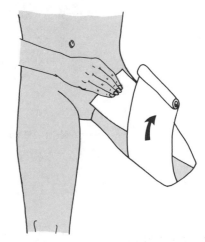

**FIGURE 44–10**  A second way to begin a figure-eight stump bandage.

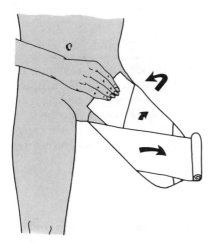

**FIGURE 44–11**  Figure-eight stump bandage applied around stump only.

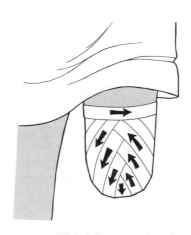

**FIGURE 44–12**  A recurrent stump bandage.

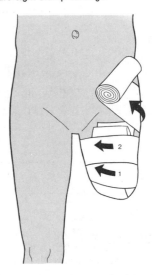

**FIGURE 44–13**  A spiral stump bandage.

| **EVALUATION FOCUS** | Adequacy of circulation to the stump (e.g., skin color for pallor or cyanosis; skin temperature; strength of pulses; presence of numbness or tingling). |
|---|---|

**SAMPLE RECORDING**

| Date | Time | Notes |
|---|---|---|
| 07/11/95 | 0930 | Figure-eight stump bandage removed as ordered. Slight serosanguineous drainage on one 4 × 4 gauze. Sterile dressing applied and figure-eight stump bandage reapplied. Wound is clean with minimal inflammation; stump skin color pink, feels warm to touch. No complaints of numbness or tingling. — Sam Fields, RN |

# 44-3 Applying a Hot Water Bottle, Electric Heating Pad, Aquathermia Pad, Commercial Hot Pack, or Perineal Heat Lamp

Before applying dry heat, determine (a) whether the client is required to sign a release for the application of dry heat (if a release is required, check the client's chart for the signed release); (b) the type of heat to be used, the temperature, and the duration and frequency of the application (check the physician's or nursing order); (c) agency protocol about the type of equipment used, the temperature recommended, and the length of heat applications; (d) at what time the heat should be applied, e.g., 1000 and 1900 hours or after a wound dressing is changed (check the nursing care plan); (e) if a heat lamp, if used, is in proper working order.

**PURPOSES**
- To warm a body part and promote comfort, relaxation, and sleep
- To increase blood circulation and promote healing and comfort
- To reduce muscle pain
- To dry the perineal tissues (heat lamp)

**ASSESSMENT FOCUS**

Any traumatic injury, signs of redness, abraded skin, swelling, or hemorrhage at the area to which the heat is to be applied; other factors contraindicating heat therapy; any discomfort experienced by the client; the client's capacity to recognize when the heat is injurious; the client's general physical condition and mental capability to cooperate with the treatment; the blood circulation to the area.

## EQUIPMENT

**Hot Water Bottle (Bag)**
- Hot water bottle with a stopper
- Cover
- Hot water and a thermometer

**Electric Heating Pad**
- Electric pad and control
- Cover, waterproof if there will be moisture under the pad

when it is applied
- Gauze ties (optional)

**Aquathermia Pad**
- Pad
- Distilled water
- Control unit
- Cover

- Gauze ties or tape (optional)

**Disposable Hot Packs**
- One or two commercially prepared disposable packs

**Heat Lamp**
- Perineal heat lamp with 60-watt bulb

▶ **Procedure 44-3** CONTINUED

**INTERVENTION**

**1. Prepare and assess the client.**

- Inspect the area to receive heat. See the Nursing Process Guide for this chapter.

- Fold down the bedclothes to expose the area to which the heat will be applied.

**Hot Water Bottle**

**2. Fill and cover the bottle.**

- Fill the hot water bottle about two-thirds full.

- Measure the temperature of the water if this was not done before the bag was filled. Follow agency practice for the appropriate temperature. Temperatures commonly used are

  a. 52° C (125° F) for a normal adult.

  b. 40.5° to 46° C (105° to 115° F) for a debilitated or unconscious adult.

  c. 40.5° to 46° C (105° to 115° F) for a child under 2 years of age.

- Expel the air from the bottle. *Air remaining in the bottle prevents it* ⚠Ⓢ *from molding to the body part being treated.*

- Secure the stopper tightly.

- Hold the bottle upside down, and check for leaks.

- Dry the bottle.

- Wrap the bottle in a towel or hot water bottle cover.

**3. Apply the bottle.**

- Support the bottle against the body part with pillows as necessary.

- Go to step 14.

**Electric Heating Pad**

**4. Prepare the client and pad for application.**

- Ensure that the body area is dry. *Electricity in the presence of mois-* ⚠Ⓢ *ture can conduct a shock.*

- Check that the electric pad is functioning and in good repair. The cord should be free from cracks, wires should be intact, heating components should not be exposed, and temperature distribution over the pad should be even.

- Place the cover on the pad. Some models have waterproof covers to be used when the pad is placed over a moist dressing. *Moisture could cause the pad to short circuit and burn or shock the client.*

- Plug the pad into the electric socket.

- Set the control dial for the correct temperature.

**5. Apply the pad.**

- After the pad has heated, place the pad *over* the body part to which heat is being applied.

- Use gauze ties instead of safety ⚠Ⓢ pins to hold the pad in place, if needed. *A pin might strike a wire, damaging the pad and giving an electric shock to the client.*

**6. Give the client the following instructions:**

- Do not insert any sharp, pointed ⚠Ⓢ object, e.g., a pin, into the pad.

- Do not lie directly on the pad. *The surface below the pad promotes heat absorption instead of normal heat dissipation.*

- To prevent injury, avoid adjust- ⚠Ⓢ ing the heat to the high setting. *The degree of heat felt shortly after application will decrease, because the body's temperature receptors quickly adapt to the temperature.*

*This adaptive mechanism can lead to tissue injury if the temperature control is adjusted to a higher setting.*

- Call the nurse if any discomfort is felt.

**Aquathermia Pad**

**7. Assemble the unit.**

- Fill the unit with distilled water until it is two-thirds full. The unit will warm the water, which circulates through the pad.

- Remove air bubbles, and secure the top.

- Regulate the temperature with the key if it has not been preset. Normal temperature is 40.5° C (105° F). Check the manufacturer's instructions.

- Cover the pad with a towel or pillowcase.

- Plug in the unit.

**8. Apply the pad to the body part.**

- Check for any leak or malfunctions of the pad before use.

- Use tape or gauze ties to hold the pad in place. Never use safety pins. *They can cause leakage.*

- If unusual redness or pain oc- ⚠Ⓢ curs, discontinue the treatment, and report the client's reaction.

**9. Give the client the following instructions:**

- Do not lie directly on the pad.

- Avoid adjusting temperature settings during the application.

- Call the nurse if any discomfort is felt.

**Disposable Hot Pack**

**10. Initiate the heating process.**

- Strike, squeeze, or knead the pack according to the manufacturer's directions.

▶

▶ **Procedure 44–3 Applying Dry Heat** *CONTINUED*

- Note the manufacturer's instructions about the length of time that heat is produced.

**Perineal Heat Lamp**

**11. Prepare the client.**

- Expose the area to be treated, and drape the client so that the body is exposed minimally.

- Clean and dry the perineum to remove all secretions, ointments, or perineal sprays. *Cleaning prevents drying of secretions, ointments, or sprays on the perineum.*

- Clean from the front (area of the symphysis pubis) to the back (area around the anus) of the perineum. *This avoids contamination between the anal area and the urethral/vaginal area, thereby preventing infection.*

**12. Position the lamp appropriately.**

- Plug in the lamp, and, with the lamp turned off, place it approx-imately 30 cm (12 in) from the perineum. (Check agency protocol.)

- Do not drape or cover the lamp. *A cover on the lamp may catch fire.*

**13. Give the client the following instructions.**

- Remain in position.

- Warn the client not to touch the bulb of the heat lamp.

- Call the nurse if any discomfort is felt.

**For All Applications**

**14. Monitor the client during the application.**

- Every 5 to 10 minutes, assess the client for any complaints of discomfort, e.g., pain, burning, and skin reaction. Frequency of assessment depends on such factors as the client's previous responses to applications and ability to report problems.

- At the first sign of pain, swelling, or excessive redness, remove the heat and report any sign to the nurse in charge.

**15. Remove the heat application.**

- Remove the heat before the rebound phenomenon begins, i.e., 20 to 30 minutes. A hot water bottle will usually stay hot for the duration of the treatment. It needs to be replaced for the next application. *Prolonged heat, e.g., 1 hour, decreases the blood flow to the area and can damage skin tissue.*

**16. Document all relevant information.**

- When the heat is applied, record the application, its purpose, the time, the method used, the site, and any nursing assessments.

- After removal, record the time and all nursing assessments.

---

**EVALUATION FOCUS**

Relief of pain or muscle tension; skin color and temperature (e.g., excessive redness); complaints of excessive heat.

**SAMPLE RECORDING**

| Date | Time | Notes |
|------|------|-------|
| 04/02/95 | 2000 | Aquathermia pad at medium setting applied to lower back for nonradiating pain aggravated by movement. Skin intact. ——————— Marilyn March, SN |
| | 2020 | Aquathermia pad removed. States pain relieved. Skin warm and pink. ——— ——————— Marilyn March, SN |

# Infant Radiant Warmer

An *infant radiant warmer* or similar device is an open heating unit. A row of long lights is positioned at a stationary height from a bedding pad below. The radiant warmer is used to prevent the loss of body heat from the newborn infant. This warming process is crucial to the immature infant who has difficulty maintaining body temperature because of insufficient subcutaneous body fat and inadequate temperature self-regulation mechanisms. If the environmental temperature is not maintained with a radiant warmer or some similar thermal device, the infant will expend significant metabolic energy, with a resultant increase in oxygen and caloric needs. Procedure 44–4 describes how to apply an infant radiant warmer.

 ## Applying an Infant Radiant Warmer

 Before applying the radiant warmer, determine (a) that the equipment is in proper working order and (b) the manufacturer's operating instructions and institutional policy regarding the temperature control process and alarm setting protocols.

**PURPOSE**

- To assist the newborn or immature infant in establishing and maintaining a stable body temperature

**ASSESSMENT FOCUS**

> The infant's initial body temperature; parental knowledge of the warmer function.

## EQUIPMENT

- ☐ Radiant warmer with appropriate skin temperature sensors and reflective sensor covers (according to institutional policy)
- ☐ Prewarmed towels and infant blankets
- ☐ Infant head cover and diaper (according to institutional policy)
- ☐ Appropriate bedding for infant warmer

## INTERVENTION

### 1. Prepare the warmer.

- Using the manual control setting, turn on the radiant warmer. *This prewarms the unit and eases the infant's transition from intrauterine to extrauterine life; it also prevents stressing of the immature infant.*

### 2. Assess and prepare the infant for the treatment.

- Wipe the blood and vernix from the newborn's head and body using the prewarmed towels. *Prewarmed towels prevent loss of the infant's body heat through evaporation.*

- Wrap the infant in the preheated blankets, transfer the infant to the mother (parents), and then return him or her to the warmer.

- Remove the blankets, and apply a diaper and a head cover (if agency protocol indicates). *This allows maximal infant exposure to the heating element.* The value of a head covering in maintaining infant body heat remains debatable.

- Apply the temperature sensor to the infant's abdomen between the umbilicus and the xiphoid process. *Thin subcutaneous tissue found over the ribcage may prevent recording of an accurate temperature.*

- Cover the temperature sensor with a reflective covering (if indicated in unit manual or institutional policy). *A reflective covering decreases functional interference of the sensor by overhead lights.*

- Turn the warmer control device to the automatic setting. *This permits the infant's body temperature to control the level of heating and prevents accidental overheating or erratic warming.*

### 3. Initiate the warming process.

- Adjust the temperature setting control to the desired goal temperature. This ranges from 35.1° C (97.0° F) to 37.0° C (98.6° F). *This prevents overheating.*

▶

▶ **Procedure 44–4 Applying an Infant Radiant Warmer** *CONTINUED*

- Turn the warmer on.

- **⚠** Set the temperature sensor alarm at the upper limit of the desired temperature range. *The alarm alerts the nurse if the infant's temperature exceeds upper limits of normal.*

### 4. Monitor the warming process.

- Check the infant's temperature sensor reading every 15 to 30 minutes (or as often as agency protocol dictates) until the infant's temperature reaches the desired level.

- Check the infant's axillary temperature every 2 to 4 hours (or according to agency protocol).

*This verifies the accuracy of the sensor probe and the effectiveness of the treatment.*

- Monitor the sensor probe site and surrounding skin for irritation or breakdown. *Early detection of skin damage facilitates early intervention.*

### 5. Terminate the warming process.

- When the infant's temperature reaches the desired level, dress the infant in a T-shirt, diaper, and head cover. Wrap the infant in two blankets, and transfer the infant from the warmer to an open crib.

- Check the infant's axillary temperature every 2 to 4 hours (or according to agency protocol). *This allows the nurse to determine the infant's ability to maintain body temperature without assistance.*

- If the infant's temperature drops below 36.1° C (97.0° F), return the infant to the warmer, remove clothing, and reinitiate the warming procedure by performing the steps above.

---

**EVALUATION FOCUS**

Temperature within acceptable range; infant's ability to maintain temperature after therapy is discontinued; vital signs other than temperature within baseline data (indicates absence of environmental stress).

**SAMPLE RECORDING**

| Date | Time | Notes |
|------|------|-------|
| 05/04/95 | 1032 | Baby Jones born by vaginal delivery. Initial temperature 96.2 F. Placed in preheated infant radiant warmer after cleaning and brief visit with parents. Temperature sensor applied to abdomen; equipment operating properly with increase noted in infant's temperature to 96.6 F after 15 minutes. No signs of distress. ———————————————————— Pearl Gunther, RN |

# Managing Clients with Hyperthermia and Hypothermia Blankets

| | |
|---|---|
| **PURPOSE** | • To increase or decrease the client's body temperature and prevent complications or extremes of temperatures |
| **ASSESSMENT FOCUS** | Vital signs as baseline data; skin condition and temperature; presence of shivering; neurologic status. |

## EQUIPMENT

- ☐ Two pairs of nonsterile gloves
- ☐ Basin of warm water, soap, washcloths, and towels (for client bath if needed)
- ☐ Hyperthermia/hypothermia control module (should come with rectal probe and blanket)
- ☐ Distilled water
- ☐ Plastic cover or thin sheet
- ☐ Lubricating jelly
- ☐ Tape
- ☐ Linen blanket (optional)

## INTERVENTION

### 1. Prepare the client.

- Don gloves.
- Bathe the client if necessary.
- Remove and discard the gloves.
- Apply towels to the extremities according to agency protocol.

### 2. Prepare the equipment.

- Connect the blanket pad to the modular unit, and inspect for adequate functioning.
- **⚠S** Inspect the pad and cords for frays or exposed wires.
- Screw (twist) the male tubing connectors of the coil blanket tubing into the inlet and outlet opening connectors on the modular unit.
- Check the solution level in the module, and fill with distilled water if necessary. *(The solution should be up to the fill line in order for the blanket temperature to be correct.)*
- Turn the modular unit on *to circulate the solution through the blanket.*

- Check for adequate filling of the coils throughout the blanket as the solution circulates throughout it. If you note leakage, obtain another blanket.
- Turn the client temperature control knob to the desired temperature, and determine whether the temperature gauge is functioning.
- Set the modular control knob or master switch to either the manual or automatic mode, and note the accuracy of the temperature settings.

**If using the automatic mode:**

- Insert the thermistor probe plug into the thermistor probe jack on modular unit.
- Check the automatic mode light to be sure it comes on.
- Set the machine to the desired temperature.
- Set the limits for the pad temperature.

**If using the manual mode:**

- Set the master temperature control knob to the desired temperature.

- Check the manual mode light to be sure it is operational.
- If the blanket is nondisposable, cover it with a plastic cover or thin sheet. If the blanket is disposable, cover it with a plastic covering to avoid excess soiling.

### 3. Apply the blanket to the client.

- Don clean gloves.
- Place the client on the blanket.
- Apply lubricating jelly to the rectal probe, insert the rectal probe 7 to 10 cm (3 to 4 in).
- Secure probe with tape. *The tape should prevent the probe from falling out.*
- Remove and discard the gloves.

### 4. Monitor the client closely.

- Take vital signs every 15 minutes for at least the first hour, every half-hour for the second hour, and every hour thereafter.
- Determine the client's neurologic status regularly as needed.
- Observe the skin for indications of burns, intactness, and color. *Heat and cold can cause burning.*

▶

► **Procedure 44–5  Managing Hyperthermia and Hypothermia Blankets** *CONTINUED*

- Determine any intolerance to the blanket. *Shivering may result from increased metabolic activity.*

**5. Maintain the therapy as required.**

- Remove and clean the rectal probe every 3 to 4 hours or when the client has a bowel movement. *When the probe is impacted with feces, the temperature reading can be distorted.*

**EVALUATION FOCUS**

| Vital signs; skin condition; presence of shivering. |
| --- |

**SAMPLE RECORDING**

| Date | Time | Notes |
| --- | --- | --- |
| 06/06/95 | 1035 | Hypothermia blanket applied. T 40 C, P 128, R 32, BP 90/40. Blanket set at 28 C. Rectal probe inserted. Skin intact, no abrasions. Hands and feet covered with towels. ———————————————————— Nancy Sun, SN |

# 44-6  Administering Hot Soaks and Sitz Baths

Before administering a hot soak or a sitz bath, determine (a) the type and temperature of the solution to be used; (b) the duration, frequency, and purpose of the soak, as indicated on the chart; and (c) agency protocol regarding the temperature and the length of time for soaks. Generally, a temperature of 40° to 43° C (105° to 110° F), as tolerated by the client, is indicated. For a hot soak, determine whether sterile technique is required.

**PURPOSES**
- To hasten suppuration, soften exudates, and enhance healing
- To apply medications to a designated area
- To clean a wound in which there is sloughing tissue or an exudate
- To promote circulation and enhance healing

**ASSESSMENT FOCUS**

Appearance of the affected area, e.g., redness, drainage (amount, color, consistency, odor), and swelling; any break in the skin; any discomfort experienced by the client; the client's mental status and ability to cooperate during the procedure; factors contraindicating heat therapy.

---

## EQUIPMENT

(Use sterile equipment and supplies for an open wound)
- Small basin, special arm or foot bath, or sitz tub or chair
- Specified solution at the correct temperature
- Thermometer
- Disposable and sterile gloves (if the client has any open areas on the skin)
- Moisture-resistant bag
- Towels
- Bath blanket
- Required dressing materials (e.g., gauze squares and roller gauze for an extremity soak, perineal pads and a T-binder for a perineal soak)

---

## INTERVENTION

### Hand or Foot Soak

**1. Prepare the soak.**

- Fill the container at least one-half full and test the temperature of the solution with a thermometer. *A temperature that is too high can cause burning and one that is too low will not produce the desired effect.*

- Pad the edge of the container with a towel. *Padding is necessary to prevent pressure on the body part that rests on the edge of the container.*

- Use sterile solution and a sterile thermometer if the client has an open wound.

**2. Prepare and assess the client.**

- Assist the client to a well-aligned, comfortable position; the position adopted will be maintained for 15 to 20 minutes. *This position helps prevent muscle strain.*

- Don disposable gloves as required, remove the dressings, and discard them in the bag. Assess the amount, color, odor, and consistency of the drainage on removed dressings.

- Inspect the appearance of the area to be soaked.

**3. Commence the soak.**

- Immerse the body part completely in the solution. *The entire affected area must be in contact with the solution.*

- If the soak is sterile, cover the open container with a sterile drape or the container wrapper. *Covering the open container helps prevent accidental contamination.*

- Place a large sheet or blanket over the soak. *This will help maintain the temperature of the solution.*

- Go to step 7.

### Sitz Bath

**4. Prepare the bath.**

- Fill the sitz bath with water at

▶ **Procedure 44–6 Administering Hot Soaks and Sitz Baths** CONTINUED

above 40° C (105° F) (The water level in a tub should be at the umbilicus.) The temperature of the water should feel comfortable to the inner aspect of the wrist.

- Pad the tub or chair with towels as required. *Padding prevents pressure on the sacrum or posterior aspects of the thighs.* When a disposable sitz bath on the toilet is used, provide a footstool. *This can prevent pressure on the back of the thighs.*

5. **Prepare the client.**

- Remove the gown, or fasten it above the waist.

- Don gloves if an open area or drainage is present.

- Remove the T-binder and perineal dressings, if present, and note the amount, color, odor, and consistency of any drainage.

- Assess the appearance of the area to be soaked for redness, swelling, odor, breaks in the skin, and drainage.

- Wrap the bath blanket around the client's shoulders and over the legs as needed. *Draping the client provides warmth and prevents chilling.*

6. **Begin the sitz bath.**

- Assist the client into the bath, and provide support for the client as needed.

- Leave a signal light within reach. Stay with the client if warranted, and terminate the bath as necessary. *Some clients may become faint or dizzy and need to be able to call a nurse or have the nurse remain with them.*

7. **Give the client the following instructions:**

- Remain in position, and call the nurse if any discomfort is felt or an untoward reaction occurs.

8. **Monitor the client.**

**Soak**

- Assess the client and test the temperature of the solution at least once during the soak. Assess for discomfort, need for additional support, and any reactions to the soak.

- If the solution has cooled, remove the body part, empty the solution, add newly heated solution, and reimmerse the body part.

**Sitz Bath**

- Assess the client during the bath in terms of discomfort, color, and pulse rate. *An accelerated pulse or extreme pallor may precede fainting.*

- Immediately report any unexpected or adverse responses to the nurse in charge.

- Test the temperature of the solution at least once during the bath. Adjust the temperature as needed.

9. **Discontinue the soak or bath.**

- At completion of a *soak*, remove the body part from the basin, and dry it thoroughly and carefully. If the soak was sterile, use a sterile towel for drying, and wear sterile gloves. *Drying prevents skin maceration.*

- Assess the appearance of the affected area carefully, and reapply a dressing if required.
  *or*
- At the completion of a *sitz bath*, assist the client out of the sitz bath, and dry the area with a towel.

- Assess the perineal area, and reapply dressings and garments as required.

10. **Document all relevant information.**

- Record the soak or sitz bath, including the duration, temperature, and type of solution. Include all assessments.

| EVALUATION FOCUS | Redness, drainage, swelling of the affected area; any discomfort; extent of healing. |
|---|---|

**SAMPLE RECORDING**

| Date | Time | Notes |
|---|---|---|
| 12/05/95 | 0900 | 43 C saline soak to (L) index finger × 20 min. 2 × 2 gauze saturated with purulent exudate. Finger measures 7 cm (down 1 cm from previous measurement) but continues to be red in color. ——— Toby N. Zacharias, NS |

**44-7** **Applying an Ice Bag, Ice Collar, Ice Glove, or Disposable Cold Pack**

Before applying dry cold, verify the order for the cold application, including when, where, why, and for how long the cold is to be applied.

**PURPOSES**
- To relieve headaches caused by vasodilation
- To prevent swelling of tissues immediately following an injury or surgery
- To prevent, decrease, or terminate bleeding following an injury or surgery
- To reduce joint pain from the pressure of accumulated fluid

**ASSESSMENT FOCUS**

Evidence of circulatory deficiencies at the area of application (e.g., bluish purplish color, feeling of cold, decreased sensation or numbness); other factors contraindicating cold therapy; any discomfort experienced by the client; swelling; client's ability to cooperate during the procedure.

## EQUIPMENT
- Ice bag, collar, glove, or cold pack
- Ice chips
- Protective covering
- Roller gauze, a binder or a towel, and tape

## INTERVENTION

**1. Prepare and assess the client.**

- Assist the client to a comfortable position, and support the body part requiring the application.

- Expose only the area to be treated, and provide warmth to avoid chilling. Privacy may or may not be necessary, depending on the location of the application and the client's wishes.

- Assess the area to which the cold will be applied. See the Assessment Focus above.

**Ice Bag, Collar, or Glove**

**2. Fill and cover the device.**

- Fill the device one-half to two-thirds full of crushed ice. *Partial filling makes the device more pliable so that it can be molded to a body part.*

- Remove excess air by bending or twisting the device. *Air inflates the device so that it cannot be molded to the body part.*

- Insert the stopper securely into an ice bag or collar, or tie a knot

at the open end of a glove. *This prevents leakage of fluid when the ice melts.*

- Hold the device upside down, and check it for leaks.

- Cover the device with a soft cloth cover, if it is not already equipped with one. *The cover absorbs moisture that condenses on the outside of the device. It is also more comfortable for the client.*

**3. Apply the cold device.**

- Apply the device for the time specified. The device is usually applied for no longer than 30 minutes because of the rebound phenomenon.

- Hold it in place with roller gauze, a binder, or a towel. Secure with tape as necessary.

**Disposable Cold Pack**

**4. Initiate the cooling process.**

- Strike, squeeze, or knead the cold pack according to the manufacturer's instructions. *The action*

*activates the chemical reaction that produces the cold.*

- Cover with a soft cloth cover, if the pack does not have a cover. Most commercially prepared cold packs have soft outer coverings to permit application directly to the body part.

**All Applications**

**5. Instruct the client as follows:**

- Remain in position for the duration of the treatment.

- Call the nurse if discomfort is felt.

**6. Monitor the client during the application.**

- Assess the client in terms of comfort and skin reaction (e.g., pallor, mottled appearance) as frequently as necessary for the client's safety, e.g., every 5 to 10 minutes. Factors such as previous responses to applications and the client's ability to report any problems need to be considered.

▶

▶ **Procedure 44–7 Applying Dry Cold** *CONTINUED*

- Report untoward reactions to the nurse in charge, and remove the application.

**7. Remove the application.**

- Remove the cold application at the designated time. *This avoids*

🔺 *the harmful effects of prolonged cold.*

**8. Document all relevant information.**

- At the time of application, document the cold application, its

purpose, the method used, the site, and nursing assessments.

- After removal, record the time and all nursing assessments.

| | |
|---|---|
| **EVALUATION FOCUS** | Presence or absence of signs of impaired blood circulation to the area; appearance of affected tissues (e.g., any swelling); any discomfort experienced by the client. |

**SAMPLE RECORDING**

| Date | Time | Notes |
|---|---|---|
| 08/10/95 | 1145 | Disposable ice pack applied to left ankle as ordered. Ankle very swollen and painful especially with weight-bearing. Skin pink. Popliteal and pedal pulses strong. —————————————————————— Roberta Victor, RN |
| | 1205 | Ice pack removed. Skin pale and slightly mottled. Ankle remains swollen. —————————————————————— Roberta Victor, RN |

**Administering a Cooling Sponge Bath**

Before administering a cooling sponge bath, determine agency protocol. Some agencies recommend sponging the entire body. To avoid chilling, others recommend sponging only the face, arms, legs, back, and buttocks (*not* the chest and abdomen).

**PURPOSE**

• To reduce a client's fever by promoting body heat loss through conduction and vaporization

**ASSESSMENT FOCUS**

> Body temperature, pulse, respirations for baseline data; other signs of fever (e.g., skin warmth, flushing, complaints of feeling hot or chilly, diaphoresis, irritability, restlessness, general malaise, or delirium).

## EQUIPMENT

- ☐ Thermometer to measure the client's temperature
- ☐ Bath blanket
- ☐ Several washcloths and bath towels (fewer are needed if ice bags or cold packs are used)
- ☐ Basin for the solution
- ☐ Bath thermometer
- ☐ Solution at the correct temperature (water or equal portions of 70% alcohol and water)
- ☐ Ice bag or cold pack (optional)
- ☐ Fan (optional)

## INTERVENTION

**1. Obtain all relevant baseline data.**

• If not already recorded prior to the sponge bath, measure the client's body temperature, pulse, and respirations to provide comparative baseline data.

• Assess the client for other signs of fever (see the Assessment Focus above).

**2. Prepare the client.**

• Remove the gown, and assist the client to a comfortable supine position.

• Place a bath blanket over the client.

• If ice bags or cold packs are not used, place bath towels under each axilla and shoulder. *Bath towels protect the lower bed sheet from getting wet.*

**3. Sponge the face.**

• Sponge the client's face with plain water only, and dry it.

• Apply an ice bag or cold pack to the head for comfort.

**4. Place cold applications in the axillae and groins.**

• Wet four washcloths; wring them out so that they are very damp but not dripping. *Washcloths need to be as moist as possible to be effective.*

• Place washcloths in the axillae and groins.
  *or*
  Place ice bags or cold packs in these areas. *The axillae and groins contain large superficial blood vessels, which aid the transfer of heat.*

• Leave washcloths in place for about 5 minutes, or until they feel warm. Rewet and replace them as required during the bath. *Washcloths warm up relatively quickly in such vascular areas.*

**5. Sponge the arms and legs.**

• Place a bath towel under one arm and sponge the arm *slowly* and *gently* for about 5 minutes or as tolerated by the client. *Slow, gen-*tle motions are indicated because firm rubbing motions increase tissue metabolism and heat production. Cool sponges given rapidly or for a short period of time tend to increase the body's heat production mechanisms by causing shivering.*

*or*

Place a saturated towel over the extremity, and rewet it as necessary. Give the client enough time to adjust to the initial reaction of chilliness and for the body to cool.

• Dry the arm, using a patting motion rather than a rubbing motion.

• Repeat the above steps for the other arm and the legs.

• When sponging the extremities, hold the washcloth briefly over the wrists and ankles. *The blood circulation is close to the skin surface in the wrists and ankles.*

**6. Reassess the client's vital signs after 15 minutes.**

▶ **Procedure 44–8 Administering a Cooling Sponge Bath** CONTINUED

---

• Compare findings with data taken before the bath. *The vital signs are checked to evaluate the effectiveness of the sponge bath.* Proceed with the bath if the temperature is above 37.7° C (100° F); discontinue if the temperature is below 37.7° C (100° F), or if the pulse rate is significantly increased and remains so after 5 minutes.

**7. (Optional) Sponge the chest and abdomen.**

• Sponge these areas for 3 to 5 minutes and pat them dry.

**8. Sponge the back and buttocks.**

• Sponge the back and buttocks for 3 to 5 minutes.

• Pat these areas dry.

**9. Remove the cold applications from the axillae and groins.**

**10. Reassess vital signs.**

**11. Document assessments, including the vital signs, as well as the type of sponge bath given.**

---

**VARIATION: Pediatric Bathing**

Cooling baths for children can be given in the tub, or the bed or crib.

Immersion of a child in a tepid tub bath for 20 to 30 minutes is a simple and effective method to reduce an elevated temperature.

**Tub**

• While the child is in the tub, firmly support the child's head and shoulders and gently squeeze water over the back and chest or gently spray water from a sprayer over the body.

• To make a tub bath more effective, lay a small infant or older child down in the water and support the head on your arm or a padded support. Small children, however, may resist any effort to place them in a horizontal position.

• For conscious children, use a floating toy or other distraction during the bath.

• Always stay with the child in a tub for safety reasons.

• Discontinue the cooling bath if there is evidence of chilling. The process of shivering generates additional heat and defeats the purpose of the bath and chilling causes vasoconstriction so that

minimal blood is carried to the skin surface.

• Dry and dress the child in lightweight clothing or only a diaper and cover the child with a light cotton blanket.

• Retake the temperature 30 minutes after removal from the tub and repeat measurement as often as indicated.

**Bed or Crib Sponge**

• Place the undressed child on an absorbent towel.

• Follow the steps above for a sponge bath, or use the following towel method:

 a. Apply a cool cloth or icebag to the forehead.

 b. Wrap each extremity in a towel moistened with tepid water.

 c. Place one towel under the back and another over the neck and torso.

 d. Change the towels as they warm.

 e. Continue the procedure for about 30 minutes.

---

| EVALUATION FOCUS | Vital signs and changes in baseline assessments. |
|---|---|

**SAMPLE RECORDING**

| Date | Time | Notes |
|---|---|---|
| 09/18/95 | 1645 | T40.2, P94, R18 and shallow. c/o "burning up," face flushed, diaphoretic. and states feels "miserable and muscles aching." Dr. Kirkpatrick notified. Cooling sponge bath given. ——————————— Jennifer Newton, RN |
| | 1700 | T39.4, P90, R16. Face less flushed. States "feels cooler." ——————————————————— Jennifer Newton, RN |
| | 1715 | T38.8, P90, R14. ——————————— Jennifer Newton, RN |

# 44-9  Cleaning a Drain Site and Shortening a Penrose Drain

Before cleaning a drain site and shortening a Penrose drain, determine (a) agency protocol about who may shorten drains; (b) that the drain is to be shortened and the length it is to be shortened, e.g., 2.5 cm (1 in); (c) whether the drain has been shortened previously (drains that have not been shortened previously are often attached to the skin by a suture, which must be removed before shortening the drain); (d) the location of the drain; and (e) the type and amount of discharge previously recorded and previous assessments of the appearance of the wound, for baseline data.

**PURPOSES**

**Cleaning a Drain Site**
- To remove any discharge from the skin, thereby reducing the danger of skin irritation
- To reduce the number of microorganisms present and therefore decrease the possibility of infection

**Shortening a Drain**
- To decrease the length of the drain a designated amount, thereby encouraging healing of the wound from the inside toward the outside

**ASSESSMENT FOCUS**

> See Procedure 44–2 in *Fundamentals of Nursing*.

## EQUIPMENT

- Moistureproof bag
- Mask for the nurse and one for the client, if necessary
- Disposable gloves
- Sterile gloves
- Sterile dressing equipment, including
  - Two pairs of forceps, including at least one hemostat
- Sterile cotton-tipped applicators
- Sterile dressing materials sufficient to cover the surgical incision and the drain site (at least two 4 × 4 gauzes are usually needed to dress the drain site, more if drainage is copious; a sterile precut gauze is needed to apply first around the drain site)
- Sterile suture scissors (if the drain has *not* been shortened previously)
- Sterile scissors
- Sterile safety pin (add this to the sterile dressing set)
- Tape, tie tapes, or other binding supplies

## INTERVENTION

**1. Verify the physician's order.**

Ⓢ • Confirm that the drain is to be shortened by the nurse and the length it is to be shortened, e.g., 2.5 cm (1 in).

**2. Prepare the client.**

- Inform the client that the drain is to be shortened and that this procedure should not be painful.

- Explain that there may be a pulling sensation for a few seconds when the drain is being drawn out before it is shortened.

- Position the client as for a dressing change.

**3. Remove dressings, and clean the incision.**

- See Procedure 44–2 in *Fundamentals of Nursing. The incision is cleaned first because it is considered cleaner than the drain site. Moist drainage facilitates the growth of resident skin bacteria around the drain.*

**4. Clean and assess the drain site.**

- Clean the skin around the drain site by swabbing in half or full circles from around the drain site outward, using separate swabs for each wipe (Figure 44–14). You may hold forceps in the nondominant hand to hold the drain erect while cleaning around it. Clean as many times as necessary to remove the drainage.

- Assess the amount and character of drainage, including odor, thickness, and color.

▶

▶ **Procedure 44–9 Shortening a Penrose Drain** *CONTINUED*

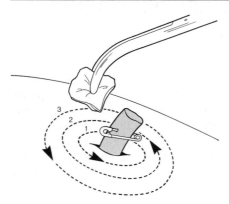

**FIGURE 44–14** Cleaning the skin around a drain site.

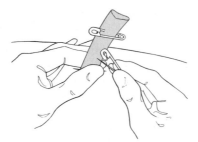

**FIGURE 44–15** Pinning a drain.

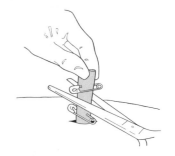

**FIGURE 44–16** Shortening a drain.

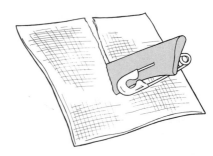

**FIGURE 44–17** Precut gauze in place around a drain.

### 5. Shorten the drain.

- If the drain has *not* been shortened before, cut and remove the suture. See Procedure 44–12. *The drain is sutured to the skin during surgery to keep it from slipping into the body cavity.*

- With a hemostat, firmly grasp the drain by its full width at the level of the skin, and pull the drain out the required length. *Grasping the full width of the drain ensures even traction.*

- Wearing sterile gloves, insert the sterile safety pin through the base of the drain as close to the skin as possible by holding the drain tightly against the skin edge and inserting the pin above your fingers (Figure 44–15). *The pin keeps the drain from falling back into the incision. Holding the drain securely in place at the skin level and inserting the pin above the fingers prevents the nurse from*

*pulling the drain further out or pricking the client during this step.*

- With the sterile scissors, cut off the excess drain so that about 2.5 cm (1 in) remains above the skin (Figure 44–16). Discard the excess in the waste bag.

### 6. Apply dressings to the drain site and the incision.

- Place a precut 4 × 4 gauze snugly around the drain (Figure 44–17), or open a 4 × 4 gauze to 4 × 8, fold it lengthwise to 2 × 8, and place the 2 × 8 around the drain so that the ends overlap. *This dressing absorbs the drainage and helps prevent it from excoriating the skin. Using precut gauze or folding it as described, instead of cutting the gauze, prevents any threads from coming loose and getting into the wound, where they could cause inflammation and provide a site for infection.*

- Apply the sterile dressings one at a time, using sterile gloved hands or sterile forceps. Take care that

the dressings do not slide off and become contaminated. Place the bulk of the dressings over the drain area and below the drain, depending on the client's usual position. *Layers of dressings are placed for best absorption of drainage, which flows by gravity.*

- Apply the final surgipad by hand; remove gloves, and dispose of them; and secure the dressing with tape or ties.

### 7. Document the procedure and nursing assessments.

| EVALUATION FOCUS | Amount of drainage and its color, clarity, thickness, and odor; degree of inflammation; pain at the incision or drain site. |
| --- | --- |

**SAMPLE RECORDING**

| Date | Time | Notes |
| --- | --- | --- |
| 12/05/95 | 1025 | Penrose drain shortened 2.5 cm. Three 4 × 4 gauzes saturated with brownish yellow drainage. Dry dressings × 4 applied. Skin intact; no redness or irritation. ———————————————— Maria L. Antonio, RN |

# Establishing and Maintaining a Closed Wound Drainage System

**PURPOSES**
- To hasten the healing process by draining excess exudate, which interferes with the formation of granulation tissue in a wound
- To maintain the patency of the wound suction

**ASSESSMENT FOCUS**

The amount, color, consistency, clarity, and odor of the drainage; discomfort around the area of the drain; clinical signs of infection (e.g., elevated body temperature).

## EQUIPMENT

- Disposable gloves
- Drainage receptacle, e.g., solution basin
- Calibrated pitcher

## INTERVENTION

**1. Establish suction if it has not been already initiated.**

- Place the evacuator bag on a solid, flat surface and don disposable gloves.
- Open the drainage plug on top of the bag, without contaminating the bag.
- Compress the bag; while it is compressed, close the drainage plug to retain the vacuum (Figure 44–18).

**2. Empty the evacuator bag.**

- When the drainage fluid reaches

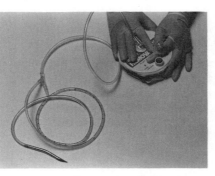

**FIGURE 44–18** Compressing the Hemovac.

the line marked "Full," don disposable gloves, and open the drainage plug.

- Invert the bag, and empty it into the collecting receptacle.
- Reestablish suction as in step 1.
- Using the calibrated pitcher, measure the amount of drainage, and note its characteristics.

**3. Document all relevant information.**

- Record the emptying of the evacuator bag and nursing assessments on the nursing progress notes.
- Record the amount and type of drainage on the intake and output record.

**EVALUATION FOCUS**

Amount of drainage and its color, clarity, consistency, and odor; increased or decreased discomfort; clinical signs of infection.

**SAMPLE RECORDING**

| Date | Time | Notes |
|------|------|-------|
| 09/09/95 | 1030 | Hemovac emptied 20 ml dark thick red drainage. Vacuum re-established. Tubing patent and suction functioning. Drain site red, small amount of thick, white discharge. Specimen to lab for culture. No odor. No discomfort. Dry dressing applied. ——————————————— Sarah J. Woo, RN |

## 44-11 Applying Moist Sterile Compresses

**PURPOSES**

**Warm Applications**
- To enhance healing
- To promote comfort
- To relieve muscle spasm or pain
- To promote reabsorption in tissues or joints

**Cold Applications**
- To prevent or minimize bleeding
- To reduce inflammation or prevent swelling
- To anesthetize tissues and reduce pain temporarily

**ASSESSMENT FOCUS**

Skin integrity; size, appearance, and type of wound or injury; redness and inflammation; swelling; abrasions; character and amount of drainage; discomfort; vital signs; neurovascular integrity (circulation, sensation, and motion) of affected area.

---

## EQUIPMENT

(Use sterile equipment and supplies for an open wound)

**Compress:**
- Container for the solution
- Solution at the strength and temperature specified by the physician or the agency
- Thermometer
- Petrolatum jelly
- Gauze squares
- Insulating towel
- Plastic or plastic underpad
- Hot water bottle or aquathermia pad (optional)
  *or*
- Ice bag (optional)

- Ties, e.g., roller gauze
- Nonsterile gloves
- Sterile gloves, forceps, and cotton applicator sticks (if compress must be sterile)

**Moist pack:**
- Flannel pieces or towel packs
- Hot-pack machine for heating the packs
  *or*
- Basin of water with some ice chips
- Insulating material, e.g., flannel or towels

- Plastic
- Hot water bottle (optional)
  *or*
- Ice bag (optional)
- Thermometer if a specific temperature is ordered for the pack
- Petrolatum jelly
- Sterile gloves or forceps (if sterility must be maintained)

---

## INTERVENTION

### 1. Prepare the client.

- Assist the client to a comfortable position.

- Expose the area for the compress or pack.

- Provide support for the body part requiring the compress or pack.

- Don nonsterile gloves, and remove the wound dressing, if present. A dry, sterile dressing is often placed over open wounds between applications of moist heat or cold.

### 2. Moisten the compress or pack.

- Place the gauze in the solution.
  *or*
- Heat the flannel or towel in a steamer, or chill it in the basin of water and ice.

### 3. Protect surrounding skin as indicated.

- With a cotton swab or an applicator stick, apply petrolatum jelly to the skin surrounding the wound, not on the wound or open areas of the skin. *Petroleum*

jelly *protects the skin from possible burns, maceration, and irritating effects of some solutions.*

### 4. Apply the moist heat.

- Wring out the gauze compress so that the solution does not drip from it. For a sterile compress, use sterile forceps or sterile gloves to wring out the gauze.

- Apply the gauze lightly and gradually to the designated area and, if tolerated by the client, mold the compress close to the body. Pack the gauze snugly against all

▶ **Procedure 44–11** *CONTINUED*

wound surfaces. *Air is a poor conductor of cold or heat, and molding excludes air.*

*or*

- Wring out the flannel (for a sterile pack, use sterile gloves).
- Apply the flannel to the body area, molding it closely to the body part.

**5. Immediately insulate and secure the application.**

- Cover the gauze or flannel quickly with a dry towel and a piece of plastic. *This step helps maintain the temperature of the application and thus its effectiveness.*
- Secure the compress or pack in place with gauze ties or tape.

- Optional: Apply a hot water bottle or aquathermia pad or ice bag over the plastic to maintain the heat or cold.

**6. Monitor the client.**

- Assess the client for discomfort at 5- to 10-minute intervals. If the client feels any discomfort, assess the area for erythema, numbness, maceration, or blistering.
- For applications to large areas of the body, note any change in the pulse, respirations, and blood pressure.
- In the event of unexpected reactions, terminate the treatment and report to the nurse in charge.

**7. Remove the compress or pack at the specified time.**

- Compresses and packs with external heat or cold usually retain their temperature anywhere from 15 to 30 minutes. Without external heat or cold, they need to be changed every 5 minutes.
- Apply a sterile dressing if one is required.

**8. Document relevant information.**

- Document the procedure, the time, and the type and strength of the solution.
- Record assessments, including the appearance of the wound and surrounding skin area.

---

**EVALUATION FOCUS**

Level of comfort; redness and inflammation; swelling; character, quality, and amount of discharge; appearance of wound and degree of healing; neurovascular integrity (circulation, sensation, and motion) of affected area; vital signs.

**SAMPLE RECORDING**

| Date | Time | Notes |
|------|------|-------|
| 5/12/95 | 0910 | Sterile normal saline compress with K-Matic 37.7 C applied to 2.5 cm open leg wound. Pink tissue surrounding wound. 1 cm diameter serosanguineous discharge on dressing. No discomfort voiced. ———————————————————— Olga R. Resnicoff, SN |
| 5/12/95 | 0940 | Compress removed. No further discharge. Wound packed with gauze and sterile dry dressing applied. ———————— Olga R. Resnicoff, SN |

# 44-12 Removing Skin Sutures

Before removing skin sutures, verify (a) the orders for suture removal (many times only *alternate* interrupted sutures are removed one day, and the remaining sutures are removed a day or two later); and (b) whether a dressing is to be applied following the suture removal. Some physicians prefer no dressing; others prefer a small, light gauze dressing to prevent friction by clothing.

| **ASSESSMENT FOCUS** | Appearance of suture line; factors contraindicating suture removal (e.g., nonuniformity of closure, inflammation, presence of drainage). |
|---|---|

## EQUIPMENT

- Moistureproof bag
- Sterile gloves
- Nonsterile gloves
- Sterile dressing equipment (see Procedure 44–2 in *Fundamentals of Nursing*), including:
  - Sterile suture scissors
  - Sterile butterfly tape (optional)
- Light sterile gauze pad
- Tape (if a dressing is to be applied)

## INTERVENTION

### 1. Prepare the client.

- Inform the client that suture removal may produce slight discomfort, such as a pulling or stinging sensation, but should not be painful.

### 2. Remove dressings, and clean the incision.

- See Procedure 44–2 in *Fundamentals of Nursing*.

- Don sterile gloves.

- Clean the suture line with an antimicrobial solution before and after suture removal. *This is generally done as a prophylactic measure to prevent infection.*

### 3. Remove the sutures.

**Plain Interrupted Sutures**

- Grasp the suture at the knot with a pair of forceps.

- Place the curved tip of the suture scissors under the suture as close to the skin as possible, either on the side opposite the knot (Figure 44–19) or directly under the knot. Cut the suture. *Sutures are cut as close to the skin as possible on one side of the visible part because the suture ma-*

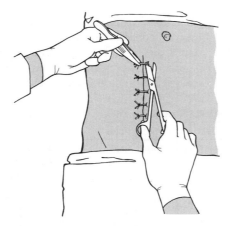

**FIGURE 44–19** Removing a plain interrupted skin suture.

*terial that is visible to the eye is in contact with resident bacteria of the skin and must not be pulled beneath the skin during removal. Suture material that is beneath the skin is considered free from bacteria.*

- With the forceps, pull the suture out in one piece. Inspect the suture carefully to make sure that all suture material is removed. *Suture material left beneath the skin acts as a foreign body and causes inflammation.*

- Discard the suture onto a piece of sterile gauze or into the moistureproof bag, being careful not to contaminate the forceps tips. Sometimes the suture sticks to the forceps and needs to be removed by wiping the tips on a sterile gauze.

- Continue to remove *alternate* sutures, i.e., the third, fifth, seventh, and so forth. *Alternate sutures are removed first so that remaining sutures keep the skin edges in close approximation and prevent any dehiscence from becoming large.*

- If no dehiscence occurs, remove the remaining sutures. If dehiscence does occur, do not remove the remaining sutures, and report the dehiscence to the nurse in charge.

- If a little wound dehiscence occurs, apply a sterile butterfly tape over the gap:

  **a.** Attach the tape to one side of the incision.

  **b.** Press the wound edges together.

▶ **Procedure 44–12** *CONTINUED*

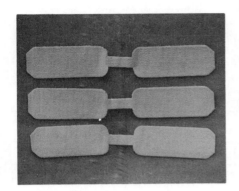

**FIGURE 44–20**  Butterfly tapes.

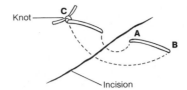

**FIGURE 44–21**  Mattress interrupted sutures.

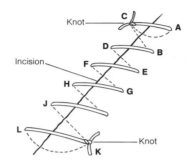

**FIGURE 44–22**  Plain continuous sutures.

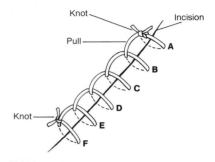

**FIGURE 44–23**  Blanket continuous sutures.

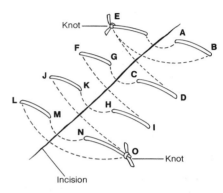

**FIGURE 44–24**  Mattress continuous sutures.

**c.** Attach the tape to the other side of the incision (Figure 44–20). *The butterfly tape holds the wound edges as close together as possible and promotes healing.*

- If a large dehiscence occurs, cover the wound with sterile gauze, and report the problem immediately to the nurse in charge or physician.

**Mattress Interrupted Sutures**

- When possible, cut the visible part of the suture close to the skin at *A* and *B* in Figure 44–21, opposite the knot, and remove this small visible piece. Discard it as described above. In some sutures, the visible part opposite the knot may be so small that it can be cut only once.

- Grasp the knot (*C*) with forceps. Remove the remainder of the suture beneath the skin by pulling out in the direction of the knot.

**Plain Continuous Sutures**

- Cut the thread of the first suture opposite the knot at *A* in Figure 44–22. Then cut the thread of the second suture on the same side at *B*.

- Grasp the knot (*C*) with the forceps, and pull. This removes the first stitch and the piece of thread beneath the skin, which is attached to the second stitch. Discard the suture.

- Cut off the visible part of the second suture at *D*, and discard it.

- Grasp the suture at *E*, and pull out the underlying loop between *D* and *E*.

- Cut the visible part at *F*, and remove it.

- Repeat the above two steps at *G* through *J*, until the last knot is reached. Note that after the first stitch is removed, each thread is cut down the same side, below the original knot.

- Cut the last suture at *L*, and pull out the last suture at *K*.

**Blanket Continuous Sutures**

- Cut the threads that are opposite the looped blanket edge; i.e., cut at *A* through *F* in Figure 44–23.

- Pull each stitch out at the looped edge.

**Mattress Continuous Sutures**

- Cut the visible suture at both skin edges opposite the knot (at *A* and *B* in Figure 44–24) and the next suture opposite the knot (at *C* and *D*). Remove and discard the visible portions as described above.

- Pull the first suture out by the knot at *E*.

- Lift the second suture between *F* and *G* to pull out the underlying suture between *G* and *C*. Cut off the visible part at *F* as close to the skin edge as possible.

- Go to the opposite side between *H* and *I*. Lift out the suture between *F* and *I*, and cut off all the visible part close to the skin at *H*.

- Lift the suture between *J* and *K* to pull out the suture between *H* and *K*, and cut the suture close to the skin at *J*.

- Repeat the above 2 steps, working from side to side of the incision, until the last suture is reached.

- Cut the visible suture opposite the knot at *L* and *M*. Pull out all remaining pieces of suture at *O*.

**5. Clean and cover the incision.**

▶

▶ **Procedure 44–12 Removing Skin Sutures** *CONTINUED*

- Clean the incision again with antimicrobial solution.
- Apply a small, light, sterile gauze dressing if any small dehiscence has occurred or if this is agency practice.

**6. Instruct the client about follow-up wound care.**

- Generally, if a wound is dry and healing well, the person can take showers in a day or two.

- Instruct the client to contact the physician if wound discharge appears.

**7. Document the suture removal and assessment data on the appropriate records.**

**EVALUATION FOCUS**

Status of suture line; any wound separation or discharge.

**SAMPLE RECORDING**

| Date | Time | Notes |
|------|------|-------|
| 12/05/95 | 1105 | Abdominal wound sutures removed. Wound dry, edges approximated closely. No signs of inflammation or dehiscence. Gauze dressing applied. — Gwen E. Owens, SN |

**45**

# Perioperative
# Nursing

## PROCEDURES

# 45-1 Preparing the Operative Site

Before commencing the surgical skin preparation, determine the surgeon's order, relevant protocols, and recorded allergies to any solutions used in the skin preparation.

**PURPOSE**

- To reduce the risks of postoperative wound infection by removing soil and transient microbes from the skin, reducing the resident microbial count to subpathogenic levels in a short time and with the least amount of tissue irritation, inhibiting rapid rebound growth of microbes

**ASSESSMENT FOCUS**

Presence of growths, moles, rashes, pustules, irritations, exudate, abrasions, bruises, or broken or ischemic areas.

## EQUIPMENT

- Adequate lighting for clear visibility of the hair on the skin
- Bath blanket

### Depilatory

- Cream hair remover with or without applicator
- Washcloth
- Gauze squares

- Lukewarm water

### Clipping

- Electric clippers with sharp heads and unbroken teeth
- Scissors for long hair, if needed
- Antimicrobial solution and applicators, if needed

### Wet Shave

- Disposable gloves
- Skin preparation set containing a disposable razor, compartmentalized basin for solutions, moistureproof drape, soap solution, sponges, and cotton-tipped applicators
- Warm water

## INTERVENTION

### 1. Drape the client appropriately.

- Expose only the area to be prepared. If using clippers or a razor, expose only small areas at a time. You will clip or shave about 15 cm (6 in) at a time.

### 2. If a depilatory is to be used, test the client's reaction to it.
*Some people may experience irritation or an allergic reaction, even after prior use without an adverse effect.*

- Apply a small amount of the depilatory on a small part of the area where hair is to be removed. Use an area at the periphery of the skin prep area or area advised by the agency policy.

- Apply the cream to the test area smoothly and thickly. Do not rub it in.

- Leave the cream on for the specified time.

- Remove the depilatory by rinsing the area thoroughly with lukewarm water and a washcloth. Do not use soap.

- Pat, rather than rub, the area dry with gauze squares.

- Wait for 24 hours, and assess the client's skin for redness or other responses.

### 3. Remove hair.

#### Depilatory

- If the client's skin appears normal after the skin test, apply the depilatory.

  a. Apply the depilatory as described above, and leave it in place for the *minimum* time specified by the manufacturer.

  b. Check a small area. If hair does not wipe off easily, wait a few minutes and check

again, but do not leave the cream on longer than the *maximum* time recommended by the manufacturer.

  c. Remove all the depilatory as described in step 2, and pat the area dry.

#### Clipping

- Make sure the area is dry.

- Remove hair with clippers; do not apply pressure. *Pressure can cause abrasions, particularly over bony prominences.*

- Move the drape, and repeat the above steps until the entire area to be prepared is clipped.

- If applying antimicrobial solution, follow step 4.

#### Wet Shave

- Don disposable gloves.

- Place the moistureproof towel under the area to be prepared.

▶ **Procedure 45–1** *CONTINUED*

- Lather the skin well with the soap solution. *Lathering makes the hair softer and easier to remove.*

- Stretch the skin taut, and hold the razor at about a 45° angle to the skin.

- Shave in the direction in which the hair grows. Use short strokes, and rinse the razor frequently. *Rinsing removes hairs and lather that can obstruct the blade.*

- Wipe excess hair off the skin with the sponges.

- Move the drape, and repeat the above steps until the entire area to be prepared is shaved.

**4. Clean and disinfect the surgical area according to agency practice.**

- This may be done in the operating room.

- Clean any body crevices, such as the umbilicus, nails, and ear canals, with applicators and solutions. Dry with swabs.

- If an antimicrobial solution is used, apply to the area immediately after it is clipped. Leave it for the designated time, then dry the area with clean swabs. Agency policy will guide you on whether to use an antimicrobial solution and, if so, which to use and how long to leave it on.

**5. Inspect the skin after hair removal.**

- Closely observe the skin for reddened or broken areas.

- Report to the nurse in charge any skin lesions.

**6. Dispose of used equipment appropriately.**

🅢 • Dispose of razor blade, if used, according to agency policy to prevent injury to others.

- Discard disposable supplies.

**7. Document all relevant information.**

- Record the procedure, area prepared, and status of skin in the skin preparation area.

---

**EVALUATION FOCUS**

| Presence of hairs on operative area; see also Assessment Focus. |
| --- |

**SAMPLE RECORDING**

| Date | Time | Notes |
| --- | --- | --- |
| 12/05/95 | 0830 | Area clipped on left lower extremity. Skin intact. Appeared tense. Stated: "I hope the scar won't show much." ———————— Eunice L. Lentz, NS |

# 45-2 Applying Antiemboli Stockings

Before applying antiemboli stockings, determine any potential or present circulatory problems and the surgeon's orders involving the lower extremities.

**PURPOSES**

- To improve arterial blood circulation to the legs and feet
- To improve venous blood circulation from the legs and feet
- To reduce or prevent edema of the legs or feet

**ASSESSMENT FOCUS**

Blood circulation to and from the feet and legs.

## EQUIPMENT

- ☐ Size chart
- ☐ Correct size of elastic stockings

## INTERVENTION

### 1. Select an appropriate time to apply the stockings.

- Apply stockings in the morning, if possible, before the client arises. *In sitting and standing positions, the veins can become distended, and edema occurs; the stockings should be applied before this happens.*

- Remove the stockings and wash the legs and feet daily. Most protocols suggest removing the stockings for a period of 30 minutes and replacing them 2–3 times a day.

- Assist the client who has been ambulating to lie down and elevate the legs for 15 to 30 minutes before applying the stockings. *This facilitates venous return and reduces swelling.*

### 2. Apply the elastic stocking to the foot.

- Assist the client to a lying position in bed.

- Dust the ankle with talcum powder, and ask the client to point the toes. *These measures ease application.*

- Turn the stocking inside out by inserting your hand into the stocking from the top and grab-

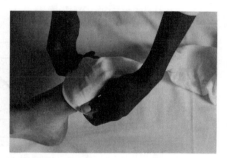

**FIGURE 45–1** Applying the inverted stocking over the client's toes.

bing the heel pocket from the inside. The foot portion should now be inside the stocking leg.

- Remove your hand, and, with the heel pocket downward, hook your index and middle fingers of both hands into the foot section.

- Face the client, and slip the foot portion of the stocking over the client's foot, toes, and heel (Figure 45–1). As you move up the foot, stretch the stocking sideways.

- Support the client's ankle with one hand while using the other hand to pull the heel pocket under the heel.

- Center the heel in the pocket.

### 3. Apply the remaining inverted portion of the stocking.

- Gather the remaining portion of the stocking up to the toes, and pull only this part over the heel. With the foot already covered, the remainder of the stocking should slide easily over it.

- At the ankle, grasp the gathered portion between your index and middle fingers, and pull the stocking up the leg to the knee. You may need to support the ankle with one hand and use the other hand to stretch the stocking and distribute it evenly.

- For *thigh-* or *waist-length stockings*, ask the client to straighten the leg while stretching the rest of the stocking over the knee.

- Ask the client to flex the knee while pulling the stocking over the thigh. Stretch the stocking from the top (front and back) to distribute it evenly over the thigh. The top should rest 2.5 to 7.5 cm (1 to 3 in) below the gluteal fold.

- For a *waist-length stocking*, ask the client to stand and continue extending the stocking up to the top of the gluteal fold.

- Apply the adjustable belt that accompanies thigh- and waist-

▶ **Procedure 45–2** *CONTINUED*

length stockings, making sure that it does not interefere with any incision or external device (e.g., drainage tube or catheter).

• Adjust the foot section by tugging on the toe section to ensure toe comfort and smoothness of the stocking. Make sure a toe window is properly positioned.

**4. Document the application of the antiemboli stockings.**

| | |
|---|---|
| **EVALUATION FOCUS** | Skin temperature and color; presence of edema; posterior tibial and dorsalis pedis pulses; pain in the calf; appearance of leg veins. |

**SAMPLE RECORDING**

| Date | Time | Notes |
|------|------|-------|
| 05/05/95 | 1800 | Both feet warm, pink color. No edema. Tibial and pedis pulses 60/bm, equal. No pain, leg veins not visible. Applied antiemboli stockings to both legs. — Rosie Blakefield, SN |

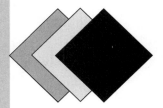

# Procedure Checklists

These Procedure Checklists are intended to be used with the procedures in this manual. Each checklist contains all the essential steps of the procedure. Students may need to adjust the procedures and the checklists in view of the needs of the individual client and according to agency protocol. These checklists can be used in a nursing skills laboratory and in client care areas to facilitate and evaluate learning.

### Procedure 21-1
### Assessing a Fetal Heart

| | | S | U | Comments |
|---|---|---|---|---|
| **1.** | **Position client appropriately.** | | | |
| | Assist woman to supine position. | | | |
| **2.** | **Locate maximum FHR intensity.** | | | |
| | Determine whether area of maximum intensity is recorded on client's chart or marked on client's abdomen. | | | |
| | or | | | |
| | Perform Leopold's maneuvers to determine fetal position and locate its posterior. | | | |
| **3.** | **Auscultate and count FHR.** | | | |
| | Warm hands and head of fetoscope before touching client's abdomen. | | | |
| | Place fetoscope or stethoscope firmly on maternal abdomen over area of maximum intensity of FHR. | | | |
| | Listen to and identify fetal heart tone. | | | |
| | Differentiate fetal heart tone from uterine souffle and from funic souffle. | | | |
| | Count FHR at least 15 seconds during gestation period before labor. | | | |
| | During labor, count FHR for 60 seconds in the relaxation period between contractions to determine baseline FHR. Then count FHR for 60 seconds during contraction and for 30 seconds immediately following a contraction. | | | |
| **4.** | **Assess rhythm and strength of heartbeat.** | | | |
| | Assist woman to listen to FHR if she wishes. | | | |
| **5.** | **Document and report pertinent assessment data.** | | | |
| | If fetal heart rate or strength is weak, report immediately to nurse in charge or physician, and initiate electronic fetal monitoring. | | | |
| *Variation:* Using a Doppler stethoscope | | | | |
| | Apply transmission gel to woman's abdomen over area where transducer is to be placed. | | | |
| | In early pregnancy, ask client to drink plenty of fluids before procedure. | | | |

| Procedure | S | U | Comments |
|---|---|---|---|

| | | | |
|---|---|---|---|
| After determining FHR, remove excess gel from abdomen and transducer. | | | |
| Clean transducer with aqueous solution. | | | |

## Procedure 21-2
## Assessing an Infant's Blood Pressure

| | | | |
|---|---|---|---|
| **1. Prepare and position infant/child appropriately.** | | | |
| Give explanation of procedure appropriate to child's age. | | | |
| Provide calm environment. Allow time for infant to recover from any activity. | | | |
| Position infants and children sitting on parent's lap if possible. | | | |
| Expose arm and support it comfortably at child's heart level. | | | |
| **2. Use auscultation method for child over 3 years of age.** | | | |
| *Auscultation method:* | | | |
| **3. Wrap deflated cuff evenly around upper arm.** | | | |
| Apply center of bladder directly over medial aspect of arm. | | | |
| **4. If client's initial examination, perform preliminary palpatory determination of systolic pressure.** | | | |
| Palpate brachial artery with fingertips. | | | |
| Close valve on pump and inflate cuff until brachial pulse is no longer felt. | | | |
| Note pressure on sphygmomanometer at which pulse is no longer felt. | | | |
| Release pressure completely in cuff, and wait 1 to 2 minutes. | | | |
| **5. Position stethoscope appropriately.** | | | |
| Place bell shaped diaphragm of the stethoscope over brachial pulse. | | | |
| **6. Auscultate client's blood pressure.** | | | |
| Inflate cuff until sphygmomanometer registers about 30 mm Hg above point where brachial pulse disappears. | | | |

| Procedure | S | U | Comments |
|---|---|---|---|
| Release valve on cuff so pressure decreases at rate of 2 to 3 mm Hg per second. | | | |
| As pressure falls, identify manometer reading at each of five phases. | | | |
| Wait 1 to 2 minutes before repeating to confirm accuracy of reading. | | | |
| **7. Remove cuff from client's arm.** | | | |
| **8. If client's initial examination, repeat procedure on client's other arm.** | | | |
| Record two pressures in form 130/80. | | | |
| Use abbreviations RA for right arm and LA for left arm. | | | |
| **9. Use palpation method, flush technique, or Doppler stethoscope when blood pressure cannot be auscultated.** | | | |
| *Palpation method:* | | | |
| Place cuff around the limb so lower edge is about 1 cm (0.4 in) above antecubital space. | | | |
| Palpate brachial pulse. | | | |
| Inflate cuff to about 30 mm Hg beyond point where brachial pulse disappears. | | | |
| Release cuff at rate of 2 to 3 mm Hg per second and identify manometer reading at point where pulse returns to brachial artery. | | | |
| *Flush technique (requires two people):* | | | |
| Place cuff on infant's wrist or ankle. | | | |
| Elevate and wrap limb distal to cuff with elastic bandage starting at fingers or toes and working up to blood pressure cuff. | | | |
| Lower extremity to heart level. | | | |
| Inflate bladder of cuff rapidly to about 200 mm Hg. | | | |
| Remove bandage and gradually release pressure at no more than 5 mm Hg per second. | | | |
| Record pressure at appearance of a flush. | | | |
| *Doppler method:* | | | |
| Plug stethoscope headset into output jack. | | | |
| Apply transmission gel to probe or client's skin. | | | |
| Hold probe at 45° angle over pulse site. | | | |

| | | S | U | Comments |
| --- | --- | --- | --- | --- |
| | Distinguish artery sounds from vein sounds. | | | |
| | After assessing pulse, remove gel. | | | |
| 10. | **Document and report pertinent assessment data.** | | | |

---

22 Procedure 22-1
Assisting with a Lumbar Puncture

---

*Preprocedure:*

| | | S | U | Comments |
| --- | --- | --- | --- | --- |
| 1. | **Explain procedure to client and support persons.** | | | |
| | Tell client what to expect during procedure. | | | |
| 2. | **Prepare client.** | | | |
| | Have client empty bladder and bowels prior to procedure. | | | |
| | Position client laterally with head bent toward chest, knees flexed to abdomen, and back to edge of bed or examining table. | | | |
| | Place small pillow under client's head. | | | |
| | Drape client, exposing only lumbar spine. | | | |
| | Open lumbar puncture set if requested to do so by physician. | | | |

*During procedure:*

| | | S | U | Comments |
| --- | --- | --- | --- | --- |
| 3. | **Support and monitor client throughout.** | | | |
| | Stand in front of client, and support back of neck and knees if client needs help in remaining still. | | | |
| | Reassure client throughout procedure by explaining what is happening. Encourage client to breathe normally and relax as much as possible. | | | |
| | Observe client's color, respirations, and pulse during lumbar puncture. | | | |
| 4. | **Handle specimen tubes appropriately.** | | | |
| | Don gloves before handling test tubes. | | | |
| | Label specimen tubes in sequence. | | | |
| 5. | **Place small sterile dressing over puncture site.** | | | |

*Postprocedure:*

| | | S | U | Comments |
| --- | --- | --- | --- | --- |
| 6. | **Ensure client's comfort and safety.** | | | |

| | | S | U | |
|---|---|---|---|---|
| | Assist client to dorsal recumbant position with only one head pillow. Determine recommended time position should be maintained. | | | |
| | Determine whether analgesics are ordered and can be given for headaches. | | | |
| 7. | **Monitor client.** | | | |
| | Observe for swelling or bleeding at puncture site. | | | |
| | Determine whether client feels faint. | | | |
| | Monitor changes in neurologic status. | | | |
| | Determine whether client is experiencing any numbness, tingling, or pain radiating down legs. | | | |
| 8. | **Transport any specimens to laboratory.** | | | |
| 9. | **Document procedure on client's chart.** | | | |

## Procedure 22-2
## Assisting with an Abdominal Paracentesis

| | | S | U | |
|---|---|---|---|---|
| *Preprocedure:* | | | | |
| 1. | **Prepare client.** | | | |
| | Explain procedure to client. | | | |
| | Have client void just before paracentesis. Notify physician if client cannot void. | | | |
| | Help client assume sitting position in bed or in chair. | | | |
| | Cover client to expose only necessary area. | | | |
| *During procedure:* | | | | |
| 2. | **Assist and monitor client.** | | | |
| | Support client verbally, and describe steps of procedure as needed, | | | |
| | Observe client closely for signs of distress and hypovolemic shock. | | | |
| | Place small sterile dressing over site of incision after cannula or aspirating needle is withdrawn. | | | |
| *Postprocedure:* | | | | |
| 3. | **Monitor client closely.** | | | |
| | Observe for hypovolemic shock. | | | |
| | Observe puncture site regularly for leakage. | | | |

| Procedure | S | U | Comments |
|---|---|---|---|
| Observe client for any scrotal edema. | | | |
| Monitor vital signs, urine output, and drainage from puncture every 15 minutes for at least two hours and every hour for four hours thereafter, or as client's condition indicates. | | | |
| Measure abdominal girth with tape measure at site it was measured during preprocedure. | | | |
| **4. Document all relevant information.** | | | |
| **5. Transport labeled specimens to laboratory.** | | | |

### Procedure 22-3
### Assisting with a Thoracentesis

| Procedure | S | U | Comments |
|---|---|---|---|
| *Preprocedure:* | | | |
| **1. Prepare client.** | | | |
| Explain procedure to client. | | | |
| Help client assume comfortable position, sitting with arms above head, or arm elevated and stretched forward, or have client lean forward over a pillow. | | | |
| Cover client as needed with bath blanket. | | | |
| *During procedure:* | | | |
| **2. Support and monitor client throughout.** | | | |
| Support client verbally and describe steps of procedure as needed. | | | |
| Observe client for signs of distress. | | | |
| **3. Place small sterile dressing over site of puncture.** | | | |
| *Postprocedure:* | | | |
| **4. Monitor client.** | | | |
| Assess pulse rate, respiratory rate, and skin color. | | | |
| Observe changes in client's cough, sputum, respiratory depth, breath sounds, and note complaints of chest pain. | | | |
| **5. Position client in accordance with agency protocol.** | | | |
| **6. Document all relevant information.** | | | |
| **7. Transport specimens to laboratory.** | | | |

| Procedure | S | U | Comments |
|---|---|---|---|

### Procedure 22-4
### Assisting with a Bone Marrow Biopsy

| | S | U | Comments |
|---|---|---|---|
| *Preprocedure:* | | | |
| **1. Prepare client.** | | | |
| Explain procedure. | | | |
| Help client assume supine position for biopsy of sternum, or prone position for biopsy of either iliac crest. Expose biopsy site. | | | |
| *During procedure:* | | | |
| **2. Monitor and support client throughout.** | | | |
| Describe steps of procedure as needed, and provide verbal support. | | | |
| Observe client for pallor, diaphoresis, and faintness due to bleeding or pain. | | | |
| **3. Place small dressing over site of puncture after needle is withdrawn. Apply direct pressure per agency protocol.** | | | |
| *Postprocedure:* | | | |
| **4. Monitor client.** | | | |
| Assess for discomfort and bleeding from site. Report any bleeding to nurse in charge. | | | |
| Provide analgesic as needed and ordered. | | | |
| **5. Document all relevant information.** | | | |
| **6. Transport specimens to laboratory.** | | | |

### Procedure 22-5
### Assisting with a Liver Biopsy

| | S | U | Comments |
|---|---|---|---|
| *Preprocedure:* | | | |
| **1. Prepare client.** | | | |
| Give preprocedural medications as ordered. | | | |
| Explain procedure to client. | | | |
| Ensure that client fasts for at least 2 hours before procedure. | | | |
| Administer appropriate sedative about 30 minutes prior or at specified time. | | | |
| Help client assume supine position, with upper right quadrant of abdomen exposed, keeping all other areas covered with bedclothes. | | | |

*During procedure:*

**2.  Monitor and support client throughout.**

Support client in supine position.

Instruct client to take a few deep inhalations and exhalations and to hold breath after final exhalation for up to 10 seconds while needle is inserted, biopsy obtained, and needle is withdrawn.

Instruct client to resume breathing when needle is withdrawn.

Apply pressure to site of puncture.

**3.  Apply small dressing to site of puncture.**

*Postprocedure:*

**4.  Position client appropriately.**

Assist client to right side-lying position with small pillow or folded towel under biopsy site. Instruct client to remain in position for several hours.

**5.  Monitor client.**

Assess client's vital signs every 15 minutes for first hour following test or until vital signs are stable. Then monitor vital signs every hour for 24 hours or as needed.

Determine whether client is experiencing abdominal pain.

Check biopsy site for localized bleeding.

**6.  Document all relevant information.**

**7.  Transport specimens to laboratory.**

---

## Procedure 27-1
## 27 Performing a Surgical Hand Scrub

**1.  Prepare for surgical hand scrub.**

Remove wristwatch and all rings.

Apply cap and face mask.

Sleeves pushed above elbows.

Uniform is well tucked in at waist.

**2.  Scrub hands.**

Hold hands above level of elbows.

Apply antimicrobial solution to hands.

| Procedure | S | U | Comments |
|---|---|---|---|

Use firm, rubbing, and circular movements to wash palms and backs of hands, wrists, and forearms.

Interlace fingers and thumbs, and move hands back and forth.

Hold hands and arms under running water to rinse thoroughly, keeping hands higher than elbows.

Apply antimicrobial solution and lather hands again. Using scrub brush, scrub each hand for 45 seconds.

Using scrub brush, scrub from wrists to 5 cm (2 in) above each elbow.

Continue to hold hands higher than elbows.

Rinse hands and arms thoroughly so that water flows from hands to elbows.

Turn off water with foot pedal.

**3.  Dry hands and arms.**

Use one sterile towel for each hand and arm. Keep hands in front and above waist.

## 29  Procedure 29-1
## Giving an Infant Sponge Bath

**1.  Prepare environment.**

Wash hands before handling a newborn.

Measure temperature of water.

**2.  Prepare infant.**

Undress infant, and bundle in supine position.

Ascertain infant's weight and vital signs.

**3.  Wash infant's head.**

Clean infant's eyes with water only wiping from inner to outer canthus.

Wash and dry infant's face using water only.

Lift infant using football hold, and position infant's head over washbasin. Lather scalp with mild soap.

Rinse and dry scalp well.

Place infant in supine position.

| Procedure | S | U | Comments |
|-----------|---|---|----------|
| **4.** **Wash infant's body.** | | | |
| Wash, rinse, and dry each arm, hand and axilla. | | | |
| Wash, rinse, and dry infant's chest and abdomen. | | | |
| Keep infant covered with bath blanket or towel between washing and rinsing. | | | |
| Clean base of umbilical cord with cotton ball dipped in 70% isopropyl alcohol. | | | |
| Wash, rinse, and dry infant's legs and feet. | | | |
| Turn infant on stomach or side. Wash, rinse, and dry back. | | | |
| **5.** **Clean genitals and anterior perineum.** | | | |
| Place infant on back. Clean and dry genitals and anterior perineal area from front to back. | | | |
| Clean folds at groin. | | | |
| *For females:* | | | |
| Separate labia, and using a clean moistened cotton ball for each stroke, clean between them wiping from front to back. | | | |
| *For males:* | | | |
| If infant is uncircumcised, retract foreskin if possible, and clean glans penis, using moistened cotton ball. After swabbing, replace foreskin. | | | |
| In infant has been recently circumcised, clean glans penis by gently squeezing cotton ball moistened with clear water over site. Note signs of bleeding or infection. | | | |
| Clean shaft of penis and scrotum. | | | |
| Apply A and D Ointment to perineum. | | | |
| **6.** **Clean posterior perineum and buttocks.** | | | |
| Grasp infant's ankles, raise feet, and elevate buttocks. | | | |
| Wash and rinse area with washcloth. | | | |
| Dry area, and apply ointment. | | | |
| **7.** **Check for dry, cracked, or peeling skin, and apply mild baby oil or lotion.** | | | |
| **8.** **Dress and position infant.** | | | |

| | Procedure | S | U | Comments |
|---|---|---|---|---|
| | Diaper and clothe infant. Cover and bundle infant with blanket. | | | |
| 9. | **Record any significant assessments.** | | | |

## Procedure 29-2
## Giving an Infant Tub Bath

| | Procedure | S | U | Comments |
|---|---|---|---|---|
| 1. | **Prepare bath area.** | | | |
| | Prepare flat, padded surface in bath area to dress and undress infant. Cover surface with a towel. | | | |
| | Place tub or basin near dressing surface. | | | |
| | Measure temperature of water. | | | |
| 2. | **Clean infant's eyes and face before placing infant in tub.** | | | |
| | Follow Procedure 29-1, step 3. | | | |
| 3. | **Place infant into tub.** | | | |
| | Gradually immerse infant into tub. | | | |
| 4. | **Wash infant.** | | | |
| | Keeping infant's head and back supported on forearm, lather scalp with mild soap. Rinse scalp well. | | | |
| | Soap and rinse infant's trunk, extremities, genitals, and perineal area with free hand. | | | |
| 5. | **Remove infant from tub, and dry infant well.** | | | |
| | Remove infant from tub, and quickly bundle baby in a towel. | | | |
| | Gently pat infant dry, giving special attention to body creases and folds. | | | |
| 6. | **Ensure infant's comfort and safety.** | | | |
| | Diaper and clothe infant. Cover and bundle infant with blanket. | | | |
| 7. | **Document all pertinent information.** | | | |

## Procedure 29-3
## Changing a Diaper

| | Procedure | S | U | Comments |
|---|---|---|---|---|
| 1. | **If using cloth diaper, fold diaper using one of three methods: rectangular, triangular, or kite.** | | | |
| 2. | **Position and handle infant appropriately.** | | | |

| | | S | U | Comments |
|---|---|---|---|---|
| | Place infant in supine position on clean, flat surface near assembled supplies. | | | |
| 3. | **Remove soiled diaper.** | | | |
| | Place fingers between infant's skin and diaper, and unpin diaper on each side. Close pins, and place them out of reach of infant. | | | |
| | Pull front of diaper down between infant's legs. | | | |
| | Grasp infant's ankles with one hand, and lift buttocks. | | | |
| | Use clean portion of diaper to wipe any excess urine or feces from buttocks. Wipe from front to back. | | | |
| | Remove diaper and lower infant's buttocks. | | | |
| 4. | **Clean buttocks and anal-genital area.** | | | |
| | Use warm water and soap or commercial cleansing tissues. | | | |
| | Clean toward posterior. Rinse and dry area well with towel. | | | |
| | Apply protective ointment or lotion to perineum, buttocks, and skin creases. | | | |
| 5. | **Apply clean diaper, and fasten it securely.** | | | |
| | Grasp infant's ankles with one hand and raise infant's legs and buttocks. Place diaper under infant so back edge is at waist level. | | | |
| | Draw diaper up between infant's legs to waist in front. | | | |
| | Fasten diaper at waist with tape provided. If using safety pins for cloth diapers, hold fingers between baby and diaper while pinning. | | | |
| | Position pins vertically or horizontally, and facing upward or outward. | | | |
| 6. | **Ensure infant comfort and safety.** | | | |
| | Clothe and return infant to crib. | | | |
| 7. | **Document all pertinent information.** | | | |
| | Record stool and/or urine observations. | | | |

## Procedure 29-4
## Care of the Client with Pediculosis

| 1. | **Remove head lice.** | | | |
|---|---|---|---|---|

| | S | U | Comments |
|---|---|---|---|
| Don gown, gloves, and surgical cap before procedure. | | | |
| Place a small damp or dry washcloth over client's eyes. | | | |
| Apply medicated shampoo and work into hair and scalp thoroughly. | | | |
| Rinse hair and scalp thoroughly. | | | |
| *Optional:* | | | |
| Remove dead lice and nits with fine-toothed comb or brush dipped in hot vinegar. | | | |
| Disinfect comb or brush with medicated shampoo. | | | |
| Repeat shampoo if indicated. | | | |
| **2. Remove body and pubic lice.** | | | |
| Don gown and gloves. | | | |
| Have client bathe in soap and water. | | | |
| Apply medicated topical cream or lotion to infested areas and allow to remain for prescribed time period. | | | |
| Clean treated areas with soap and water to remove dead lice and medication. | | | |
| If eyelashes are involved, use a prescribed opthalmic ointment as ordered. Remove nits manually. | | | |
| **3. Dispose of linens and clothing appropriately.** | | | |
| Place used towel, gowns, and bed linens into label isolation bag. | | | |
| Provide clean gown and bed linens for client. | | | |
| **4. Document any pertinent information.** | | | |

## Procedure 29-5
## Braiding the Hair

| | S | U | Comments |
|---|---|---|---|
| **1. Brush and comb hair, and remove any tangles.** | | | |
| **2. Braid hair.** | | | |
| For one braid, divide hair into three even sections. For two braids, part hair down middle, and then divide hair into three strands. | | | |

| Procedure | S | U | Comments |
|---|---|---|---|
| Hold left strand in left hand, center strand between second finger and thumb of left hand, and right strand in right hand. | | | |
| Lay right strand (3) over middle strand (2). Transfer strand 3 to left hand and strand 2 to right hand. Strand 3 is now middle strand, and strand 2 is right strand. | | | |
| Holding strands tautly, cross left strand (1) over middle strand (3). Strand 1 is now middle strand, and strand 3 is left strand. Left hand holds strand 3, right fingers hold strand 1, and right hand holds strand 2. | | | |
| Cross right strand (2) over center strand (1). Cross left strand(3) over middle strand (2). | | | |
| Continue crossing side strands over center strand, alternating right and left sides until ends of strands are reached. | | | |
| Firmly secure end of braid with covered elastic band or ribbon. | | | |
| Braid other side of hair if second braid is needed. | | | |

## Procedure 29-6
## Inserting Contact Lenses

| Procedure | S | U | Comments |
|---|---|---|---|
| **1. Take client's lens storage case, and select correct lens for eye.** | | | |
| Start with right eye. | | | |
| *Hard lenses:* | | | |
| **2. Lubricate lens.** | | | |
| Put a few drops of sterile wetting solution on right lens. | | | |
| Spread wetting solution on both surfaces of lens by using thumb and index finger. | | | |
| **3. Insert lens.** | | | |
| Ask client to tilt head backward. | | | |
| Place lens convex side down on tip of dominant index finger. | | | |
| Separate upper and lower eyelids of right eye with thumb and index finger of nondominant hand. | | | |
| Place lens gently on cornea, directly over iris and pupil. | | | |

| Procedure | S | U | Comments |
|---|---|---|---|

Repeat above steps for left lens.

**4.  If lens is off center, center lens.**

*Soft lenses:*

**5.  Keep dominant finger dry for insertion.**

Remove lens from saline-filled storage case with nondominate hand.

**6.  Position lens correctly for insertion.**

*For a regular soft lens:*

Hold lens at edge between thumb and index finger.

Flex lens slightly, edges point inward.

*For an ultrathin soft lens:*

Put lens on placement finger and allow it to dry for a few seconds.

Inspect lens to see whether edges turn upward.

**7.  Wet lens with saline solution using non-dominant fingers.**

**8.  Insert lens.**

Ensure placement finger is dry.

Insert lens in same manner as hard lenses.

**9.  Document pertinent information.**

## Procedure 29-7
## Removing Contact Lenses

**1.  Locate position of lens.**

Ask client to tilt head backward.

Retract upper eyelid with index finger, and ask client to look up, down, and from side to side. Repeat with lower eyelid.

Reposition displaced lens.

*Hard lenses:*

**2.  Separate upper and lower eyelids.**

Use both thumbs or index fingers to separate upper and lower eyelids of one eye until they are beyond edges of lens.

or

Use middle finger to retract upper eyelid and thumb of same hand to retract lower lid.

**3. Remove lens.**

Gently move margins of both lower and upper eyelid toward lens.

Hold top eyelid stationary at edge of lens, and lift bottom edge of lens by pressing lower lid at its margin firmly under lens.

After lens is slightly tipped, slide lens off and out of eye by moving both eyelids toward each other.

Grasp lens with index finger and thumb, and place in palm of hand.

Place first lens in its designated cup in storage case.

Repeat above steps for other lens.

*Soft lenses:*

**4. Separate upper and lower eyelids.**

Ask client to look upward and keep eye opened wide.

Retract lower or upper lid with one or two fingers of nondominant hand.

Using index finger of dominant hand, move lens down to inferior part of sclera.

**5. Remove lens.**

Gently pinch lens between pads of thumb and index finger of dominant hand.

Place lens in palm of hand.

Repeat above step for other lens.

**6. Clean and store lenses appropriately.**

Place lens in correct slot in its storage case.

**7. Document all relevant information.**

## Procedure 29-8
## Removing, Cleaning, and Inserting an Artificial Eye

**1. Remove eye.**

Assist client to a sitting or supine position.

Pull lower eyelid down over infraorbital bone with dominant thumb, and exert slight pressure below eyelid.

| Procedure | S | U | Comments |
|---|---|---|---|
| Compress small rubber bulb, and apply tip directly on eye. Gradually decrease finger pressure on bulb, and draw eye out of socket. | | | |
| Grasp eye and place it carefully in lined container. | | | |
| **2. Clean eye and socket.** | | | |
| Clean socket with soft gauze or cotton wipes and normal saline. Pat area dry. | | | |
| Wash and dry tissue around eye, stroking from inner to outer canthus using fresh gauze for each wipe. | | | |
| Wash artificial eye gently with warm normal saline. Dry it with dry wipes. | | | |
| If eye is not to be reinserted, place it in lined container filled with water or saline, close lid, label container with client's name and room number. | | | |
| **3. Reinsert eye.** | | | |
| Ensure eye is moistened with water or saline. | | | |
| Using thumb and index finger, retract eyelids, exerting pressure on supraorbital and infraorbital bones. | | | |
| With thumb and index finger of other hand, hold eye so front of it is toward palm of hand. Slip eye gently into socket, and release lids. | | | |
| **4. Document pertinent information.** | | | |

### Procedure 32-1
### Teaching Progressive Relaxation

| Procedure | S | U | Comments |
|---|---|---|---|
| **1. Ensure environment is quiet, peaceful, and at a temperature that promotes client comfort.** | | | |
| **2. Tell client how progressive relaxation works.** | | | |
| Provide rationale for procedure. | | | |
| Ask client to identify stressors operating in client's life and reactions to these stressors. | | | |
| Demonstrate method of tensing and relaxing muscles. | | | |
| **3. Assist client to comfortable position.** | | | |

| | Procedure | S | U | Comments |
|---|---|---|---|---|
| | Ensure all body parts are supported and joints are slightly flexed, with no strain or pull on muscles. | | | |
| 4. | **Encourage client to rest the mind.** | | | |
| | Ask client to gaze slowly across ceiling, down wall, along window curtain, around fabric pattern, and back up wall. | | | |
| 5. | **Instruct client to tense and relax each muscle group.** | | | |
| | Progress through each muscle group in order starting with dominant side: <br> a. hand and forearm <br> b. upper arm <br> c. forehead <br> d. central face <br> e. lower face and jaw <br> f. neck <br> g. chest, shoulders, and upper back <br> h. abdomen <br> i. thigh <br> j. calf muscles <br> k. foot | | | |
| | Encourage client to breathe slowly and deeply during entire procedure. | | | |
| | Encourage client to focus on each muscle group being tensed and relaxed. | | | |
| | Speak to client in soothing voice that encourages relaxation. | | | |
| 6. | **Ask client to state whether any tension remains after all muscle groups have been tensed and relaxed.** | | | |
| | Repeat procedure for muscle groups not relaxed. | | | |
| 7. | **Terminate relaxation exercise slowly by counting backward from 4 to 1.** | | | |
| | Ask client to move body slowly, first hands and feet, then arms and legs, and finally head and neck. | | | |
| 8. | **Document client's response to exercise.** | | | |

## Procedure 32-2
## Assisting with Guided Imagery

| | Procedure | S | U | Comments |
|---|---|---|---|---|
| 1. | **Provide comfortable, quiet environment free of distraction.** | | | |

| Procedure | S | U | Comments |
|---|---|---|---|

**2.** Explain rationale and benefits of imagery.

**3.** Assist client to reclining position.

Use touch only if non-threatening to client.

**4.** Implement actions to induce relaxation.

Use client's preferred name.

Speak clearly in calming and neutral tone of voice.

Ask client to take slow, deep breaths and to relax all muscles.

Use progressive relaxation exercises as needed to assist client to achieve total relaxation.

For pain or stress management, encourage client to "go to a place where you have previously felt very peaceful."

or

For internal imagery, encourage client to focus on meaningful image of power and to use it to control specific problem.

**5.** Assist client to elaborate on description of image.

Ask client to use all senses when describing image.

**6.** Ask client to describe physical and emotional feelings elicited by image.

Direct client to explore response to image.

**7.** Provide client with continuous feedback.

Comment on signs of relaxation and peacefulness.

**8.** Take client out of image.

Slowly count backward from 5 to 1. Tell client there will be feelings of restfulness when eyes are opened.

Remain until client is alert.

**9.** Following experience, discuss client's feelings about experience.

Identify anything that could enhance experience.

**10.** Encourage client to practice imagery technique.

| Procedure | S | U | Comments |
|---|---|---|---|

### Procedure 34-1
### Using a Hydraulic Lift

| | Procedure | S | U | Comments |
|---|---|---|---|---|
| 1. | **Prepare client.** | | | |
| | Explain procedure, and demonstrate lift. | | | |
| 2. | **Prepare equipment.** | | | |
| | Lock wheels of client's bed. | | | |
| | Raise bed to high position, put up side rail on opposite side of bed, and lower side rail on near side. | | | |
| | Position lift close to client. | | | |
| | Place chair that is to receive client beside bed. | | | |
| | Lock wheels of chair. | | | |
| 3. | **Position client on sling.** | | | |
| | Roll client on side. | | | |
| | Place canvas seat or sling under client, with wide lower edge under client's thighs and the narrow edge up under client's shoulders. | | | |
| | Raise bed rail on near side of bed, and lower opposite side rail. | | | |
| | Roll client to opposite side, and pull canvas sling through. | | | |
| | Roll client to supine position on top of canvas sling. | | | |
| 4. | **Attach sling to swivel bar** | | | |
| | Wheel lift into position, on side where chair is positioned. Lock wheels of lifter. | | | |
| | Lower side rail. | | | |
| | Lower horizontal bar or mast boom to sling level. | | | |
| | Attach lifter straps or hooks. | | | |
| 5. | **Lift client gradually.** | | | |
| | Elevate head of bed to place client in sitting position. | | | |
| *Nurse 1:* | | | | |
| | Close pressure valve, and gradually pump jack handle until client is above bed surface. | | | |

| Procedure | S | U | Comments |
|---|---|---|---|
| *Nurse 2:* | | | |
|     Assume broad stance, and guide client with hands as client is lifted. | | | |
|     Check placement of sling before moving client away from bed. | | | |
| **6.**  **Move client over chair.** | | | |
| *Nurse 1:* | | | |
|     With pressure valve securely closed, slowly roll lift until client is over chair. | | | |
| *Nurse 2:* | | | |
|     Guide movement with hands until client is directly over chair. | | | |
| **7.**  **Lower client into chair.** | | | |
| *Nurse 1:* | | | |
|     Release pressure valve gradually. | | | |
| *Nurse 2:* | | | |
|     Guide client into chair. | | | |
| **8.**  **Ensure client comfort and safety.** | | | |
|     Remove hooks from canvas seat. Leave seat in place. | | | |
|     Align client appropriately in sitting position. | | | |
|     Apply seatbelt or other restraint as needed. | | | |
|     Place call bell within reach. | | | |

## Procedure 34-2
## Providing Passive Range-of-Motion Exercises

| Procedure | S | U | Comments |
|---|---|---|---|
| **1.**  **Prior to initiating exercises, review any possible restrictions with physician or physical therapist. Also refer to agency protocol.** | | | |
| **2.**  **Assist client to supine position and expose body parts requiring exercise.** | | | |
|     Place client's feet together, place arms at sides, and leave space around head and feet. | | | |
| **3.**  **Return to starting position after each motion. Repeat each motion three time on affected limb.** | | | |

| | Procedure | S | U | Comments |
|---|---|---|---|---|

*Shoulder and elbow movement:*

Begin each exercise with client's arm at client's side. Grasp arm beneath elbow with one hand and beneath wrist with other hand.

**4.** **Flex, externally rotate, and extend shoulder.**

Move arm up to ceiling and toward head of bed.

**5.** **Abduct and externally rotate shoulder.**

Move arm away from body and toward client's head until hand is under head.

**6.** **Abduct shoulder.**

Move arm over body until hand touches client's other hand.

**7.** **Rotate shoulder internally and externally.**

Place arm out to side at shoulder level (90° abduction) and bend elbow so forearm is at right angle to mattress.

Move forearm down until palm touches mattress and then up until back of hand touches bed.

**8.** **Flex and extend elbow.**

Bend elbow until fingers touch chin, then straighten arm.

**9.** **Pronate and supinate forearm.**

Grasp client's hand as for handshake, turn palm downward and upward, ensuring only forearm moves.

*Wrist and hand movement:*

Flex client's arm at elbow until forearm is at right angle to mattress. Support wrist joint with one hand while other hand manipulates joint and fingers.

**10.** **Hyperextend wrist and flex fingers.**

Bend wrist backward, and at same time, flex fingers, moving tips of fingers to palm of hand.

Align wrist in straight line with arm, place fingers over client's fingers to make fist.

**11.** **Flex wrist and extend fingers.**

| Procedure | S | U | Comments |
|---|---|---|---|
| Bend wrist forward, and at same time extend fingers. | | | |
| **12. Abduct and oppose thumb.** | | | |
| Move thumb away from fingers and then across hand toward base of little finger. | | | |
| *Leg and hip movement:* | | | |
| During leg and hip exercises, place one hand under client's knee and other under ankle. | | | |
| **13. Flex and extend knee and hip.** | | | |
| Lift leg and bend knee, moving knee up toward chest as far as possible. Bring leg down, staighten knee, and lower leg to bed. | | | |
| **14. Abduct and adduct leg.** | | | |
| Move leg to side, away from client and back across in front of other leg. | | | |
| **15. Rotate hip internally and externally.** | | | |
| Roll leg inward, then outward. | | | |
| *Ankle and foot movement:* | | | |
| Place hands in positions described, depending on motion to be achieved. | | | |
| **16. Dorsiflex foot and stretch Achilles tendon.** | | | |
| Place one hand under client's heel, resting inner forearm against bottom of client's foot. | | | |
| Place other hand under knee to support it. | | | |
| Press forearm against foot to move it upward toward leg. | | | |
| **17. Invert and evert foot.** | | | |
| Place one hand under client's ankle and one hand over arch of foot. | | | |
| Turn foot inward, then turn it outward. | | | |
| **18. Plantar flex foot, and extend and flex toes.** | | | |
| Place one hand over arch of foot to push foot away from leg. | | | |
| Place fingers of other hand under toes to bend toes upward, and then over toes to push toes downward. | | | |
| *Neck movement:* | | | |
| Remove client's pillow. | | | |

| Procedure | S | U | Comments |
|---|---|---|---|
| **19.**   **Flex and extend neck.** | | | |
| Place palm of hand under client's head and palm of other hand on client's chin. | | | |
| Move head forward until chin rests on chest, then back to resting supine position without head pillow. | | | |
| **20.**   **Laterally flex neck.** | | | |
| Place heels of hands on each side of client's cheeks. | | | |
| Move top of head to right and to left. | | | |
| *Hyperextension movements:* | | | |
| **21.**   **Assist client to prone or lateral position on closest side of bed, but facing away.** | | | |
| **22.**   **Hyperextend shoulder.** | | | |
| Place one hand on shoulder and other under client's elbow. | | | |
| Pull upper arm up and backward. | | | |
| **23.**   **Hyperextend hip.** | | | |
| Place one hand on hip. With other hand, cradle lower leg in forearm, and cup knee joint with hand. | | | |
| Move leg backward from hip joint. | | | |
| **24.**   **Hyperextend neck.** | | | |
| Remove pillow. With client's face down, place one hand on forehead and other on back of skull. | | | |
| Move head backward. | | | |
| *Following exercise:* | | | |
| **25.**   **Assess client's pulse and endurance of exercise.** | | | |
| **26.**   **Report to nurse in charge any unexpected problems or notable changes in client's movements.** | | | |
| **27.**   **Document exercise and assessments.** | | | |

## Procedure 34-3
## Applying a Continuous Passive Motion Device to the Knee

| Procedure | S | U | Comments |
|---|---|---|---|
| **1.**   **Check safety test date.** | | | |
| **2.**   **Verify physician's orders and agency protocol.** | | | |

| Procedure | S | U | Comments |
|---|---|---|---|
| Determine degrees of flexion, extension, and speed initially prescribed. | | | |
| **3.**   **Set up machine.** | | | |
| Remove egg crate mattress if indicated, place machine on bed. | | | |
| Apply supportive sling to movable cradle. | | | |
| Attach machine to Balkan frame using traction equipment. | | | |
| Connect control box to machine. | | | |
| **4.**   **Set prescribed levels of flexion, extension, and speed.** | | | |
| Check that machine is functioning properly by running it through complete cycle. | | | |
| **5.**   **Position client and place leg in machine.** | | | |
| Place client in supine position, with head of bed slightly elevated. | | | |
| Support leg, and with client's help, lift leg and place it in padded cradle. | | | |
| Lengthen or shorten appropriate sections of frame to fit machine to client. | | | |
| Adjust footplate so foot is supported in neutral position or slight dorsiflexion. | | | |
| Ensure leg is neither internally nor externally rotated. | | | |
| Apply restraining straps around thigh, top of foot, and cradle, allowing enough space to fit several fingers under it. | | | |
| **6.**   **Start machine.** | | | |
| When machine reaches fully extended position, stop machine, and verify degree of flexion with goniometer. | | | |
| Restart machine, and observe a few cycles of flexion and extension to ensure proper functioning. | | | |
| **7.**   **Ensure continued client safety and comfort.** | | | |
| Raise side rails. | | | |
| Stay with confused or sedated client while machine is on. | | | |
| Instruct mentally alert client how to operate on/off switch. | | | |

| Procedure | S | U | Comments |
|---|---|---|---|
| Loosen straps and check client's skin at least twice per shift. | | | |
| Wash perineal area at least once per shift, and keep it dry. | | | |
| Drape towel over groin of a male client. | | | |
| **8.**   **Document all relevant information.** | | | |

## Procedure 34-4
## Assisting a Client to Use a Cane

| Procedure | S | U | Comments |
|---|---|---|---|
| **1.**   **Prepare client for walking.** | | | |
| Ask client to hold cane on stronger side of body. | | | |
| Position tip of cane about 15 cm (6 in) to side and 15 cm (6 in) in front of near foot, so elbow is slightly flexed. | | | |
| **2.**   **When maximum support is required, instruct client to move as follows:** | | | |
| Move cane forward about 30 cm (1 ft), or distance that is comfortable while body weight is on both legs. | | | |
| Move unaffected leg forward ahead of cane and weak leg while weight is on cane and weak leg. | | | |
| **3.**   **When client requires less support, instruct client to follow these steps:** | | | |
| Move cane and weak leg forward at same time, while weight is on stronger leg. | | | |
| Move stronger leg forward while weight is on cane and weak leg. | | | |
| **4.**   **Ensure client safety.** | | | |
| Walk beside client on affected side for specified time and distance on nursing care plan. | | | |

## Procedure 34-5
## Assisting a Client to Use Crutches

| Procedure | S | U | Comments |
|---|---|---|---|
| **1.**   **Prepare client.** | | | |
| Verify correct length for crutches and placement of handpieces. | | | |
| Ensure client is wearing supportive, nonskid shoes. | | | |
| **2.**   **Assist client to assume tripod position.** | | | |

| Procedure | S | U | Comments |
|---|---|---|---|
| Ask client to stand and place tips of crutches 15 cm (6 in) in front of feet and out laterally about 15 cm (6 in). | | | |
| Make sure feet are slightly apart. | | | |
| Ensure posture is erect and elbows extended. | | | |
| Stand slightly behind and on client's affected side. | | | |
| If client is unsteady, place walking belt around client's waist, and grasp belt from above. | | | |
| **3. Teach client appropriate crutch gait.** | | | |
| *Four-point alternate gait:* | | | |
| Ask client to | | | |
| a. Move right crutch forward 10 to 15 cm (4 to 6 in). b. Move left foot forward to level of crutch. c. Move left crutch forward. d. Move right foot forward. | | | |
| *Three-point gait:* | | | |
| Ask client to | | | |
| a. Move crutches and weaker leg forward. b. Move stronger leg forward. | | | |
| *Two-point gait:* | | | |
| Ask client to | | | |
| a. Move left crutch and right foot forward together. b. Move right crutch and left foot ahead together. | | | |
| *Swing-to gait:* | | | |
| Ask client to | | | |
| a. Move both crutches ahead together. b. Lift body by arms and swing *to* crutches. | | | |
| *Swing-through gait:* | | | |
| Ask client to | | | |
| a. Move both crutches forward together. b. Lift body weight by arms and swing *through and beyond* crutches | | | |
| **4. Teach client to get into and out of chair.** | | | |
| *Getting into a chair:* | | | |
| Instruct client to | | | |
| a. Stand with back of unaffected leg centered against chair. | | | |

b. Transfer crutches to hand on affected side, hold crutches by hand bars, and grasp arm of chair with hand on unaffected side.

c. Lean forward, flex knees and hips, and lower into chair.

*Getting out of chair:*

Instruct client to

a. Move forward to edge of chair and place unaffected leg slightly under or at edge of chair.

b. Grasp crutches by hand bars on affected side, and grasp arm of chair by hand on unaffected side.

c. Push down on crutches and chair armrest while elevating body out of chair.

d. Assume tripod position before moving.

**5.  Teach client to go up and down stairs.**

*Going up stairs:*

Stand at position behind client and slightly to affected side.

Ask client to

a. Assume tripod position at bottom of stairs.

b. Transfer body weight to crutches and move unaffected leg onto step.

c. Transfer body weight to unaffected leg on step and move crutches and affected leg up to step.

*Going down stairs:*

Stand one step below client on affected side.

Ask client to

a. Assume tripod position at top of stairs.

b. Shift body weight to unaffected leg, and move crutches and affected leg down onto next step.

c. Transfer body weight to crutches, and move unaffected leg to that step.

or

Ask client to

a. Hold both crutches in outside hand and grasp hand rail with other hand for support.

b. Move as in steps b and c above.

**6.  Document teaching and all assessments.**

| | Procedure 36-1 Managing Pain with a Transcutaneous Electric Nerve Stimulation Unit (TENS) | S | U | Comments |
| --- | --- | --- | --- | --- |
| 1. | Explain purpose and application procedure to client and family. | | | |
| 2. | Prepare equipment. | | | |
| | Insert battery into TENS unit to test status of functioning. | | | |
| | With TENS unit off, plug in lead wires. | | | |
| 3. | Clean application area. | | | |
| | Wash, rinse, and dry designated area with soap and water. | | | |
| 4. | Apply electrodes to client. | | | |
| | If electrodes are not prejelled, moisten with small amount of water or apply gel. | | | |
| | Place electrodes on clean, unbroken skin area. Choose area according to location, nature and origin of pain. | | | |
| | Ensure electrodes make full surface contact with skin. | | | |
| | Secure electrodes with hypoallergenic tape. | | | |
| 5. | Turn unit on. | | | |
| | Ascertain amplitude control is set at 0. | | | |
| | Slowly increase intensity of amplitude until client notes slight increase in discomfort, then slowly decrease until client notes a pleasant sensation. | | | |
| 6. | Monitor the client for discomfort. | | | |
| 7. | Provide client teaching. | | | |
| | Review with client instructions for use, and verify that client understands. | | | |
| | Have client demonstrate use of TENS unit. | | | |
| | Instruct client not to submerge unit in water. | | | |
| 8. | Document all relevant information. | | | |

| | Procedure 37-1 Assisting an Adult to Eat | | | |
| --- | --- | --- | --- | --- |
| 1. | Check client's chart or kardex for diet order. | | | |

| Procedure | S | U | Comments |
|-----------|---|---|----------|
| **2.**    **Prepare client and overbed table.** | | | |
| Assist client in washing hands prior to meal. Assist with oral hygiene as needed. | | | |
| Clear and arrange overbed table close to the bedside to allow client to see food. | | | |
| **3.**    **Position client and self appropriately.** | | | |
| Assist client to comfortable position. | | | |
| Assume sitting position, if possible, beside client. | | | |
| **4.**    **Assist client as required.** | | | |
| Check tray for client's name, type of diet, and completeness. Confirm client's name by checking wristband before leaving tray. | | | |
| Encourage client to eat independently, assisting as needed. | | | |
| Remove food covers, pour liquids, cut foods into smaller pieces, and butter bread if needed. | | | |
| For blind client, identify placement of food by using a clock system. | | | |
| **5.**    **After meal, ensure client comfort.** | | | |
| Assist client to clean mouth and hands. | | | |
| Reposition client. | | | |
| Replace food covers, and remove food tray from bedside. | | | |
| **6.**    **Document all relevant information.** | | | |
| Note how much and what type of food was eaten, and amount of fluid intake. If client is not eating, notify nurse in charge. | | | |

## Procedure 37-2
## Bottle-Feeding an Infant

| Procedure | S | U | Comments |
|-----------|---|---|----------|
| **1.**    **Obtain and verify orders before feeding.** | | | |
| **2.**    **Prepare bottle, nipple, and formula.** | | | |
| If formula is refrigerated, warm to room temperature. | | | |
| Test size of nipple holes by turning bottle upside down. | | | |
| **3.**    **Ensure infant comfort.** | | | |

| Procedure | S | U | Comments |
|---|---|---|---|
| Check whether infant needs diaper change. | | | |
| Sit comfortably in chair with infant. | | | |
| Tuck bib or clean cloth under infant's chin. | | | |
| **4. Position infant appropriately.** | | | |
| Cradle baby in arms, with head slightly elevated. Support head and neck. | | | |
| **5. Insert nipple, and feed baby.** | | | |
| Insert nipple gently along infant's tongue and hold bottle at 45° angle. | | | |
| **6. Remove bottle periodically and burp baby.** | | | |
| Place baby either over shoulder, in supported sitting position on lap, or in prone position on lap. | | | |
| Rub or pat infant's back gently. | | | |
| **7. Continue with feeding until formula is finished and/or baby is satisfied.** | | | |
| **8. Ensure infant safety and comfort after feeding. Return infant to crib or isolate.** | | | |
| Check whether diaper needs changing, and change if necessary. | | | |
| Position infant on side. | | | |
| Ensure crib sides are elevated before leaving infant. | | | |
| Assess infant for signs of allergic reaction. | | | |
| **9. Document all relevant information.** | | | |

## Procedure 37-3
## Feeding Solid Foods to an Infant

| Procedure | S | U | Comments |
|---|---|---|---|
| **1. Prepare infant for meal.** | | | |
| Change diaper if damp or soiled. | | | |
| Put bib on infant, and place infant on lap, in infant seat or highchair. | | | |
| **2. Promote acceptance and digestion of food.** | | | |
| Gently hold infant's arms or give infant something to hold to control infant's hands. | | | |
| Offer plain foods before sweet ones. | | | |

| Procedure | S | U | Comments |
|---|---|---|---|
| Place small spoonfuls of food well back on infant's tongue. | | | |
| Scrape up any food that is pushed back out of mouth, and refeed it. | | | |
| Talk to infant throughout meal. | | | |
| **3. Provide follow-up care as needed.** | | | |
| Wash and dry infant's face and hands. | | | |
| Change diaper, if needed. | | | |
| Place infant in safe position in crib. Ensure crib sides are elevated before leaving infant. | | | |
| **4. Document all relevant information.** | | | |

## 38 · Procedure 38-1
### Using a Dial-A-Flo In-line Device

| Procedure | S | U | Comments |
|---|---|---|---|
| **1. Attach Dial-A-Flo device appropriately.** | | | |
| Connect Dial-A-Flo device to end of tubing. | | | |
| Connect insertion spike of IV tubing to solution container. | | | |
| **2. Prime tubing.** | | | |
| Adjust regulator on Dial-A-Flo to open position. | | | |
| Open all clamps and infusion flow regulators on IV tubing. | | | |
| Remove protective cap at end of tubing, and allow fluid to run through tubing. | | | |
| Reclamp tubing to prevent continued flow. | | | |
| **3. Establish infusion.** | | | |
| Attach primed tubing to venipuncture needle or catheter hub. | | | |
| Open IV tubing flow regulator. | | | |
| Align Dial-A-Flo regulator to arrow indicating desired volume of fluid to infuse over 1 hour. | | | |
| **4. Confirm appropriate drip rate.** | | | |
| Count drip rate for 15 seconds and multiply by 4. | | | |
| Recheck after 5 minutes and again after 15 minutes. | | | |
| If drip rate does not coincide with that calculated, adjust height of IV pole. | | | |

| Procedure | S | U | Comments |
|-----------|---|---|----------|
| 5. Monitor volume of fluid infused at least every hour, and compare it with time tape on IV container. | | | |
| 6. Document all relevant information. | | | |

## Procedure 38-2
## Using an Infusion Controller or Pump

| Procedure | S | U | Comments |
|-----------|---|---|----------|
| *Infusion controller:* | | | |
| 1. Attach controller to IV pole below and in line with IV container. | | | |
| 2. Set up IV infusion. | | | |
| Open IV container, maintaining sterility of port, and spike container with administration set | | | |
| Place IV container on pole, and position drip chamber 76 cm (30 in) above venipuncture site. | | | |
| Fill drip chamber of IV tubing one-third full. | | | |
| Rotate drip chamber. | | | |
| Prime tubing, and close clamp. | | | |
| 3. Attach IV drop sensor, and insert IV tubing into controller. | | | |
| Attach IV drop sensor to drip chamber below drip orifice and above fluid level in drip chamber. | | | |
| Make sure sensor is plugged into controller. | | | |
| Insert tubing into controller. | | | |
| 4. Initiate infusion. | | | |
| Perform a venipuncture or connect tubing to primary IV tubing and catheter. | | | |
| Open IV control clamp completely. | | | |
| 5. Set volume dials for appropriate volume per hour. | | | |
| Set dials on front of controller to appropriate infusion rate and volume. | | | |
| Press power and start button. | | | |
| Count drops for 15 seconds and multiply result by 4. | | | |
| *Optional:* | | | |
| 6. Set alarm. | | | |

| | Procedure | S | U | Comments |
|---|---|---|---|---|
| **7.** | **Monitor infusion.** | | | |
| | Check volume of fluid infused at least every hour, and compare it with time tape on IV container. | | | |

*Infusion pump:*

| | Procedure | S | U | Comments |
|---|---|---|---|---|
| **8.** | **Attach pump at eye level on IV pole.** | | | |
| **9.** | **Set up infusion.** | | | |
| | Open IV container, maintaining sterility of port, and spike container with administration set. | | | |
| | Place IV container on IV pole above pump. | | | |
| | Fill drip chamber, and rotate it. | | | |
| | Prime tubing, and close clamp. | | | |
| **10.** | **Attach IV drop sensor and insert IV tubing into pump.** | | | |
| | Position drop sensor, if required, on drip chamber. | | | |
| | Load machine and ensure correct pressure is set. | | | |
| **11.** | **Initiate infusion.** | | | |
| **12.** | **Set dials for required drops per minute or millimeters per hour.** | | | |
| | Close door to pump and ensure IV tubing clamps are open. | | | |
| **13.** | **Set alarm and monitor infusion.** | | | |
| **14.** | **Document relevant information.** | | | |

## Procedure 38-3
## Using an Implantable Venous Access Device (IVAD)

| | Procedure | S | U | Comments |
|---|---|---|---|---|
| **1.** | **Assemble equipment.** | | | |
| | Attach IV tubing to infusion or transfusion container. | | | |
| | Prime infusion tubing with saline. | | | |
| | Prepare syringes of normal saline and heparinized saline. | | | |
| **2.** | **Position client appropriately and locate implant port.** | | | |
| | Position client in either a supine or sitting position. | | | |

| Procedure | S | U | Comments |
|---|---|---|---|
| Locate IVAD, and grasp it between two fingers of nondominant hand to stabilize it. Palpate and locate septum. | | | |
| **3. Prepare site.** | | | |
| Wash hands, and don sterile gloves. | | | |
| *Optional:* | | | |
| Insert 2% lidocaine subcutaneously in injection site. | | | |
| Prepare skin and let area dry. | | | |
| **4. Insert Huber needle.** | | | |
| Grasp device and palpate septum for injection. | | | |
| Insert needle at a 90° angle to septum, and push firmly through skin and septum until it contacts base of IVAD chamber. | | | |
| **5. Secure needle and ensure proper placement of IVAD catheter.** | | | |
| Aspirate blood when needle contacts base of septum. | | | |
| Support Huber needle with 2 x 2 dressing and Steristrips. | | | |
| Infuse saline flush and priming solution. | | | |
| **6. After use, flush system with heparinized saline.** | | | |
| When flushing, maintain positive pressure, and clamp tubing as soon as flush is finished. | | | |
| **7. Attach IV-lock to Huber needle.** | | | |
| **8. Prevent manipulation or dislodgment of needle.** | | | |
| Apply occlusive transparent dressing to needle sit. | | | |
| Apply povidone or antibiotic ointment to site before dressings are applied. | | | |
| **9. Document all relevant information.** | | | |
| *Variation:* Obtaining a blood specimen | | | |
| Withdraw 10 ml of blood and discard it. | | | |
| Draw up required amount of blood and transfer it to appropriate containers. | | | |
| Slowly instill 20 ml of normal saline over a 5 minute period. | | | |

| | Procedure | S | U | Comments |
|---|---|---|---|---|
| | Inject 5 ml of heparinized saline. | | | |

## Procedure 38-4
## Obtaining a Capillary Blood Specimen and Measuring Blood Glucose

| | Procedure | S | U | Comments |
|---|---|---|---|---|
| 1. | **Prepare equipment.** | | | |
| | Obtain reagent strip from container. | | | |
| | Insert strip into meter, and make any required adjustments. | | | |
| | Remove reagent strip from meter, and place it on clean, dry paper towel. | | | |
| 2. | **Select and prepare puncture site.** | | | |
| | Clean site with antiseptic swab, and permit it to dry. | | | |
| 3. | **Obtain blood specimen.** | | | |
| | Don gloves. | | | |
| | Place injector, if used, against site and release needle, permitting it to pierce skin. Make sure lancet is perpendicular to site. | | | |
| | or | | | |
| | Prick site with a lancet or needle, using a darting motion. | | | |
| | Wipe away first drop of blood with cotton ball. | | | |
| | Gently squeeze site until large drop of blood forms. | | | |
| | Hold reagent strip under puncture site until enough blood covers indicator squares. | | | |
| | Ask client to apply pressure to skin puncture site with cotton ball. | | | |
| 4. | **Expose blood to test strip for period of time and in manner specified by manufacturer.** | | | |
| | Press timer on glucose meter and monitor time. | | | |
| 5. | **Measure and document blood glucose.** | | | |
| | Place strip into meter according to manufacturer's instructions. | | | |

| Procedure | S | U | Comments |
|---|---|---|---|
| At desired time, activate meter to display glucose reading. | | | |
| Turn off meter and discard test strip and cotton balls. | | | |
| Document method of testing and results on client's record. If indicated, report results to physician. | | | |

## Procedure 38-5
## Obtaining a Venous Blood Specimen from an Adult by Venipuncture

| | Procedure | S | U | Comments |
|---|---|---|---|---|
| 1. | **Verify physician's orders for tests to be obtained, and obtain correct test tubes for specific test ordered.** | | | |
| 2. | **Identify client appropriately.** | | | |
| 3. | **Don gloves and perform venipuncture.** | | | |
| 4. | **Obtain specimen.** | | | |
| | *Using sterile syringe and needle:* | | | |
| | When needle is in vein, gently pull back on syringe plunger until appropriate amount of blood is obtained. | | | |
| | Remove tourniquet when sufficient blood is obtained, and remove needle from vein. Place a sterile 2 x 2 gauze over site and ask client to firmly hold it in place 2 to 3 minutes, if able. | | | |
| | Transfer specimens to tubes by removing top from laboratory test tube. Then remove needle from blood-filled syringe, and insert blood down one side of tube. | | | |
| | Replace test tube stopper. <br> or <br> Insert needle directly through stopper of blood tube, and allow vacuum to fill tube with blood. | | | |
| | For all blood tubes containing additives, gently rotate or invert test tube several times. | | | |
| | *Using a vacucontainer system:* | | | |
| | Once venipuncture needle is positioned in vein, hold plastic adapter securely, and press vacuum tube firmly into short needle until it pierces top of tube. | | | |
| | Fill vacucontainer with blood, release it, and set it aside. | | | |

| | | | | |
|---|---|---|---|---|
| | Insert another vacucontainer if more blood is required. | | | |
| 5. | **Ensure client comfort and safety.** | | | |
| | Assess client's venipuncture site. | | | |
| | When bleeding is minimized, apply a Band-Aid over site. | | | |
| 6. | **Label test tubes appropriately and send them to laboratory.** | | | |
| 7. | **Document and report relevant information.** | | | |
| *Variation:* *Collecting a blood specimen for culture* | | | | |
| | Gather equipment, including two paired sets of culture media bottles with povidone-iodine. | | | |
| | Collect 5 ml of blood from vein that does not have an IV running into it. | | | |
| | Remove venipuncture needle, and replace it with a sterile needle. | | | |
| | Swab tops of blood culture bottles. Insert needle through tops, and carefully inject 2.5 to 5 ml of blood into one or both bottles. | | | |
| | Collect second specimen after 15 minutes, and place second sample in set of paired culture bottles. | | | |

## Procedure 38-6
## Assisting with the Insertion of a Central Venous Catheter

| | | | | |
|---|---|---|---|---|
| 1. | **Prepare client.** | | | |
| | Describe procedure and explain purpose of catheter and procedures involved in care and maintenance of line. | | | |
| | Before commencing, ensure client has given informed consent. | | | |
| | Instruct client on how to perform Valsalva's maneuver. Encourage client to practice before procedure, unless contraindicated by client's condition. | | | |
| | If client is unable to perform Valsalva's maneuver: | | | |
| | a. Ask client to hold breath at end of deep inspiration or during expiratory phase of respiratory cycle and/or | | | |

| | Procedure | S | U | Comments |
|---|---|---|---|---|
| | b. Have assistant compress client's abdomen with both hands. | | | |
| **2.** | **Prepare IV infusion equipment for attachment to catheter.** | | | |
| | Connect in sequence: | | | |
| | a. Infusion tubing spike into port of normal saline or 5% dextrose in water solution container, using surgical aseptic technique. | | | |
| | b. Filter. | | | |
| | c. Extention tubing. Place filter between infusion and extension tubing. | | | |
| | Tape tubing connections. | | | |
| | Start flow of solution, place tubing protector cap on end of tubing and hang tubing on IV pole. | | | |
| **3.** | **Position client appropriately.** | | | |
| | Assist client to a Trendelenburg position. If client cannot tolerate this position, use supine or modified Trendelenburg position with only feet elevated 45° to 60°. | | | |
| | For subclavian insertion, place rolled bath blanket under client's back between shoulders. | | | |
| | For jugular insertion, place rolled bath blanket under opposite shoulder, turning client's head to opposite side. | | | |
| | For peripheral vein insertion in brachiocephalic vein or superior vena cava, place client supine with dominant arm at 90° angle to trunk. | | | |
| **4.** | **Clean and shave insertion area.** | | | |
| | Open skin preparation equipment and don gloves. | | | |
| | Wash and dry insertion site with soap and water. | | | |
| | Shave client's neck and upper thorax if ordered. | | | |
| | Discard gloves. | | | |
| | Don mask and sterile gloves. | | | |
| | Clean site with povidone-iodine sponges for 2 minutes or, if using 70% alcohol, for 10 minutes or according to agency protocol. Use circular motion, working outward. | | | |
| **5.** | **Support and monitor client.** | | | |

| | Explain procedure to client, and provide support. | | | |
|---|---|---|---|---|
| | Maintain client in position. | | | |
| | Monitior client for signs of respiratory distress, complaints of chest pain, tachycardia, pallor, or cyanosis. | | | |
| **6.** | **Attach primed IV tubing to catheter.** | | | |
| | While physician removes stylet from catheter, quickly attach IV tubing to catheter, and simultaneously ask client to perform Valsalva's maneuver as practiced. | | | |
| **7.** | **After infusion is attached, apply temporary dressing to site.** | | | |
| | Put on second pair of sterile gloves. | | | |
| | Apply povidone-iodine ointment to site if agency protocol dictates. | | | |
| | Apply 4 x 4 sterile gauze dressing or transparent occulsive dressing according to agency protocol. | | | |
| **8.** | **After x-ray examination or fluoroscopy confirms position of catheter, secure dressing with tape.** | | | |
| | Tape IV tubing to catheter. | | | |
| | Label dressing with date and time of insertion and length of catheter. | | | |
| **9.** | **Establish appropriate infusion.** | | | |
| **10.** | **Document all relevant information.** | | | |

## Procedure 38-7
## Maintaining and Monitoring a CVC System

| **1.** | **Label each lumen of multilumen catheters.** | | | |
|---|---|---|---|---|
| | Mark each lumen or port with description of its purpose, or use color code established by agency. | | | |
| **2.** | **Monitor tubing connections.** | | | |
| | Ensure all tubing connections are taped or secured according to agency protocol. | | | |
| | Check connections every 2 hours. | | | |
| | Tape cap ends if agency protocol indicates. | | | |

| Procedure | S | U | Comments |
|---|---|---|---|
| **3. Change tubing according to agency policy.** | | | |
| **4. Change catheter site dressing according to agency policy.** | | | |
| **5. Administer all infusions as ordered.** | | | |
| Use controller or pump for all fluids. | | | |
| Prime all tubing to remove air. | | | |
| Maintain fluid flow at prescribed rate. | | | |
| Whenever line is interrupted for any reason, instruct client to do Valsalva's maneuver. If client is unable to perform Valsalva's maneuver, place client in supine position, and clamp lumen of catheter with soft-tipped clamp. Place piece of tape over catheter before applying clamp. | | | |
| **6. Cap lumens without continuous infusions, and flush regularly.** | | | |
| Cap ports not in use with an intermittent infusion cap. | | | |
| Clean adapter caps with alcohol or povidone-iodine swab before penetration. | | | |
| Flush noninfusing tubings with 1 or 2 ml of heparin flush solution every eight hours or according to agency protocol. | | | |
| Aspirate for blood before flushing tubings. | | | |
| Use #25 gauge 5/8-inch needle to penetrate adapter cap when flushing catheter. | | | |
| **7. Administer medications as ordered.** | | | |
| Flush catheter line with 5 to 10 ml of normal saline according to agency protocol. | | | |
| After medication is instilled through port, inject normal saline, then heparin flush solution according to agency protocol. | | | |
| **8. Monitor client for complications.** | | | |
| Assess client's vital signs, skin color, mental alertness, appearance of catheter site, and presence of adverse symptoms at least every 4 hours. | | | |
| If air embolism is suspected, give client 100% oxygen by mask, place person in left Trendelenburg position, and notify physician. | | | |

| | S | U | Comments |
|---|---|---|---|
| If sepsis is suspected, replace infusion with 5% or 10% dextrose solution, and change IV tubing and dressing. Save remaining solution for lab analysis, record lot number of solution and any additives, and notify physician immediately. When changing dressing, take culture of catheter site as ordered by physician or according to agency protocol. | | | |
| **9.**   **Document all relevant information.** | | | |

## Procedure 38-8
## Changing a CVC Tubing and Dressing

| | S | U | Comments |
|---|---|---|---|
| *Tubing change:* | | | |
| **1.**   **Prepare client.** | | | |
| Assist client to supine position. | | | |
| **2.**   **Prepare equipment.** | | | |
| Prepare solution container, attach new IV tubing, and prime tubing. | | | |
| Remove tape securing tubing to dressing and catheter hub connection. | | | |
| Don sterile gloves and mask. | | | |
| Place sterile gauze underneath connection site of catheter and tubing. Clean junction of catheter and tubing with antiseptic, if required by agency protocol. | | | |
| **3.**   **Change tubing.** | | | |
| Ask client to perform Valsalva's maneuver. If client is unable to perform Valsalva's maneuver, place client in supine position, and clamp lumen of catheter with soft-tipped clamp. Place tape over catheter before applying clamp. | | | |
| Quickly attach new primed IV tubing to TPN catheter, ensuring tight seal. | | | |
| Release soft-tipped clamp, if used. | | | |
| Open clamp on new tubing and adjust flow to rate ordered. | | | |
| Secure tubing to catheter with tape if Luer-Lok connection is not present. | | | |
| Loop and tape tubing over dressing. | | | |
| **4.**   **Label tubing and document tubing change.** | | | |

| Procedure | S | U | Comments |
|---|---|---|---|
| Mark date and time of tubing change on new IV tubing or drip chamber. | | | |
| Document tubing change and all assessments. | | | |

*Dressing change:*

**5. Prepare client.**

| Procedure | S | U | Comments |
|---|---|---|---|
| Assist client to supine or semi-Fowler's position. | | | |
| Don mask, have client don mask (if tolerated or as agency protocol), and/or ask client to turn head away from insertion site. | | | |

**6. Prepare equipment.**

| Procedure | S | U | Comments |
|---|---|---|---|
| Wash hands before handling sterile supplies and if agency policy indicates, apply alcohol, and allow hands to air dry. | | | |
| Open sterile supplies. | | | |

**7. Change dressing.**

| Procedure | S | U | Comments |
|---|---|---|---|
| Remove soiled dressing by pulling tape slowly and gently from skin. | | | |
| Inspect skin for signs of irritation or infection. Inspect catheter for signs of leakage or other problems. If infection is suspected, take swab of drainage for culture, label it, send it to laboratory, and notify physician. | | | |
| Don sterile gloves. | | | |
| Clean catheter insertion site with sterile gauze sponges soaked in solvent such as 10% acetone. Clean in circular motion, moving from insertion site outward to edge of adhesive border. Take new sponge for each wipe. Repeat until sponge is unstained after use. | | | |
| Using above method, clean insertion site with povidone-iodine solution. If using alcohol as a substitute for iodine, clean area for 5 minutes. | | | |
| Apply precut sterile drain gauze around catheter or cut sterile 2 x 2 with sterile scissors. Apply sufficient sterile gauze dressings to cover catheter and skin. | | | |
| or | | | |
| If using Elastoplast dressing, apply tincture of benzoin to skin surrounding dressing gauzes, and allow it to air dry about 1 minute. | | | |
| Remove gloves. | | | |

**8.** **Secure dressing and tubing.**

Ask client to abduct arm and turn head away from dressing site. Tape dressing securely to skin with transparent occlusive dressing or Elastoplast.

Loop and tape IV tubing over occlusive dressing.

Label dressing with date, time, and initials.

**9.** **Document tubing and dressing change, including all nursing assessments.**

## Procedure 38-9
## Removing a Central Venous Catheter

**1.** **Prepare equipment.**

Open sterile suture removal set and establish sterile field.

Open sterile packages.

Place some povidone-iodine ointment on one sterile gauze square if ointment is to be used. Check agency protocol.

Don mask, and put one on client if necessary.

Close clamp on infusion.

**2.** **Position client appropriately.**

Place client in supine or slight Trendelenberg position.

Loosen and remove dressing.

Don sterile gloves.

Remove any sutures that secure catheter.

**3.** **Remove catheter.**

Ask client to perform Valsalva's maneuver during removal.

Grasp catheter hub or needle, and carefully withdraw it, maintaining direction of vein.

Inspect catheter to make sure it is intact. If it is not, immediately place client in left lateral Trendelenburg position and notify nurse in charge or physician immediately.

**4.** **Immediately after catheter removal, apply pressure with an air-occlusve dressing over subclavian site.**

| | | | |
|---|---|---|---|
| When bleeding is controlled, replace dressing with air-occlusive dressing while client again performs Valsalva's maneuver. | | | |
| Completely cover insertion site with povi-done-iodine ointment, if used, sterile pads, and moisture-proof tape.<br><br>or<br><br>If agency protocol indicates, use sterile transparent air-occlusive dressing. | | | |
| Leave air-occlusive dressing in place for 24 to 48 hours, or length of time agency protocol recommends. | | | |
| **5. Ensure client safety.** | | | |
| Ask client to remain flat and supine for a short time after subclavian catheter is removed. | | | |
| Observe client for signs of air embolism. | | | |
| If an air embolism is suspected, immediately place client in left lateral Trendelenburg position, and administer 100% oxygen by face mask. | | | |
| **6. Document all pertinent information including time of removal, and size, length, and condition of catheter.** | | | |

## Procedure 38-10
## Measuring Central Venous Pressure

| | | | |
|---|---|---|---|
| **1. Prepare client.** | | | |
| Place client in supine position without pillow unless this position is contraindicated. If client feels breathless, elevate head of bed slightly; note exact position. | | | |
| Locate level of client's right atrium at 4th intercostal space on midaxillary line. | | | |
| Mark site with indelible pen or piece of non-allergenic tape. | | | |
| **2. Prepare equipment.** | | | |
| Prepare IV tubing and infusion, prime tubing, and then close clamp on tubing. | | | |
| When using separate manometer and stopcock, attach manometer to stopcock. Manometer is attached to vertical arm of stopcock. | | | |

| Procedure | S | U | Comments |
|---|---|---|---|
| If using one-piece manometer and stopcock, attach them to IV pole. | | | |
| Attach IV tubing to left side of three-way stopcock. | | | |
| **3.** **Flush manometer and stopcock.** | | | |
| Do not attach stopcock to client's catheter until it is flushed free of air. | | | |
| Turn stopcock to IV-container-to-manometer position. | | | |
| Open IV tubing clamp and fill manometer with IV solution to level of about 18 to 20 cm. | | | |
| Close IV tubing clamp. | | | |
| Turn stopcock to IV-container-client position and flush stopcock. | | | |
| Close IV tubing clamp. | | | |
| **4.** **Attach manometer to central catheter.** | | | |
| Place sterile 4 x 4 gauze under catheter hub. | | | |
| Ask client to perform Valsalva's maneuver and to turn head away. Quickly attach manometer tubing to catheter. | | | |
| Turn stopcock so that IV runs into client. | | | |
| **5.** **Measure central venous pressure.** | | | |
| Check that level of client's right atrium is aligned with zero point on manometer scale. If an adjustment is required, first raise or lower bed, second readjust manometer on IV pole. | | | |
| Adjust stopcock to manometer-to-client setting. | | | |
| Observe fall in fluid level in manometer tube. Also, note slight fluctuations in fluid level with client's inspiration and expiration. If fluid level does not fluctuate, ask client to cough. | | | |
| Lightly tap manometer tube with index finger when fluid level stablizes. | | | |
| Take reading at end of an expiration or according to agency protocol. Inspect column at eye level, and take CVP reading from base of meniscus. If manometer contains small floating ball, take reading from its midline. | | | |
| Refill manometer, and take another reading of CVP. | | | |

| Procedure | S | U | Comments |
|---|---|---|---|
| Readjust stopcock to IV-container-to-client position and adjust infusion to ordered rate of flow. | | | |
| **6.** | **Return client to a comfortable position.** | | | |
| **7.** | **Document CVP.** | | | |
| Report changes in CVP as ordered. | | | |

### Procedure 39-1
### Collecting a Sputum Specimen

| Procedure | S | U | Comments |
|---|---|---|---|
| **1.** | **Give client following information and instructions:** | | | |
| Purpose of test and how to provide sputum specimen. | | | |
| Not to touch inside of sputum container. | | | |
| To expectorate sputum directly into sputum container. | | | |
| To keep outside of container free of sputum, if possible. | | | |
| How to hold pillow firmly against abdominal incision if client finds it painful to cough. | | | |
| Amount of sputum required. | | | |
| **2.** | **Provide necessary assistance to collect specimen.** | | | |
| Assist client to standing or sitting position. | | | |
| Ask client to hold sputum cup on outside. For client who is not able to do so, don gloves and hold cup for client. | | | |
| Ask client to breathe deeply and then cough up secretions. | | | |
| Hold cup so that client can expectorate into it, making sure sputum does not come into contact with outside of container. | | | |
| Assist client to repeat coughing until sufficient amount of sputum has been collected. | | | |
| Cover container with lid immediately after sputum is in container. | | | |
| If spillage occurs on outside of container, clean outer surface with disinfectant. | | | |
| **3.** | **Ensure client comfort.** | | | |
| Assist client to rinse mouth with mouthwash as needed. | | | |

| | Procedure | S | U | Comments |
|---|---|---|---|---|
| | Assist client to position of comfort that allows maximum lung expansion as required. | | | |
| 4. | **Label and transport specimen to laboratory.** | | | |
| | Ensure specimen label and laboratory requisition carry correct information. Attach securely to specimen. | | | |
| | Arrange for specimen to be sent to laboratory immediately or refrigerated. | | | |
| 5. | **Document all relevant information.** | | | |

## Procedure 39-2
## Obtaining Nose and Throat Specimens

| | | S | U | Comments |
|---|---|---|---|---|
| 1. | **Prepare client and equipment.** | | | |
| | Assist client into sitting position. | | | |
| | Don gloves if client's mucosa will be touched. | | | |
| | Remove cap from one culture tube. Lay cap on firm surface, inner side upward. | | | |
| | Remove one sterile applicator, and hold by stick end, keeping remainder sterile. | | | |
| 2. | **Collect specimen.** | | | |
| *For throat specimen:* | | | | |
| | Ask client to open mouth, extend tongue, and say *ah*. | | | |
| | If posterior pharynx cannot be seen, adjust light, and depress tongue with tongue blade. Depress tongue firmly without touching throat. | | | |
| | Insert swab into mouth, not touching any areas on pharynx that are particularly erythematous or contain exudate. | | | |
| | Remove swab without touching mouth or lips. | | | |
| | Insert swab into correctly labeled sterile tube, without touching outside of container. | | | |
| | Place top securely on tube without touching inside of cap. | | | |
| | Discard tongue blade in waste container. | | | |
| *For nasal specimen:* | | | | |
| | Gently insert lighted nasal speculum in one nostril. | | | |

| Procedure | S | U | Comments |
|---|---|---|---|
| Insert sterile swab through speculum without touching edges. | | | |
| Wipe along reddened areas or areas with most exudate. | | | |
| Remove swab without touching speculum and place it into sterile tube. | | | |
| Repeat steps for other nostril. | | | |
| **3.** **Label and transport specimens to laboratory.** | | | |
| **4.** **Document all relevant information.** | | | |

## Procedure 39-3
## Assisting a Client to Use a Sustained Maximal Inspiration (SMI) Device

| Procedure | S | U | Comments |
|---|---|---|---|
| **1.** **Prepare client.** | | | |
| Explain procedure. | | | |
| Assist client into upright position in bed or chair. | | | |
| *For Flow-Oriented SMI:* | | | |
| **2.** **Set spirometer.** | | | |
| If spirometer has inspiratory volume-level pointer, set pointer at prescribed level. | | | |
| **3.** **Instruct client to use spirometer as follows:** | | | |
| Hold spirometer in upright position. | | | |
| Exhale normally. | | | |
| Seal lips tightly around mouthpiece and take in slow, deep breath to elevate balls. Then, hold breath for 2 seconds initially, increasing to 6 seconds keeping balls elevated if possible. Instruct client to avoid brisk, low-volume breaths that snap balls to top of chamber. | | | |
| Remove mouthpiece and exhale normally. | | | |
| Cough productively, if possible, after using spirometer. | | | |
| Relax, and take several deep breaths before using spirometer again. | | | |
| Repeat procedure several times, and then, four or five times hourly. | | | |

| Procedure | S | U | Comments |
|---|---|---|---|

*For Volume-Oriented SMI:*

**4. Set spirometer to predetermined volume. Check physician's or respiratory therapist's order.**

**5. Instruct client to use spirometer as follows:**

Exhale normally.

Seal lips tightly around mouthpiece, and take slow, deep breath until piston is elevated to predetermined level.

Hold breath for 6 seconds.

Remove mouthpiece, and exhale normally.

Cough productively, if possible, after using spirometer.

Relax, and take several normal breaths before using spirometer again.

Repeat procedure several times, then four to five times hourly.

*For all devices:*

**6. Clean and put away equipment.**

Clean mouthpiece with sterile water, and shake dry. Label mouth piece and disposable SMI with client's name, and store in bedside unit. Change disposable mouthpiece every 24 hours.

**7. Document all relevant information.**

## Procedure 39-4
## Administering Percussion, Vibration, and Postural Drainage (PVD) to Adults

**1. Prepare client.**

Provide visual and auditory privacy.

Explain positions client will need to assume, as well as percussion and vibration techniques.

**2. Assist client to appropriate position for postural drainage.**

Use pillows to support client comfortably in required positions.

**3. Percuss affected area.**

Ensure area to be percussed is covered by towel or gown.

254

| Procedure | S | U | Comments |
|---|---|---|---|
| Ask client to breathe slowly and deeply. | | | |
| Cup hands, relax wrist, and flex elbows. | | | |
| With both hands cupped, alternately flex and extend wrists rapidly to slap chest. | | | |
| Percuss each affected lung segment for 1 to 2 minutes. Percussing action should produce hollow, popping sound. | | | |
| **4. Vibrate affected area.** | | | |
| Place flattened hands, one over other (or side by side) against affected chest area. | | | |
| Ask client to inhale deeply through mouth and exhale slowly through pursed lips or nose. | | | |
| During exhalation, straighten elbows, lean slightly against client's chest while tensing arm and shoulder muscles in isometric contractions. | | | |
| Vibrate during five exhalations over one affected lung segment. | | | |
| Encourage client to cough and expectorate secretions into sputum container. Offer client tissues and mouthwash. | | | |
| Auscultate client's lungs, and compare findings to baseline data. | | | |
| **5. Label and transport specimen, if obtained.** | | | |
| Arrange for specimen to be sent to laboratory immediately, or refrigerate. | | | |
| **6. Document percussion, vibration, and postural drainage and assessments.** | | | |

## Procedure 39-5
## Administering Percussion, Vibration, and Postural Drainage (PVD) to Infants and Children

| Procedure | S | U | Comments |
|---|---|---|---|
| **1. Prepare infant or child.** | | | |
| Provide explanation suitable to child's age. | | | |
| Assist child to appropriate position for postural drainage. | | | |
| Use pillows to support client comfortably in required positions. | | | |
| **2. Percuss affected area using percussion device if appropriate, or three finger-tips flexed and held together.** | | | |

| Procedure | S | U | Comments |
|---|---|---|---|
| Vibrate affected area as appropriate, using vibrator appropriate to child's age. | | | |
| Instruct child to sit up, and encourage deep breathing and coughing to remove loosened secretions.<br><br>or<br><br>Suction airway. | | | |
| Repeat percussion, vibration, deep breathing, and coughing for each lobe requiring drainage. | | | |
| **3.** **Document PVD and all assessments.** | | | |

## Procedure 39-6
## Bulb Suctioning an Infant

| Procedure | S | U | Comments |
|---|---|---|---|
| **1.** **Position infant appropriately for procedure.** | | | |
| Bundle infant in large towel or blanket to restrain arms, or cradle child with arm, tucking infant's near arm behind back and holding other arm securely with hand. | | | |
| Put bib or towel under infant's chin. | | | |
| **2.** **Suction oral and nasal cavities.** | | | |
| Compress bulb of syringe with thumb before inserting syringe. | | | |
| Keeping bulb compressed, insert tip of syringe into infant's nose or mouth. | | | |
| Release bulb compression gradually, and slowly move it outward to aspirate secretions. | | | |
| Remove syringe, hold tip over waste receptacle, and compress bulb again. | | | |
| Repeat until infant's nares and mouth are clear of secretions and breathing sounds are clear. | | | |
| **3.** **Ensure infant comfort and safety.** | | | |
| Cuddle and soothe infant as necessary. Place infant in side-lying or prone position. | | | |
| **4.** **Ensure availability of equipment for next suction.** | | | |
| Rinse syringe and waste receptacle. | | | |
| Place syringe in clean folded towel at cribside. | | | |

| Procedure | S | U | Comments |
|---|---|---|---|

**5.** Document all relevant information.

*Variation:*

    DeLee suction Device (Mucus Trap).

## Procedure 39-7
## Administering Oxygen by Humidity Tent

**1.** Verify physician's order.

**2.** Prepare child.

    Provide an explanation appropriate to age of child.

    Cover child with gown or cotton blanket.

**3.** Prepare humidity tent.

    Close zippers on each side of tent.

    Fan-fold front part of canopy into bedclothes or into an overlying drawsheet, and ensure all sides of canopy are tucked well under mattress.

    If cool mist is ordered, fill trough with ice to depth indicated by line.

    Ensure drainage tube for trough is in place.

    Fill water jar with sterile distilled water.

    Connect tent to wall oxygen or compressed air.

    Flood tent with oxygen by setting flow meter at 15 liters per minute for about 5 minutes. Adjust flow meter according to orders.

    Open damper valve for about 5 minutes to increase humidity.

**4.** Place child in tent and assess child's respiratory status.

    Assess vital signs, skin color, breathing, and chest movements.

**5.** Provide required care for child.

    Change bedding and clothing when damp.

    Place small pillow or rolled towel at head of tent.

**6.** Monitor functioning of humidity tent.

**7.** Document relevant data.

### Procedure 39-8
### Inserting and Maintaining a Pharyngeal Airway

| Procedure | S | U | Comments |
|---|---|---|---|
| **1. Insert airway.** | | | |
| *Oropharyngeal airway:* | | | |
| Place client in supine position with neck hyperextended or with pillow placed under shoulders. | | | |
| Don disposable gloves, open client's mouth, and place tongue depressor on anterior half of tongue. | | | |
| Remove dentures, if present. | | | |
| Lubricate airway with water-soluble lubricant or with cool water. | | | |
| Turn airway upside down, with curved end upwards or sideways, and advance it along roof of mouth. | | | |
| When airway passes uvula, rotate airway until curve of airway follows natural curve of tongue. | | | |
| Remove excess lubricant from client's lips. | | | |
| *Nasopharyngeal airway:* | | | |
| Assess patency of each naris. | | | |
| Ask client, if conscious, to blow nose. | | | |
| Lubricate entire tube with a topical anesthetic, if ordered. | | | |
| Hold airway by wide end and insert narrow end into naris, applying gentle inward and downward pressure when advancing airway. | | | |
| Advance airway until external horn fits against outer naris. | | | |
| Remove excess lubricant from nares. | | | |
| **2. Tape airway in position, if required.** | | | |
| **3. Ensure client's comfort and safety.** | | | |
| *Oropharyngeal tube:* | | | |
| Maintain client in lateral or semiprone position. | | | |
| Suction secretions as required. | | | |
| Provide mouth care as required. | | | |

|  | S | U | Comments |
|---|---|---|---|
| Remove airway once client has regained consciousness and has swallow, gag, and cough reflexes. | | | |
| *Nasopharyngeal tube:* | | | |
| Remove tube, clean it with warm, soapy water, and insert in other nostril at least every 8 hours, or as ordered. | | | |
| Provide nasal hygiene every 4 hours or more if needed. | | | |
| **4.** **Document all relevant information.** | | | |

### Procedure 39-9
### Deflating and Inflating a Cuffed Tracheostomy Tube

|  | S | U | Comments |
|---|---|---|---|
| **1.** **Position client appropriately.** | | | |
| Assist client into semi-Fowler's position unless contraindicated. | | | |
| Place clients receiving positive pressure ventilation in supine position. | | | |
| **2.** **Deflate cuff.** | | | |
| Suction oropharyngeal cavity. | | | |
| Discard catheter. | | | |
| Attach 5 or 10 ml syringe to distal end of inflation tube, making sure seal is tight. | | | |
| While client inhales, slowly withdraw amount of air from cuff indicated by manufacturer, or as orders indicate, while providing positive pressure breath with manual resuscitator. | | | |
| Keep syringe attached to tubing. | | | |
| If cough reflex is stimulated during cuff-deflation, suction lower airway with sterile catheter. | | | |
| Assess client's respirations and suction client as needed. If client experiences breathing difficulties, immediately reinflate cuff. | | | |
| **3.** **Reinflate cuff to minimal occluding volume (MOV) using minimal air leak technique (MLT).** | | | |
| Use stethoscope over client's neck, adjacent to trachea while inflating cuff. | | | |
| Inflate cuff on inhalation, and inject least amount of air needed (usually 2 to 5 ml) to achieve tracheal seal. | | | |

| | | | |
|---|---|---|---|
| Stop cuff inflation when there is no audible air leak on auscultation. | | | |
| Establish minimum air leak by listening to client's neck with stethoscope and aspirating small amount of air until slight leak is detected. | | | |
| Note exact amount of air used to inflate cuff to achieve minimal air leak. | | | |
| Remove syringe. | | | |
| **4.** **Measure cuff pressure.** | | | |
| Make sure client is in same position for each pressure cuff reading. | | | |
| Attach cuff's pilot port to cuff pressure manometer tubing. | | | |
| Read dial on manometer. Pressure should not exceed 15 to 20 mm Hg or 25 cm $H_2O$. | | | |
| Remove syringe. | | | |
| **5.** **Ensure client comfort and safety.** | | | |
| Check cuff pressure every 8 to 12 hours. Note whether MOV increases or decreases. | | | |
| Make sure client is comfortable and call signal and communication aids are within easy reach. | | | |
| **6.** **Document all relevant information.** | | | |
| *Variation:* Using a stopcock to measure cuff pressure | | | |
| Attach ends of stopcock to manometer tubing, syringe, and pilot port of cuff. | | | |
| Make sure stopcock dial to pilot is in "off" position. | | | |
| Ensure tight seal at all connections. | | | |
| Turn stopcock dial to "off" position to syringe. | | | |
| Note pressure reading on manometer as client exhales. | | | |
| Turn stopcock dial to "off" position to pilot balloon, and disconnect apparatus. | | | |

## Procedure 39-10
## Plugging a Tracheostomy Tube

| | | | |
|---|---|---|---|
| **1.** **Position client.** | | | |

|  |  |  |
|---|---|---|
| Assist client into semi-Fowler's position unless contraindicated. |  |  |

**2. Suction airways.**

|  |  |  |
|---|---|---|
| Suction client's nasopharynx if there are any secretions present. |  |  |
| Change suction catheters and suction tracheostomy. |  |  |

**3. Deflate tracheal cuff if ordered.**

|  |  |  |
|---|---|---|
| Suction tracheostomy tube again if secretions are present. |  |  |

**4. Insert tracheostomy plug.**

|  |  |  |
|---|---|---|
| Using sterile gloves, fit tracheostomy plug into either inner or outer cannula, depending on whether tracheostomy tube has double or single cannula. |  |  |
| Monitor client closely for 10 minutes for signs of respiratory distress. At first signs of respiratory distress, remove plug, and suction tracheostomy if necessary. |  |  |
| Clean inner cannula, if it was removed. |  |  |
| Observe client frequently while tube is plugged. |  |  |

**5. Remove plug at designated time.**

|  |  |  |
|---|---|---|
| After removing plug, suction tracheostomy if indicated, and replace inner cannula if removed. |  |  |
| Reinflate cuff if ordered. |  |  |

**6. Document all relevant information.**

## Procedure 39-11
## Assisting with the Insertion of a Chest Tube

**1. Prepare client.**

|  |  |  |
|---|---|---|
| Explain placement and rationale for chest tube(s) to client and family. |  |  |
| Assist client into lateral position with area to receive tube facing upward. Determine from physician whether to have bed in supine position or semi-Fowler's. |  |  |

**2. Prepare equipment.**

|  |  |  |
|---|---|---|
| Open chest tube tray and sterile gloves on overbed table. |  |  |

| | Procedure | S | U | Comments |
|---|---|---|---|---|
| | Pour antiseptic solution onto sponges. | | | |
| | Cleanse stopper of local anesthetic with alcohol swab and invert vial and hold it for physician to aspirate medication. | | | |
| | Maintain sterile technique. | | | |
| 3. | **Provide emotional support and monitor client as required.** | | | |
| 4. | **Provide airtight dressing.** | | | |
| | After tube insertion: Don sterile gloves and wrap piece of sterile petrolatum gauze around chest tube. Place drain gauzes around insertion site. Place several 4 x 4 gauze squares over them. | | | |
| | Tape dressings, covering them completely. | | | |
| 5. | **Secure chest tube appropriately.** | | | |
| | Tape chest tube to client's skin away from insertion site. | | | |
| | Tape connections of chest tube to drainage tube and to drainage system. | | | |
| | Coil drainage tubing and secure it to bed linen, ensuring enough slack for client movement. | | | |
| 6. | **When all drainage connections are completed, ask client to:** | | | |
| | Take deep breath and hold it for a few seconds and then slowly exhale. | | | |
| 7. | **Ensure client safety.** | | | |
| | Place rubber-tipped chest tube clamps at bedside. | | | |
| | Assess client regularly for signs of pneumothorax and subcutaneous emphysema. | | | |
| | Assess client's vital signs every 15 minutes for first hour, then as ordered. | | | |
| | Auscultate lungs every 4 hours. | | | |
| | Check for intermittent bubbling in water-seal bottle or chamber. | | | |
| 8. | **Prepare client for portable chest X-ray.** | | | |
| 9. | **Document all relevant information.** | | | |

| Procedure | S | U | Comments |
|---|---|---|---|

**Procedure 39-12**
**Monitoring a Client with Chest Drainage**

**1. Assess client.**

Assess vital signs every 4 hours or more often, as indicated.

Determine ease of respirations, breath sounds, respiratory rate, and chest movement.

Monitor client for signs of pneumothorax.

Inspect dressing for excessive and abnormal drainage. Palpate around dressing site, and listen for crackling sound.

Assess level of discomfort.

**2. Implement all necessary safety precautions.**

Keep two 15- to 18-cm (6- to 7-in) Kelly clamps within reach at bedside.

Keep one sterile petrolatum gauze within reach at bedside.

Keep extra drainage system available in client's room. In emergency situations such as malfunction or breakage:

a. Clamp chest tube close to insertion site with two rubber-tipped clamps placed in opposite directions.
b. Reestablish water-sealed drainage system.
c. Remove clamps and notify physician.

Keep drainage system below chest level and upright at all times, unless chest tubes are clamped.

**3. Maintain patency of drainage system.**

Check that all connections are secured with tape.

Inspect drainage tubing for kinks or loops dangling below entry level of drainage system.

Coil drainage tubing and secure to bed linen, ensuring enough slack for client movement.

Inspect air vent in system periodically for occlusions.

Milk or strip chest tubing as ordered and only in accordance with agency protocol.

|  | To milk chest tube, follow these steps: | | | |
|---|---|---|---|---|
|  | a. Lubricate about 10 to 20 cm (4 to 8 in) of drainage tubing. | | | |
|  | b. With one hand, securely stabilize and pinch tube at insertion site. | | | |
|  | c. Compress tube with thumb and forefinger of hand and milk it by sliding down tube, moving away from insertion site. | | | |
|  | d. If entire tube is to be milked, reposition hands farther along tubing, and repeat steps **a** through **c** in progressive overlapping steps, until end of tubing is reached. | | | |
| **4.** | **Assess any fluid level fluctuation and bubbling in drainage system.** | | | |
|  | In gravity drainage systems, check for fluctuation (tidaling) of fluid level in water-seal glass tube in bottle system or water-seal chamber in commercial system as client breathes. | | | |
|  | To check for fluctuation in suction systems, temporarily turn off suction and observe fluctuation. | | | |
|  | Check for intermittent bubbling in water of water-seal bottle or chamber. | | | |
|  | Check for gentle bubbling in suction-control bottle or chamber. | | | |
| **5.** | **Assess drainage.** | | | |
|  | Inspect drainage in collection container at least every 30 minutes during first two hours after chest tube insertion, and every 2 hours thereafter. | | | |
|  | Every 8 hours mark time, date, and drainage level on adhesive tape and affix to container, or mark it directly on disposable container. | | | |
|  | Note any sudden change in amount or color of drainage. If drainage exceeds 100 ml per hour or if color change indicates hemorrhage, notify physician immediately. | | | |
| **6.** | **Watch for dislodgement of tubes and remedy problem promptly.** | | | |
|  | If chest tube become disconnected from drainage system: | | | |
|  | a. Have client exhale fully. | | | |

b. Clamp chest tube close to insertion site with two rubber-tipped clamps in opposite direction.

c. Quickly clean ends of tubing with an antiseptic, reconnect, and tape securely.

d. Unclamp tube as soon as possible.

e. Assess client closely for respiratory distress.

f. Check vital signs every 10 minutes.

If chest tube becomes dislodged from insertion site:

a. Remove dressing, and immediately apply pressure with petrolatum gauze, hand or towel.

b. Cover site with sterile 4 x 4 gauze squares.

c. Tape dressing with air-occlusive tape.

d. Notify physician immediately.

e. Assess client for respiratory distress every 10 to 15 minutes or as client condition indicates.

If drainage system is accidentally tipped over:

a. Immediately return it to upright position.

b. Ask client to take several deep breaths.

c. Notify nurse in charge and physician.

d. Assess client for respiratory distress.

7. **If continuous bubbling persists in water-seal collection chamber, indicating an air leak, determine its source.**

To detect an air leak, follow next steps sequentially:

a. Check tubing connection sites. Tighten and retape any that appear loose.

b. If bubbling continues, clamp chest tube near insertion site and determine if bubbling stops while client takes several deep breaths.

c. If bubbling stops, proceed with next step. Source of air leak is above clamp. It may be at insertion site or inside client.

d. If bubbling continues, source of air leak is below clamp. See next step below.

To determine if air leak is at insertion site or inside of client:

a. Unclamp tube and palpate gently around insertion site. If bubbling stops, leak is at insertion site. Apply a petrolatum gauze and 4 x 4 gauze around insertion site, and secure dressings with adhesive tape.

b. If leak is not at insertion site, it is inside client. Leave tube unclamped, notify physician, and monitor client for signs of respiratory distress.

To locate air leak below chest tube clamp:

a. Move clamp a few inches down and keep moving it downward a few inches at a time. Each time clamp is moved, check water-seal collection chamber for bubbling.
b. When leak is located, seal leak by applying tape to that portion of drainage tube.
c. If bubbling continues after entire length of tube is clamped, air leak is in drainage device. Replace drainage system according to agency protocol.

**8. Take specimen of chest drainage as required.**

Specimens of chest drainage are taken from disposable systems through self-sealing port. If specimen is required:

a. Use a povidone-iodine swab to wipe self-sealing diaphragm on back of drainage collection chamber. Allow to dry.
b. Attach sterile #18 or #20 gauge needle to 3- or 5-ml syringe and insert needle into diaphragm.
c. Aspirate specimen, label syringe, and send to laboratory with appropriate requisition form.

**9. Ensure essential client care.**

Encourage deep-breathing and coughing exercises every 2 hours if indicated. Have client sit upright to perform exercises, and splint tube insertion site with pillow or hand.

While client takes deep breaths, palpate chest for thoracic expansion. Note whether chest expansion is symmetric.

Reposition client every 2 hours. When client is lying down on affected side, place rolled towels beside tubing.

Assist client with range-of-motion exercises of affected shoulder three times per day.

When transporting and ambulating client:

a. Attach rubber-tipped forceps to client's gown.
b. Keep water-seal unit below chest level and upright.

| Procedure | S | U | Comments |
|---|---|---|---|

    c. If necessary to clamp tube, remove clamp as soon as possible or in accordance with client's condition.

    d. Disconnect drainage system from suction apparatus before moving client and make sure air vent is open.

**10.**   **Document all relevant information.**

---

## Procedure 39-13
## Assisting with the Removal of a Chest Tube

**1.**   **Prepare client.**

Administer analgesic, if ordered, 30 minutes before tube is removed.

Ensure chest tube is securely clamped.

Assist client into semi-Fowler's position or to lateral position on unaffected side.

Put absorbent pad under client beneath chest tube.

Instruct client to perform Valsalva's maneuver when physician removes chest tube.

**2.**   **Prepare sterile field and sterile air-tight gauze.**

Open sterile packages and prepare sterile field.

Don sterile gloves and place sterile petrolatum gauze on 4 x 4 gauze square.

**3.**   **Remove soiled dressing.**

While wearing gloves, be careful not to dislodge tube when removing underlying gauzes.

**4.**   **Prepare strips of air-occlusive tape.**

While physician is removing tube, prepare three 15 cm (6 in) strips of air-occlusive tape.

After petrolatum gauze dressing is applied over insertion site immediately after removal, completely cover it with air-occlusive tape.

**5.**   **Provide emotional support and monitor client's response to chest tube removal.**

**6.**   **Assess client.**

Monitor vital signs and assess quality of respirations as ordered or as condition indicates.

| | | | |
|---|---|---|---|
| Auscultate client's lungs every 4 hours. | | | |
| Assess client regularly for signs of pneumothorax, subcutaneous emphysema, and infection. | | | |
| **7.** Prepare client for chest X-ray if ordered. | | | |
| **8.** Document relevant information. | | | |

### Procedure 39-14
### Clearing an Obstructed Airway

| | | | |
|---|---|---|---|
| *Abdominal thrusts: standing or sitting victim* | | | |
| **1.** Identify yourself as a trained rescuer. | | | |
| Stand behind victim and wrap arms around person's waist. | | | |
| Direct bystander to call EMS. | | | |
| **2.** Give abdominal thrusts. | | | |
| Make fist with one hand, tuck thumb inside of fist, place flexed thumb just above victim's navel and below xiphoid process. | | | |
| With other hand, grasp fist and press it into person's abdomen with firm, quick upward thrust. | | | |
| Deliver successive thrusts as separate and complete movements until victim's airway clears or victim becomes unconscious. | | | |
| *Abdominal thrusts: unconscious victim lying on ground* | | | |
| **1.** Direct bystander to call EMS. | | | |
| **2.** Airway management. | | | |
| Tilt victim's head back, lift chin, and pinch nose shut. | | | |
| Give two slow breaths. If unable to ventilate, re-tilt head and repeat breaths. | | | |
| **3.** Give abdominal thrusts. | | | |
| Straddle one or both of victim's legs. | | | |
| Place heel of one hand slightly above victim's navel and well below xiphoid process. | | | |
| Place other hand directly on top of first; shoulders are over victim's abdomen and elbows are straight. | | | |
| **4.** Foreign object check. | | | |

| Procedure | S | U | Comments |
|---|---|---|---|
| Using fingers and thumb, lift victim's lower jaw and tongue. Slide one finger down inside cheek and attempt to hook object out. In children, perform finger sweep only if object can be seen. | | | |
| Repeat abdominal thrusts, airway maneuvers, and foreign object checks until airway is clear or victim breathes. | | | |

*Chest thrusts: conscious standing or sitting person*

| Procedure | S | U | Comments |
|---|---|---|---|
| **1.**   **Identify yourself as a trained rescuer.** | | | |
| Stand behind victim with arms under victim's armpits and encircling victim's chest. | | | |
| Direct bystander to call EMS. | | | |
| Place thumb side of fist on middle of victim's breastbone. | | | |
| **2.**   **Deliver thrusts.** | | | |
| Grab fist with other hand and deliver quick backward thrust. | | | |
| Repeat thrusts until obstruction is relieved or victim become unconscious. | | | |

*Chest thrusts: unconscious victim lying flat*

| Procedure | S | U | Comments |
|---|---|---|---|
| **1.**   **Airway management.** | | | |
| Tilt victim's head back, lift chin, and pinch nose shut. | | | |
| Give two slow breaths. If unable to ventilate, re-tilt head and repeat breaths. | | | |
| **2.**   **Deliver thrusts.** | | | |
| Position victim supine and kneel close to side of victim's trunk. | | | |
| Position hands as for cardiac compression with heel of hand on lower half of sternum. | | | |
| **3.**   **Foreign object check.** | | | |
| Using fingers and thumb, lift victim's lower jaw and tongue. Slide one finger down inside cheek and attempt to hook object out. In children, perform finger sweep only if object can be seen. | | | |
| Repeat chest thrusts, airway maneuvers, and foreign object checks until airway is clear or victim breathes. | | | |

*Back blows and chest thrusts for infants*

| Procedure | S | U | Comments |
|---|---|---|---|
| **1.**   **Deliver back blows.** | | | |

269

| Procedure | S | U | Comments |
|---|---|---|---|
| Straddle infant over forearm with head lower than trunk. | | | |
| Support head by firmly holding jaw in hand. | | | |
| With heel of free hand, deliver five sharp blows to infant's back over spine between shoulder blades. | | | |
| **2. Deliver chest thrusts.** | | | |
| Turn infant as a unit to supine postion. | | | |
| Place free hand on infant's back. | | | |
| While continuing to support jaw, neck, and chest with other hand, turn and place infant on thigh with head lower than trunk. | | | |
| Using two fingers, administer five chest thrusts over sternum, one finger width below nipple line. | | | |
| In conscious infant, continue chest thrusts and back blows until airway is cleared or infant becomes unconscious. | | | |
| If infant is unconscious, assess airway and give two breaths. If unable to ventilate, re-tilt infant's head and give two breaths. If air does not go in, give back blows and chest thrusts. | | | |
| Lift jaw and tongue and check for foreign object. If object is seen, sweep it out with finger. | | | |
| Repeat sequence of foreign object checks, breaths, back blows, and chest thrusts until airway clears or infant begins to breathe. | | | |
| *Finger sweep* | | | |
| **1. Don disposable gloves.** | | | |
| **2. Open victim's mouth by grasping tongue and lower jaw between thumb and fingers, and lifting jaw upward.** | | | |
| **3. Insert index finger of free hand along inside of victim's cheek and deep into throat.** | | | |
| With finger hooked, use sweeping motion to try to dislodge and lift out foreign object. | | | |
| If measures fail, try abdominal thrusts in adults and children. With infant, give back blows and chest thrusts. | | | |
| **4. After removing foreign object, clear out liquid material with a scooping motion using two fingers wrapped with tissue or cloth.** | | | |

| | Procedure | S | U | Comments |
|---|---|---|---|---|
| 5. | After maneuver, assess air exhange. | | | |
| 6. | Document relevant information. | | | |

### Procedure 39-15
### Administering Oral Resuscitation

| | Procedure | S | U | Comments |
|---|---|---|---|---|
| 1. | **Clear mouth and throat of obstructive material and position victim appropriately.** | | | |
| | Clear mouth and throat using finger sweep. | | | |
| | If victim is lying on one side or face down, turn victim as a unit supporting head and neck, onto back and kneel beside head. | | | |
| 2. | **Open airway.** | | | |
| | Use head-tilt, chin-lift maneuver or jaw-thrust maneuver. Use modified jaw-thrust for persons with suspected neck injury. | | | |
| | *Head-tilt, chin-lift maneuver:* | | | |
| | Place one hand palm down on forehead. | | | |
| | Place fingers of other hand on bony part of lower jaw near chin. | | | |
| | Simultaneously press down on forehead and lift victim's chin. | | | |
| | Open victim's mouth by pressing lower lip downward with thumb after tilting head. | | | |
| | Remove dentures if they cannot be maintained in place. | | | |
| | *Jaw-thrust maneuver:* | | | |
| | Kneel at top of victim's head. | | | |
| | Grasp angle of mandible directly below earlobe between thumb and forefinger on each side of victim's head. | | | |
| | While tilting head backward, lift lower jaw until it juts forward and is higher that upper jaw. | | | |
| | Rest elbows on surface which victim is lying. | | | |
| | Retract lower lip with thumbs prior to giving artificial respiration. | | | |
| | *Modified jaw-thrust maneuver:* | | | |
| | Perform first two steps for jaw-thrust. | | | |
| | Do not tilt head backward while lifting lower jaw forward. | | | |

| Procedure | S | U | Comments |
|---|---|---|---|

Support head carefully without hyperextending it or moving it from side to side.

**3. Determine victim's ability to breathe.**

Place ear and cheek to victim's mouth and nose.

Look at chest and abdomen for rising and falling movement.

Listen for air escaping during exhalation.

Feel for air escaping against cheek.

**4. If no breathing is evident, provide rescue breathing if required.**

Use mouth-to-mouth, mouth-to-nose, mouth-to-mask, or hand-compressible breathing bag method.

*Mouth-to-mouth:*

Put on mouth shield.

Maintain open airway.

Pinch victim's nostrils with index finger and thumb.

Take deep breath, and place mouth opened widely around victim's mouth. Ensure airtight seal.

Deliver two full breaths of 1-1/2 seconds each into victim's mouth.

Ensure adequate ventilation by observing victim's chest rise and fall.

If initial ventilation attempt is unsucessful, reposition victim's head and repeat rescue breathing. If victim still cannot be ventilated, proceed to clear airway of any foreign objects by using finger sweep, abdominal thrusts, or chest thrusts.

*Mouth-to-nose:*

Maintain head-tilt and chin-lift.

Close victim's mouth by pressing hand against victim's chin.

Put on mouth shield.

Take deep breath, seal lips around victim's nose.

Deliver two full breaths of 1-1/2 seconds each.

|  |  |  |  |
|---|---|---|---|
| Remove mouth from victim's nose and allow to exhale passively. |  |  |  |
| *Mouth-to-mask:* |  |  |  |
| Remove mask from case and push out dome. |  |  |  |
| Connect one-way valve to mask. |  |  |  |
| Kneel at top of victim's head, and open airway using jaw-thrust maneuver. |  |  |  |
| Place bottom rim of mask between victim's lower lip and chin. Place rest of mask over face using thumbs on each side to hold mask in place. |  |  |  |
| Perform jaw-thrust manuever to tilt head backward. Use three fingers of both hands behind angles of jaw, and grasp victim's temples with palm of hands. |  |  |  |
| Maintain head position while blowing intermittently into mouth piece. |  |  |  |
| *Hand-compressible breathing bag:* |  |  |  |
| Stand at victim's head. |  |  |  |
| Use one hand to secure mask and to hold victim's jaw forward. Use other hand to squeeze and release bag. |  |  |  |
| **5.** **Determine whether victim's breathing is restored.** |  |  |  |
| **6.** **Determine presence of carotid pulse.** |  |  |  |
| Take about 5 to 10 seconds for this pulse check. |  |  |  |
| **7.** **Assess airway patency, rate, rhythm, and quality of respirations; level of consciouness; breath sounds; and vital signs.** |  |  |  |
| **8.** **Document relevant information.** |  |  |  |

## Procedure 39-16
## Administering External Cardiac Compressions

|  |  |  |  |
|---|---|---|---|
| **1.** **Survey scene for safety hazards, presence of bystanders, and other victims.** |  |  |  |
| **2.** **Assess victim's level of consciousness, patency of airway, presence/absence of breathing, and pulse.** |  |  |  |
| Ask victim "Are you alright?" |  |  |  |

| | Procedure | S | U | Comments |
|---|---|---|---|---|
| | If victim does not respond, in a health care facility call a "code" or follow agency protocol. If alone outside of health care facility, call for help and have another person call for EMS or 911. | | | |
| **3.** | **Position victim appropriately.** | | | |
| | Place victim in supine position. If in a health care facility, place cardiac board under victim's back, or place victim on floor if necessary. | | | |
| | If victim must be turned, turn body as a unit while supporting head and neck. | | | |
| | Have a bystander elevate lower extremities, if possible. | | | |
| **4.** | **Assess airway, breathing, and circulation.** | | | |
| | *Airway:* | | | |
| | Clear and open airway, if necessary. | | | |
| | *Breathing:* | | | |
| | Assess breathing: look, listen, and feel for air flow. | | | |
| | Ventilate victim if breathing is not restored. | | | |
| | Deliver two full breaths into victim's mouth. | | | |
| | If unable to ventilate, reposition victim's head and repeat two breaths. | | | |
| | If still unsuccessful, follow procedures for obstructed airway. | | | |
| | *Circulation:* | | | |
| | Assess carotid pulse for 5 to 10 seconds. | | | |
| | If pulse is present, continue rescue breathing at 12 breaths per minute while monitoring pulse. | | | |
| | If pulse is absent, begin external chest compressions. | | | |
| **5.** | **Position hands on sternum.** | | | |
| | Use middle and index fingers to locate lower margin of rib cage. | | | |
| | Move fingers up rib cage to notch where lower ribs meet sternum. | | | |
| | Place heel of other hand along lower half of victim's sternum. | | | |

| Procedure | S | U | Comments |
|---|---|---|---|
| Place first hand on top of second hand, and extend or interlace fingers. | | | |
| Lock elbows, straighten arms, and position shoulders directly over hands. | | | |
| For each compression, thrust straight down on sternum. For adult, depress sternum 3.8 to 5.0 cm (1.5 to 2 in). | | | |
| Completely release compression pressure, but do not lift or move hands. | | | |
| Provide external cardiac compressions at rate of 80 to 100 per minute. Count "one and, two and," and so on. | | | |
| Administer 5 or 15 external compressions depending on number of rescuers, and coordinate with rescue breathing. | | | |
| *CPR performed by one rescuer:* | | | |
| If there is no bystander, and rescuer is alone, summon help and then perform CPR. | | | |
| Perform two rescue breaths. | | | |
| Perform 15 external chest compressions at rate of 80 to 100 per minute. Counting "one and, two and," up to 15. | | | |
| Alternate rescue breathing and external compressions for four complete cycles. | | | |
| Assess victim's carotid pulse after four cycles. If there is no pulse, continue CPR, checking pulse every few minutes. | | | |
| *CPR performed by two rescuers:* | | | |
| Second rescuer, identified as a trained rescuer, verifies that EMS has been notified. | | | |
| First rescuer completes cycle of compression with two breaths. Second rescuer gets into position to give compressions. | | | |
| First rescuer assesses carotid pulse for five seconds, and if pulse is absent, gives one breath and then states, "No pulse, continue CPR." | | | |
| Second rescuer then provides compressions, and paces by counting aloud, "one and, two and, three and, four and, five and, ventilate." | | | |
| First rescuer provides one ventilation after every five chest compressions, and observes each breath for effectiveness. | | | |

| Procedure | S | U | Comments |
|---|---|---|---|
| First rescuer assesses carotid pulse frequently between breaths for effectiveness of cardiac compressions. Also observes for overinflation of lungs by watching for abdominal distention. | | | |
| When second rescuer becomes fatigued, position change is indicated by stating, "Change one and, two and, three and, four and, five and . . ." Then moves to victim's head and counts pulse for 5 seconds. | | | |
| Person ventilating gives breath and moves into position to provide compressions. | | | |
| If no pulse is present, original person compressing states, "No pulse, start compression," gives one full breath, and CPR is again initiated. | | | |
| *CPR for children and infants:* | | | |
| In children, find hand position for compression by running index and middle finger up ribs to sternal notch. Look at location of index finger and lift fingers off sternum and put heel of same hand just above location of index finger. | | | |
| Other hand remains on child's forehead to keep airway open. | | | |
| Use heel of one hand for compressions, keeping fingers off chest. Compression depth is 2.5 to 3.8 cm (1 to 1-1/2 in). | | | |
| Give compressions at rate of 100 per minute with cycles of five compressions to one breath. | | | |
| For infants, when ventilating, cover infant's mouth and nose. | | | |
| For pulse checks, use brachial pulse site. | | | |
| Find position for compressions, place index finger on sternum at nipple line. Place middle and ring fingers on sternum next to index finger, then lift index finger. | | | |
| Compress chest 1.25 to 2.5 cm (1/2 to 1 in) straight down using two fingers while other hand remains on forehead to maintain open airway. | | | |
| *When relieved from CPR:* | | | |
| Stand by to assist, and provide support to victim's family and any bystanders. | | | |

*Terminating CPR:*

Terminate CPR only when another trained individual takes over, when heartbeat and breathing have been reestablished, when adjunctive life-support measures are initiated, when a physician states victim is dead and to discontinue CPR, or when rescuer is exhausted and there is no one else to take over.

**6.  Document relevant information.**

---

**40**  Procedure 40-1
Obtaining and Testing a Specimen of Feces

**1.  Give ambulatory clients following information and instructions.**

Purpose of stool specimen and how client can assist collecting it.

Defecate in clean or sterile bedpan or bedside commode.

If possible, do not contaminate specimen by urine or menstrual discharge. Void before specimen collection.

Do not place toilet tissue in bedpan after defecation.

Notify nurse as soon as possible after defecation.

**2.  Assist clients who need help.**

Assist client to bedside commode or bedpan placed on bedside chair or under toilet seat in bathroom.

After client has defecated, cover bedpan or commode.

Don gloves and clean client as required. Inspect skin around anus.

**3.  Transfer required amount of stool to stool specimen container.**

Use one or two tongue blades to transfer some or all stool to specimen container.

or

For a culture, dip sterile swab into specimen and place swab in sterile test tube using sterile technique.

Maintain universal precautions when disposing of tongue blades.

|  | Place lid on container as soon as specimen is in container. | | | |
| **4.** | **Ensure client comfort.** | | | |
|  | Empty and clean bedpan or commode, and return it to its place. | | | |
|  | Provide air freshener for any odors if needed. | | | |
| **5.** | **Label and send specimen to laboratory.** | | | |
|  | Ensure specimen label and requisition form have correct information and are securely attached to specimen container. | | | |
|  | Arrange for specimen to be taken to laboratory immediately or follow instructions on specimen container. | | | |
|  | To test stool for oocult blood, follow manufacturer's directions. <br> a. For Guaiac test, smear thin layer of feces on paper towel or filter paper with tongue blade. Drop reagents onto smear as directed. <br> b. For Hematest, smear thin layer of feces on filter paper, place tablet in middle of specimen, and add two drops of water as directed. <br> c. For Hemoccult slide, smear thin layer of feces over circle inside envelope, and drop reagent solution onto smear. | | | |
|  | Note reaction. For all tests, blue color indicates positive result. | | | |
| **6.** | **Document all relevant information.** | | | |

## Procedure 40-2
## Siphoning an Enema

| **1.** | **Position client appropriately.** | | | |
|  | Assist client to right side-lying position. | | | |
| **2.** | **Prepare equipment.** | | | |
|  | Place bedpan on chair at side of bed near client's hip. | | | |
|  | Attach open end of rectal tube partially filled enema set. | | | |
|  | Lubricate rectal tube. | | | |
| **3.** | **Siphon enema solution.** | | | |

| Procedure | S | U | Comments |
|---|---|---|---|
| Fill tube with solution, pinch it and gently insert it into rectum. | | | |
| Hold enema container about 10 cm (4 in) above anus, release pinched rectal tube, and quickly lower enema container. | | | |
| **4.** **Document all relevant information.** | | | |

## Procedure 40-3
## Removing a Fecal Impaction Digitally

| Procedure | S | U | Comments |
|---|---|---|---|
| **1.** **Prepare client** | | | |
| Explain procedure to client. | | | |
| Assist client to right lateral or Sims' position. | | | |
| Cover client with bath blanket. | | | |
| **2.** **Prepare equipment.** | | | |
| Place disposable bedpan under client's hips, and arrange top bedclothing so it falls obliquely over hips, exposing only buttocks. | | | |
| Place bedpan and toilet tissue nearby on bed or bedside chair. | | | |
| Don gloves and lubricate gloved index finger. | | | |
| **3.** **Remove impaction.** | | | |
| Gently insert index finger into rectum, moving toward umbilicus. | | | |
| Gently massage around stool. | | | |
| Work finger into hardened mass of stool to break it up. | | | |
| Work stool down to anus, remove it in small pieces, and place them in bedpan. | | | |
| Assess client for signs of pallor, feelings of faintness, shortness of breath, and perspiration. Stop procedure if these occur. | | | |
| Assist client to position on clean bedpan, commode, or toilet. | | | |
| **4.** **Assist client with hygienic measures as needed.** | | | |
| Wash rectal area with soap and water and dry gently. | | | |
| **5.** **Document procedure and all assessments.** | | | |

## Procedure 40-4
## Irrigating a Colostomy

| Procedure | S | U | Comments |
|-----------|---|---|----------|
| **1.**    **Prepare client.** | | | |
|     Assist client who must remain in bed to side-lying position. Place disposable bedpad on bed in front of client, and place bedpan on top of pad beneath stoma. | | | |
|     Assist ambulatory client to sit on toilet or commode. Ensure client is not unduly exposed. | | | |
|     Throughout procedure, provide explanations and encourage client to participate. | | | |
| **2.**    **Prepare equipment.** | | | |
|     Fill solution bag with 500 ml warm tap water or other solution as ordered. | | | |
|     Hang solution bag on IV pole, bottom level with client's shoulder, or 12 to 18 inches above stoma. | | | |
|     Attach colon catheter securely to tubing. | | | |
|     Open regulator clamp and run fluid through tubing to expel all air. Close clamp until ready for irrigation. | | | |
| **3.**    **Remove colostomy bag and position irrigation drainage sleeve.** | | | |
|     Remove soiled colostomy bag and place in moisture-resistant bag. | | | |
|     Center irrigation drainage sleeve over stoma and attach snugly. | | | |
|     Direct lower, open end of drainage sleeve into bedpan or between client's legs into toilet. | | | |
| **4.**    **If ordered, dilate stoma.** | | | |
|     Don gloves and lubricate tip of little finger. | | | |
|     Gently insert finger into stoma, using a massaging motion. | | | |
|     Repeat using progressively larger fingers until maximum dilation is achieved. | | | |
| **5.**    **Insert stoma cone or colon catheter.** | | | |
|     Lubricate tip of stoma cone or colon catheter. | | | |

| Procedure | S | U | Comments |
|---|---|---|---|
| Using rotating motion, insert through opening in top of irrigation drainage sleeve and gently through stoma. | | | |
| Insert catheter 7 cm (3 in) or stoma cone until it fits snugly. Do not apply force. | | | |
| **6.**   **Irrigate colon.** | | | |
| Open tubing clamp and allow fluid to flow. If cramping occurs, stop flow until cramping subsides, then resume flow. | | | |
| After fluid is instilled, remove catheter or cone and allow colon to empty. | | | |
| **7.**   **Seal drainage sleeve and allow complete emptying of colon.** | | | |
| Clean base of irrigation drainage sleeve and seal bottom with drainage clamp. | | | |
| Encourage ambulatory client to ambulate for about 30 minutes. | | | |
| **8.**   **Empty and remove irrigation sleeve.** | | | |
| **9.**   **Ensure client comfort.** | | | |
| Clean area around stoma and dry thoroughly. | | | |
| Put colostomy appliance on client as needed. | | | |
| **10.**   **Document and report relevant information.** | | | |

## 41 — Procedure 41-1
## Collecting a Routine Urine Specimen from an Adult or Child Who Has Urinary Control

| Procedure | S | U | Comments |
|---|---|---|---|
| **1.**   **Give ambulatory clients information and instructions.** | | | |
| Explain purpose and how client can assist. | | | |
| Explain all specimens must be free of fecal contamination. | | | |
| Instruct all female clients to discard toilet tissue in toilet or waste bag rather than in bedpan. | | | |
| Give client specimen container and direct client to void 120 ml (4 oz) in bathroom. | | | |
| **2.**   **Assist clients who are seriously ill, physically incapacitated, or disoriented.** | | | |
| Provide required assistance in bathroom, or help client use bedpan or urinal. | | | |

| Procedure | S | U | Comments |
|---|---|---|---|

| | | | |
|---|---|---|---|
| Wear gloves when assisting client to void in bedpan or urinal, and when transferring urine to specimen container. | | | |
| Empty bedpan or urinal. | | | |
| **3.** **Ensure specimen is sealed and container clean.** | | | |
| **4.** **Label and transport specimen to laboratory immediately or refrigerate.** | | | |
| **5.** **Document all relevant information.** | | | |

## Procedure 41-2
## Collecting a Timed Urine Specimen

| | | | |
|---|---|---|---|
| **1.** **Prepare and give client procedure instructions.** | | | |
| **2.** **Start collection period.** | | | |
| Ask client to void in toilet, bedpan, or urinal. Discard urine and document time test starts with discarded specimen. Collect all subsequent urine specimens, including one at end of period. | | | |
| Ask client to ingest required amount of liquid for certain tests or restrict fluid intake. Follow test instructions. | | | |
| Instruct client to void all subsequent urine into bedpan or urinal and to notify nursing staff when each specimen is provided. | | | |
| Number specimen containers sequentially. | | | |
| Place alert signs in client's unit. | | | |
| **3.** **Collect all required specimens.** | | | |
| Place each specimen into appropriately labeled container. | | | |
| If outside of specimen container is contaminated with urine, clean it with soap and water. | | | |
| Ensure each specimen is refrigerated throughout timed collection period. | | | |
| Measure amount of each specimen. | | | |
| Ask client to provide last specimen 5 to 10 minutes before end of collection period. | | | |
| **4.** **Document all relevant information.** | | | |

| Procedure | S | U | Comments |
|---|---|---|---|

### Procedure 41-3
### Collecting a Urine Specimen from an Infant

| Procedure | S | U | Comments |
|---|---|---|---|
| **1. Prepare parents and infant.** | | | |
| Remove infant's diaper and clean perineal-genital area with soap and water and then with an antiseptic. | | | |
| *For girls:* | | | |
| Separate labia and wash, rinse, and dry perineal area from front to back on each side of urinary meatus, and then over meatus. Repeat using antiseptic solution to clean, sterile water to rinse, and dry cotton balls to dry. | | | |
| *For boys:* | | | |
| Clean and disinfect both penis and scrotum. Wash penis in circular motion from tip toward scrotum, and wash scrotum last. Retract foreskin of an uncircumcised boy. | | | |
| **2. Apply specimen bag.** | | | |
| Remove protective paper from bottom half of adhesive backing of collection bag. | | | |
| Spread infant's legs apart. | | | |
| Place opening of collection bag over urethra or penis and scrotum. Base of opening needs to cover vagina or to fit well up under scrotum. | | | |
| Press adhesive portion firmly against infant's skin, starting at perineum. | | | |
| Remove protective paper from top half of adhesive backing, and press it firmly in place, working from top center outward. | | | |
| Elevate head of crib mattress to semi-Fowler's position. | | | |
| **3. Remove bag, and transfer specimen.** | | | |
| After child has voided desired amount, gently remove bag from skin. | | | |
| Empty urine from bag through opening at its base into specimen container. | | | |
| Discard urine bag. | | | |
| Tightly apply lid to specimen container. | | | |
| **4. Ensure client comfort.** | | | |

| | | S | U | Comments |
|---|---|---|---|---|
| | Apply infant's diaper. | | | |
| | Leave infant in comfortable and safe position held by parent or in a crib. | | | |
| **5.** | **Transport specimen.** | | | |
| | Ensure specimen label and laboratory requisition have correct information. Attach them securely to specimen. | | | |
| | Arrange for specimen to be sent to laboratory immediately or refrigerate it. | | | |
| **6.** | **Document all relevant information.** | | | |

## Procedure 41-4
## Changing a Urinary Diversion Ostomy Appliance

| | | S | U | Comments |
|---|---|---|---|---|
| **1.** | **Determine need for appliance change.** | | | |
| | Assess appliance for leakage of urine. | | | |
| | Ask client about any discomfort at or around stoma. | | | |
| | Drain pouch into graduated cylinder when one-third to one-half full and prior to removing pouch. | | | |
| | With evidence of leakage or discomfort at or around stoma, change appliance. | | | |
| **2.** | **Communicate acceptance and support of client throughout procedure.** | | | |
| **3.** | **Select appropriate time.** | | | |
| **4.** | **Prepare client and support persons.** | | | |
| | Explain procedure to client and support persons. | | | |
| | Provide privacy, preferably in bathroom. | | | |
| | Assist client into comfortable standing, sitting, or lying position. | | | |
| | Don gloves and unfasten belt, if worn. | | | |
| **5.** | **Shave peristomal skin of well-established ostomies as needed.** | | | |
| **6.** | **Remove emptied ostomy appliance.** | | | |
| | Assess volume and character of output. | | | |
| | Peel bag off slowly while holding client's skin taut. | | | |
| **7.** | **Clean and dry peristomal skin and stoma.** | | | |

| Procedure | S | U | Comments |
|---|---|---|---|
| Using cotton balls, wash peristomal skin with warm water and mild soap if needed. | | | |
| Pat dry skin with towel or cotton balls. | | | |
| Place rolled gauze or tampon to wick urine from stoma. | | | |
| **8. Assess stoma and peristomal skin.** | | | |
| Inspect color, size, and shape. Note any bleeding. | | | |
| Inspect peristomal skin for redness, ulcerations, or irritation. | | | |
| **9. If using Skin Prep liquid or wipes:** | | | |
| Cover stoma with gauze pad. | | | |
| Wipe Skin Prep evenly around peristomal skin, or use an applicator to apply thin layer of liquid to area. | | | |
| Allow to dry until it no longer feels tacky. | | | |
| **10. If using wafer- or disc-type barrier:** | | | |
| Use according to manufacturer's directions. | | | |
| Use stoma measuring device and trace a circle on backing of skin barrier. | | | |
| Make a template of stoma pattern and cut out traced pattern. | | | |
| Remove backing on one side of skin barrier and apply to faceplate of ostomy appliance. | | | |
| **11. Prepare clean appliance.** | | | |
| For disposable pouch with adhesive square, trace and cut a circle no larger than 2 – 3 cm (1/8 in) stoma size on appliance adhesive square. Peel off backing, and attach seal to disc-type skin barrier or if liquid product was used, apply to client's peristomal skin. | | | |
| For reusable pouch with faceplate attached, apply either adhesive cement or double-faced adhesive disc to faceplate. | | | |
| For reusable pouch with detachable faceplate, remove protective paper strip from one side of disc, and apply to back of faceplate. Remove remaining protective paper strip from other side, and attach faceplate to disc-type skin barrier or, if liquid product was used, apply to client's peristomal skin. | | | |
| **12. Apply clean appliance.** | | | |

| Procedure | S | U | Comments |
|---|---|---|---|
| For a disposable pouch, remove gauze pad or tampon over stoma, and gently press adhesive backing onto skin and smooth out wrinkles. Remove air from pouch, and attach spout to urinary drainage system or cap. | | | |
| For a reusable pouch with faceplate attached, insert coiled paper guidestrip into faceplate opening leaving strip protruding slightly. Using guidestrip, center faceplate over stoma, and firmly press adhesive seal to peristomal skin. Place deodorant in bag if desired, and close spout with cap. | | | |
| For reusable pouch with detachable faceplate, press and hold faceplate against client's skin for a few minutes, and tape to client's abdomen using four or eight 7.5 cm (3 in) strips of tape. Stretch opening on back of pouch and position it over base of faceplate, easing over faceplate flange. Place lock ring between pouch and back of pouch and faceplate flange, and close spout of pouch with cap. | | | |
| **13. Adjust client's teaching plan and nursing care plan as needed.** | | | |
| **14. Document relevant information.** | | | |

## 43 Procedure 43-1
## Administering Dermatologic Medications

| Procedure | S | U | Comments |
|---|---|---|---|
| **1. Verify order.** | | | |
| Compare medication record with most recent order. | | | |
| Determine label on medication tube or jar with medication record. | | | |
| **2. Prepare client.** | | | |
| Provide privacy and expose area of skin to be treated. | | | |
| **3. Prepare area for medication.** | | | |
| Wash hands and don gloves. | | | |
| Determine whether area is to be washed before applying medication. If it is, wash it gently, and pat it dry with gauze pads. | | | |
| **4. Apply medication and dressing as ordered.** | | | |
| Place small amount of cream on tongue blade, and spread it evenly on skin. | | | |

| Procedure | S | U | Comments |
|---|---|---|---|
| or | | | |
| Pour some lotion on gauze, and pat skin area with it. | | | |
| or | | | |
| If a liniment is used, rub it into skin with hands using long, smooth strokes. | | | |
| Repeat application until area is completely covered. | | | |
| Apply sterile dressing as necessary. | | | |
| or | | | |
| Apply prepackaged transdermal patch as directed. | | | |
| 5.  Provide client comfort. | | | |
| Provide clean gown or pajamas after application if medication will come in contact with clothing. | | | |
| 6.  Document all relevant assessments and interventions. | | | |

## Procedure 43-2
## Administering Nasal Installations

| Procedure | S | U | Comments |
|---|---|---|---|
| 1.  Verify medication or irrigation order. | | | |
| 2.  Prepare client. | | | |
| If secretions are excessive, ask client to blow nose to clear nasal passages. | | | |
| Inspect discharge on tissues for color, odor, and thickness. | | | |
| 3.  Assess client. | | | |
| Assess congestion of mucous membranes and any obstruction to breathing. Ask client to hold one nostril closed and blow out gently through other nostril. Listen for any sound of obstruction to air. Repeat for other nostril. | | | |
| Assess signs of distress when nares are occluded. Block each naris of an infant or young child and observe for signs of greater distress when naris is obstructed. | | | |
| Assess facial discomfort. | | | |
| Using nasal speculum, assess any crusting, redness, bleeding, or discharge of mucous membranes of nostrils. | | | |
| 4.  Position client appropriately. | | | |

| Procedure | S | U | Comments |
|---|---|---|---|
| *Eustachian tube:* | | | |
| Have client assume back-lying position. | | | |
| *Ethmoid and sphenoid sinuses:* | | | |
| Have client take a back-lying position with head over edge of bed or a pillow under shoulders so head is tipped backward. | | | |
| *Maxillary and frontal sinuses:* | | | |
| Have client assume back-lying position with head over edge of bed or a pillow under shoulders and head turned toward side to be treated. | | | |
| **5. Administer medication.** | | | |
| Draw up required amount of solution into dropper. | | | |
| Hold tip of dropper just above nostril, and direct solution laterally toward midline of superior concha of ethmoid bone as client breathes through mouth. | | | |
| Repeat for other nostril if indicated. | | | |
| Ask client to remain in position for 5 minutes. | | | |
| Discard any remaining solution in dropper, and dispose of soiled supplies appropriately. | | | |
| **6. Document all relevant information.** | | | |

## Procedure 43-3
## Administering an Intradermal Injection

| Procedure | S | U | Comments |
|---|---|---|---|
| **1. Verify order.** | | | |
| Check physician's order for medication, dosage, and route. | | | |
| **2. Prepare medication from ampule or vial.** | | | |
| **3. Identify and prepare client for injection.** | | | |
| Check client's arm band and ask client's name. | | | |
| Explain that medication will produce small bleb. | | | |
| **4. Select and clean site.** | | | |
| Don gloves and clean site with swab moistened with alcohol or other colorless antiseptic. Start at center of site and widen circle outward. | | | |

5.  **Prepare syringe for injection.**

    Remove needle cap while waiting for site to dry.

    Expel any bubbles from syringe.

    Grasp syringe in dominant hand, holding it between thumb and four fingers, with palm upward. Hold needle at 15° angle to skin surface, with bevel of needle up.

6.  **Inject fluid.**

    With nondominant hand, pull skin taut, and thrust needle tip firmly through epidermis. Do not aspirate.

    Inject medication carefully so it produces small bleb on skin.

    Withdraw needle quickly while providing countertraction on skin, and apply Band-Aid if indicated. Do not massage area.

    Dispose of syringe and needle safely in *sharps* container.

7.  **Document all relevant information.**

8.  **Assess client's response to testing substance in 24 or 48 hours, depending on test.**

---

## 44 Procedure 44-1
## Basic Bandaging

---

1.  **Position and prepare client.**

    Provide client with chair or bed, and arrange support for area to be bandaged.

    Make sure area to be bandaged is clean and dry.

    Align part to be bandaged with slight flexion of joint, unless contraindicated.

2.  **Apply bandage.**

    *Circular turns:*

    Hold bandage in dominant hand, keeping roll uppermost, and unroll bandage about 8 cm (3 in).

    Apply end of bandage to part of body to be bandaged.

| Procedure | S | U | Comments |
|---|---|---|---|
| Encircle body part a few times with each turn covering previous turn. | | | |
| Secure end of bandage with metal clip, tape, or safety pin over uninjured area. | | | |
| *Spiral turns:* | | | |
| Make two circular turns. | | | |
| Continue spiral turns at 30° angle, each overlapping preceeding one by two-thirds width of bandage. | | | |
| Terminate bandage with two circular turns, and secure ends. | | | |
| *Spiral reverse turns:* | | | |
| Anchor bandage with two circular turns, bring bandage upward at 30° angle. | | | |
| Place thumb of free hand on upper edge of bandage. | | | |
| Unroll bandage about 15 cm (6 in), turn hand so that bandage falls over itself. | | | |
| Continue bandage around limb, overlapping each previous turn by two-thirds width of bandage. | | | |
| Terminate bandage with two circular turns and secure end. | | | |
| *Recurrent turns:* | | | |
| Anchor bandage with two circular turns. | | | |
| Fold bandage back on itself, and bring it centrally over distal end to be bandaged. | | | |
| Holding it with other hand, bring bandage back over end to right of center bandage but overlapping it by two-thirds width of bandage. | | | |
| Bring bandage back on left side, overlapping first turn by two-thirds width of bandage. | | | |
| Continue pattern of alternating right and left until area is covered. | | | |
| Terminate bandage with two circular turns and secure. | | | |
| *Figure-eight turns:* | | | |
| Anchor bandage with two circular turns. | | | |
| Carry bandage above joint, around it, and below it, making a figure-eight. | | | |

| | | | |
|---|---|---|---|
| Continue above and below joint, overlapping previous turn by two-thirds width of bandage. | | | |
| Terminate bandage above joint with two circular turns and secure end. | | | |
| *Thumb spica:* | | | |
| Anchor bandage with two circular turns around wrist. | | | |
| Bring bandage down to distal aspect of thumb, and encircle thumb. Leave tip of thumb exposed if possible. | | | |
| Bring bandage back up and around wrist, then back down and around thumb, overlapping previous turn by two-thirds width of bandage. | | | |
| Repeat last two steps, working up thumb and hand until thumb is covered. | | | |
| Anchor bandage with two circular turns around wrist and secure. | | | |
| **3.** **Document all relevant information.** | | | |

## Procedure 44-2
## Applying a Stump Bandage

| | | | |
|---|---|---|---|
| **1.** **Position client appropriately.** | | | |
| Assist client to semi-Fowler's position in bed or to sitting position on edge of bed. | | | |
| Clean skin or stump wound and apply sterile dressing as needed. | | | |
| **2.** **Apply bandage.** | | | |
| *Figure-eight bandage:* | | | |
| Anchor bandage with two circular turns around hips. | | | |
| Bring bandage down over stump and then back up and around hips. | | | |
| Bring bandage down again, overlapping previous turn, and making figure-eight around stump and back up around hips. | | | |
| Repeat, working bandage up stump. | | | |
| Anchor bandage around hips with two circular turns. | | | |
| Secure bandage with adhesive tape, safety pins, or clips. | | | |
| or | | | |

| Procedure | S | U | Comments |
|---|---|---|---|
| Place end of elastic bandage at top of anterior surface of leg and have client hold it in place. Bring bandage diagonally down toward end of stump. | | | |
| Applying even pressure, bring bandage diagonally upward toward groin area. | | | |
| Make figure-eight turn behind top of leg, downward again over and under stump, and back up to groin area. | | | |
| Repeat figure-eight turns at least twice. | | | |
| Anchor bandage around hips with two circular turns, and secure. | | | |
| *Recurrent bandage:* | | | |
| Anchor bandage with two circular turns around stump. | | | |
| Cover stump with recurrent turns. | | | |
| Anchor recurrent bandage with two circular turns, and secure. | | | |
| *Spiral bandage:* | | | |
| Make recurrent turns to cover end of stump. | | | |
| Apply spiral turns from distal aspect of stump toward body. | | | |
| Anchor bandage with two circular turns and hips, and secure. | | | |
| **3.** **Document all relevant information.** | | | |

## Procedure 44-3
## Applying a Hot Water Bottle, Electric Heating Pad, Commercial Hot Pack, or Perineal Heat Lamp

| Procedure | S | U | Comments |
|---|---|---|---|
| **1.** **Prepare and assess client.** | | | |
| Inspect area to receive heat. | | | |
| Fold down bedclothes to expose area where heat will be applied. | | | |
| *Hot water bottle:* | | | |
| **2.** **Fill and cover bottle.** | | | |
| Fill hot water bottle about two-thirds full. | | | |
| Measure temperature of water. | | | |
| Expel air from bottle. | | | |

| Procedure | S | U | Comments |
|---|---|---|---|
| Secure stopper tightly, hold bottle upside down, and check for leaks. | | | |
| Dry bottle, and wrap in towel, or hot water bottle cover. | | | |
| **3.**    **Apply bottle.** | | | |
| Support bottle against body part with pillows as necessary. | | | |
| *Electric heating pad:* | | | |
| **4.**    **Prepare client and pad for application.** | | | |
| Ensure body area is dry. | | | |
| Check that electric pad is functioning and in good repair. | | | |
| Place cover on pad and plug into electric socket. | | | |
| Set control dial for correct temperature. | | | |
| **5.**    **Apply pad.** | | | |
| After pad has heated, place pad over body area. Only use gauze ties to hold pad in place. | | | |
| **6.**    **Give client safety instructions.** | | | |
| *Aquathermia pad:* | | | |
| **7.**    **Assemble unit.** | | | |
| Fill unit with distilled water two-thirds full. | | | |
| Remove air bubbles and secure top. | | | |
| Cover pad with towel or pillowcase, and plug in unit. | | | |
| **8.**    **Apply pad to body part.** | | | |
| Check for any leaks or malfunctions before use. | | | |
| Use tape or gauze ties to hold pad in place. | | | |
| If unusual redness or pain occurs, discontinue treatment, and report client's reaction. | | | |
| **9.**    **Give client instructions.** | | | |
| *Disposable hot pack:* | | | |
| **10.**    **Initiate heating process.** | | | |
| Strike, squeeze, or knead pack according to manufacturer's directions. | | | |
| Apply hot pack to body part, and observe client's reaction. | | | |

| Procedure | S | U | Comments |
|---|---|---|---|

*Perineal heat lamp:*

**11. Prepare client.**

Expose area to be treated, and drape client so body is exposed minimally.

Clean and dry perineum, wiping from front to back.

**12. Position lamp appropriately.**

Plug in lamp, and, with lamp turned off, place it approximately 30 cm (12 in) from perineum.

**13. Give client safety instructions.**

*For all applications:*

**14. Monitor client during application.**

Every 5 to 10 minutes, assess client for any complaints of discomfort.

At first sign of pain, swelling, or excessive redness, remove heat and report to nurse in charge.

**15. Remove heat application.**

**16. Document all relevant information.**

## Procedure 44-4
## Applying an Infant Radiant Warmer

**1. Prepare warmer.**

Using manual control setting, turn on radiant warmer.

**2. Assess and prepare infant for treatment.**

Wipe blood and vernix from newborn's head and body using prewarmed towels.

Wrap infant in preheated blankets, transfer infant to mother (parents), and return infant to warmer.

Remove blankets, apply diaper and head cover.

Apply temperature sensor to infant's abdomen between umbilicus and xiphoid process.

Cover temperature sensor with reflective covering.

| | Turn warmer control device to automatic setting. | | | |
|---|---|---|---|---|
| 3. | **Initiate warming process.** | | | |
| | Adjust temperature setting control to desired goal temperature. | | | |
| | Turn warmer on and set temperature sensor alarm at upper limit of desired temperature range. | | | |
| 4. | **Monitor warming process.** | | | |
| | Check infant's temperature sensor reading every 15 to 30 minutes. | | | |
| | Check infant's axillary temperature every 2 to 4 hours. | | | |
| | Monitor sensor probe site and surrounding skin for irritation or breakdown. | | | |
| 5. | **Terminate warming process.** | | | |
| | When infant's temperature reaches desired level, dress infant in T-shirt, diaper, and head cover. Wrap infant in two blankets, and transfer infant from warmer to an open crib. | | | |
| | Check infant's axillary temperature every 2 to 4 hours. | | | |
| | If infant's temperature drops below 36.1° C (97.0° F), return infant to warmer, remove clothing, and reinitiate warming procedure. | | | |
| 6. | **Document all relevant information.** | | | |

## Procedure 44-5
## Managing Clients with Hyperthermia and Hypothermia Blankets

| 1. | **Prepare client.** | | | |
|---|---|---|---|---|
| | Don gloves and bathe client if necessary. | | | |
| | Remove gloves and apply towels to extremities. | | | |
| 2. | **Prepare equipment.** | | | |
| | Connect blanket pad to modular unit and inspect for adequate functioning. | | | |
| | Inspect pad and cords for frays or exposed wires. | | | |
| | Twist male tubing connectors of coil blanket tubing into inlet and outlet opening connectors on modular unit. | | | |

| Procedure | S | U | Comments |
|---|---|---|---|
| Check solution level in module and fill with distilled water if necessary. | | | |
| Turn on unit, and check for adequate filling of coils throughout blanket as solution circulates. | | | |
| Turn client temperature control knob to desired temperature and determine whether temperature gauge is functioning. | | | |
| Set modular control knob or master switch to either manual or automatic mode, and note accuracy of temperature settings. | | | |
| *If using automatic mode:* | | | |
| Insert thermistor probe plug into thermistor probe jack on modular unit. | | | |
| Check automatic mode light. | | | |
| Set machine to desired temperature. | | | |
| Set limits for pad temperature. | | | |
| *If using manual mode:* | | | |
| Set master temperature control knob to desired temperature. | | | |
| Check manual mode light. | | | |
| If blanket is nondisposable, cover it with plastic cover or thin sheet. | | | |
| **3.  Apply blanket to client.** | | | |
| Don clean gloves and place client on blanket. | | | |
| Apply lubricating jelly to rectal probe, insert 7 to 10 cm (3 to 4 in). | | | |
| Secure probe with tape. | | | |
| **4.  Monitor client closely.** | | | |
| Take vital signs every 15 minutes for first hour, every 30 minutes for second hour, and every hour thereafter. | | | |
| Determine client's neurological status regularly as needed. | | | |
| Observe skin for indications of burns, intactness, and color. | | | |
| Determine any intolerance to blanket. | | | |
| **5.  Maintain therapy as required.** | | | |
| Remove and clean rectal probe every 3 to 4 hours or when client has bowel movement. | | | |

| Procedure | S | U | Comments |
|---|---|---|---|

### Procedure 44-6
### Administering Hot Soaks and Sitz Baths

*Hand or foot soak:*

**1. Prepare soak.**

Fill container half full and test temperature of solution with thermometer.

Pad edge of container with towel.

Use sterile solution and sterile thermometer if client has an open wound.

**2. Prepare and assess client.**

Assist client to well-aligned, comfortable position.

Don disposable gloves as required, remove dressings, and discard them in bag. Assess amount, color, odor, and consistency of drainage on removed dressings.

Inspect appearance of area to be soaked.

**3. Commence soak.**

Immerse body part completely in solution.

If soak is sterile, cover open container with sterile drape or container wrapper.

Place large sheet or blanket over soak. Proceed to step 7.

*Sitz bath:*

**4. Prepare bath.**

Fill sitz bath with water at 40° C (105° F).

Pad tub or chair with towel as required.

**5. Prepare client.**

Remove gown, or fasten it above waist.

Don gloves if an open area or drainage are present.

Remove T-binder and perineal dressings if present, and note amount, color, odor, and consistency of any drainage.

Assess appearance of area to be soaked for redness, swelling, odor, breaks in skin, and drainage.

Wrap blanket around client's shoulders and over legs as needed.

| Procedure | S | U | Comments |
|-----------|---|---|----------|
| **6.**    **Begin sitz bath.** | | | |
| Assist client into bath and provide support for client as needed. | | | |
| Leave signal light within reach. Stay with client if warranted, and terminate bath if necessary. | | | |
| **7.**    **Monitor client.** | | | |
| *Soak:* | | | |
| Assess client and test temperature of solution at least once per soak. Assess for discomfort, need for additional support, and any reactions to soak. | | | |
| If solution has cooled, remove body part, empty solution, add newly heated solution, and reimmerse body part. | | | |
| *Sitz bath:* | | | |
| Assess client during bath for discomfort, color, and pulse rate. | | | |
| Immediately report any unexpected or adverse responses to nurse in charge. | | | |
| Test temperature of solution at least once during bath. Adjust temperature as needed. | | | |
| **8.**    **Discontinue soak or bath.** | | | |
| At completion of soak, remove body part from basin, and dry it thoroughly and carefully. If soak was sterile, use sterile towel for drying and wear sterile gloves. | | | |
| Assess appearance of affected area carefully, and reapply dressing if required. | | | |
| or | | | |
| At completion of sitz bath, assist client out of bath and dry area with towel. | | | |
| Assess perineal area and reapply dressings and garments as required. | | | |
| **9.**    **Document all relevant information.** | | | |

## Procedure 44-7
## Applying an Ice Bag, Ice Collar, Ice Glove, or Disposable Cold Pack

| Procedure | S | U | Comments |
|-----------|---|---|----------|
| **1.**    **Prepare and assess client.** | | | |
| Assist client to comfortable position, and support body part requiring application. | | | |

| | | | |
|---|---|---|---|
| Expose only area to be treated, and provide warmth to avoid chilling. | | | |
| Assess area to which cold will be applied. | | | |

*Ice bag, collar, or glove:*

| | | | |
|---|---|---|---|
| **2.**   **Fill and cover device.** | | | |
| Fill device one-half to two-thirds full of crushed ice. | | | |
| Remove excess air, insert stopper into ice bag or collar, or tie knot at open end of glove. | | | |
| Hold device upside down and check for leaks. | | | |
| Cover device with soft cloth cover. | | | |
| **3.**   **Apply cold device.** | | | |
| Apply device for time specified, usually not longer than 30 minutes. | | | |
| Hold it in place with roller gauze, binder, or towel. Secure with tape as necessary. | | | |

*Disposable cold pack:*

| | | | |
|---|---|---|---|
| **4.**   **Initiate cooling process.** | | | |
| Strike, squeeze, or knead cold pack according to manufacturer's instructions. | | | |
| Cover with soft cloth. | | | |

*All applications:*

| | | | |
|---|---|---|---|
| **5.**   **Instruct client to remain in position and call nurse if discomfort is felt.** | | | |
| **6.**   **Monitor client during application.** | | | |
| Assess client for comfort and skin reactions every 5 to 10 minutes. | | | |
| Report reactions to nurse in charge and remove application. | | | |
| **7.**   **Remove application.** | | | |
| **8.**   **Document all relevant information.** | | | |

## Procedure 44-8
## Administering a Cooling Sponge Bath

| | | | |
|---|---|---|---|
| **1.**   **Obtain all relevant baseline data.** | | | |
| Assess client for other signs of fever. | | | |
| **2.**   **Prepare client.** | | | |

|  | Remove gown and assist client to comfortable supine position. |  |  |  |
|  | Place bath blanket over client. |  |  |  |
|  | If ice bags or cold packs are not used, place bath towels under each axilla and shoulder. |  |  |  |
| 3. | **Sponge face with plain water and dry it.** |  |  |  |
|  | Apply ice bag or cold pack to head for comfort. |  |  |  |
| 4. | **Place cold applications in axillae and groins.** |  |  |  |
|  | Wet four washcloths, wring them out so they are very damp, but not dripping. |  |  |  |
|  | Place washcloths, ice bags or cold packs in axillae and groins. |  |  |  |
|  | Leave washcloths in place for about five minutes, or until they feel warm. Rewet and replace as required. |  |  |  |
| 5. | **Sponge arms and legs.** |  |  |  |
|  | Place bath towel under one arm and sponge arm for about 5 minutes. or Place saturated towel over extremity rewetting as necessary. |  |  |  |
|  | Pat arm dry and repeat steps for other arm and legs. |  |  |  |
|  | When sponging extremities, hold washcloth briefly over wrists and ankles. |  |  |  |
| 6. | **Reassess client's vital signs after 15 minutes.** |  |  |  |
|  | Compare findings and evaluate effectiveness of sponge bath. |  |  |  |
|  | Continue sponge bath if client's temperature is above 37.7° C (100° F), discontinue if below, or if pulse rate is significantly increased and remains so after five minutes. |  |  |  |
| 7. | **(Optional) Sponge chest and abdomen for 3 to 5 minutes and pat areas dry.** |  |  |  |
| 8. | **Sponge back and buttocks 3 to 5 minutes and pat areas dry.** |  |  |  |
| 9. | **Remove cold applications from axillae and groins.** |  |  |  |
|  | Reassess vital signs. |  |  |  |

| Procedure | S | U | Comments |
|---|---|---|---|
| Document assessments, including all vital signs, and type of sponge bath given. | | | |
| *Variation: Pediatric bathing* | | | |
| Cooling baths for children can be given in tub, bed, or crib. | | | |
| *Tub:* | | | |
| Immerse child in tepid water for 20 to 30 minutes. | | | |
| Firmly support child's head and shoulders. Gently squeeze water over back and chest or spray water from sprayer over body. | | | |
| Use a floating toy or other distraction for conscious child. | | | |
| Discontinue bath if there is evidence of chilling. | | | |
| Dry and dress child in light-weight clothing or diaper and cover with light cotton blanket. | | | |
| Take temperature 30 minutes after bath. | | | |
| *Bed or crib sponge:* | | | |
| Place undressed child on absorbent towel. | | | |
| Follow adult sponge bath method or use following towel method:<br>a. Apply cool bath or icebag to forehead.<br>b. Wrap each extremity in towel moistened with tepid water.<br>c. Place one towel under back and another over neck and torso.<br>d. Change towels as they warm.<br>e. Continue procedure for about 30 minutes. | | | |

## Procedure 44-9
## Cleaning a Drain Site and Shortening a Penrose Drain

| Procedure | S | U | Comments |
|---|---|---|---|
| 1. **Verify physician's order.** | | | |
| Confirm drain is to be shortened by nurse and length it is to be shortened. | | | |
| 2. **Prepare client.** | | | |
| Explain procedure to client and that there may be a pulling sensation for a few seconds when drain is being drawn out, but this procedure should not be painful. | | | |
| Position client for dressing change. | | | |

| | Procedure | S | U | Comments |
|---|---|---|---|---|
| 3. | **Remove dressings and clean incision and drain site.** | | | |
| | Clean incision site first. | | | |
| | Clean skin around drain site by swabbing in half or full circles from drain site outward, using separate swabs for each wipe. Clean until all drainage is removed. | | | |
| | Assess amount, odor, thickness, and color of drainage. | | | |
| 4. | **Shorten drain.** | | | |
| | If drain has not been shortened before, remove suture. | | | |
| | With hemostat, grasp drain by its full width, and pull out required length. | | | |
| | Wearing sterile gloves, insert sterile safety pin through base of drain as close to skin as possible. | | | |
| | With sterile scissors, cut off excess drain leaving 2.5 cm (1 in) above skin. | | | |
| 5. | **Apply dressings to drain site and incision.** | | | |
| | Apply sterile dressings one at a time using sterile gloved hands or sterile forceps. | | | |
| | Apply final surgipad by hand. Remove gloves and secure dressing with tape or tie. | | | |
| 6. | **Document procedure and nursing assessments.** | | | |

## Procedure 44-10
## Establishing and Maintaining a Closed Wound Drainage System

| | Procedure | S | U | Comments |
|---|---|---|---|---|
| 1. | **Establish suction if it has not been already initiated.** | | | |
| | Place evacuator bag on solid, flat surface and don gloves. | | | |
| | Open drainage plug on top of bag. | | | |
| | Compress bag; while it is compressed, close drainage plug. | | | |
| 2. | **Empty evacuator bag.** | | | |
| | When drainage fluid reaches "Full" line. Don gloves and open drainage plug. | | | |

| Procedure | S | U | Comments |
|---|---|---|---|
| Invert bag and empty into collecting receptacle. | | | |
| Reestablish suction. | | | |
| Using calibrated pitcher, measure amount of drainage, and note characteristics. | | | |
| **3.** **Document all relevant information.** | | | |

## Procedure 44-11
## Applying Moist Sterile Compresses

| Procedure | S | U | Comments |
|---|---|---|---|
| **1.** **Prepare client.** | | | |
| Assist client to comfortable position. | | | |
| Expose area for compress or pack. | | | |
| Provide support for body part requiring compress or pack. | | | |
| Don disposable gloves and remove wound dressing, if present. | | | |
| **2.** **Moisten compress or pack.** | | | |
| Place gauze in solution. or Heat flannel towel in steamer, or chill it in basin of water and ice. | | | |
| **3.** **Protect surrounding skin as indicated.** | | | |
| With cotton swab or applicator stick, apply petrolatum jelly to skin surrounding wound. | | | |
| **4.** **Apply moist heat.** | | | |
| Wring out gauze compress and appy gauze lightly to designated area, and if tolerated by client, mold compress close to body. Pack gauze snugly against all wound surfaces. or Wring out flannel and apply to body area, molding it closely to body part. | | | |
| For sterile pack, use sterile gloves. | | | |
| **5.** **Immediately insulate and secure application.** | | | |
| **6.** **Monitor client.** | | | |
| Assess client for discomfort at 5 to 10 minute intervals. If client feels any discomfort, assess for erythema, numbness, maceration, or blistering. | | | |

| Procedure | S | U | Comments |
|---|---|---|---|
| For applications over large body areas, note any change in pulse, respirations, and blood pressure. With unexpected reaction, terminate treatment and report to nurse in charge. | | | |
| **7. Remove compress or pack at specified time.** | | | |
| Apply sterile dressing if one is required. | | | |
| **8. Document relevant information.** | | | |

## Procedure 44-12
## Removing Skin Sutures

| Procedure | S | U | Comments |
|---|---|---|---|
| **1. Prepare client.** | | | |
| Inform client suture removal may produce slight discomfort, such as pulling or stinging, but should not be painful. | | | |
| **2. Remove dressings and clean incision.** | | | |
| Don sterile gloves and clean suture line with antimicrobial solution before and after suture removal. | | | |
| **3. Remove sutures.** | | | |
| *Plain interrupted sutures:* | | | |
| Grasp sutures at knot with forceps. | | | |
| Place curved tip of suture scissors under suture as close to skin as possible and cut suture. | | | |
| With forceps, pull suture out in one piece, Inspect suture carefully to make sure all suture material is removed. | | | |
| Discard suture onto piece of sterile gauze or into moisture-proof bag. Do not contaminate forcep tips. | | | |
| Continue to remove alternate sutures. | | | |
| If no dehiscence occurs, remove remaining sutures. If dehiscence does occur, do not remove remaining sutures. Report to nurse in charge. | | | |
| With small dehiscence, apply sterile butterfly tape over gap, after pressing wound edges together. | | | |
| With large dehiscence, cover wound with sterile gauze and immediately report to nurse in charge or physician. | | | |

| Procedure | S | U | Comments |
|---|---|---|---|
| *Mattress interupted sutures:* | | | |
| Cut visible part of suture close to skin opposite knot, and remove small piece. | | | |
| Grasp knot with forceps and pull. | | | |
| *Plain continuous sutures:* | | | |
| Cut thread of first suture opposite knot. Then cut thread of second suture on same side as first thread. | | | |
| Grasp knot with forceps and pull. | | | |
| Cut off visible part left on second suture. | | | |
| Grasp third suture next to skin opposite beginning knot side and pull underlying thread out between second and third suture. | | | |
| Cut remaining thread off from third suture. | | | |
| Repeat last two steps for remaining sutures until last knot is reached. Note after first stitch is removed, each thread is cut down same side, below original knot. | | | |
| Cut last suture opposite ending knot and pull out last suture. | | | |
| *Blanket continuous sutures:* | | | |
| Cut threads that are opposite looped blanket edge. | | | |
| Pull each stitch out at looped edge. | | | |
| *Mattress continuous sutures:* | | | |
| Cut visible suture at both skin edges opposite beginning knot and next suture opposite knot. Remove visible portions of sutures. | | | |
| Pull first suture out by knot. | | | |
| Lift second suture on beginning knot side to pull out underlying suture in center. | | | |
| Go to third suture opposite beginning knot side, lift out suture and cut off all visible parts close to skin. | | | |
| Go to knot side of third suture and pull out underlying center thread and cut remaining portion of third suture thread close to skin. | | | |
| Repeat last two steps, working from side to side of incision, until last suture is reached. | | | |
| Cut visible suture opposite knot. Go to knot and pull out remaining pieces. | | | |

| 5. | **Clean and cover incision.** | | | |
|----|-------------------------------|---|---|---|
| | Clean incision with antimicrobial solution. | | | |
| | Apply small, light, sterile dressing. | | | |
| 6. | **Instruct client about follow-up wound care.** | | | |
| | If wound is dry and healing well, client can usually take a shower in a day or two. | | | |
| | Instruct client to contact physician if wound discharge appears. | | | |
| 7. | **Document suture removal and assessment data on appropriate records.** | | | |

### ◆45◆ Procedure 45-1
### Preparing the Operative Site

| 1. | **Drape client appropriately.** | | | |
|----|--------------------------------|---|---|---|
| | Expose only area to be prepared. | | | |
| 2. | **If depilatory is to be used, test client's reaction to it.** | | | |
| | Apply small amount of depilatory on small part of area where hair is to removed. | | | |
| | Apply cream to test area smoothly and thickly. Do not rub in. | | | |
| | Leave cream on specified time. | | | |
| | Remove depilatory by rinsing with lukewarm water and washcloth. Do not use soap. | | | |
| | Pat area dry with gauze squares. | | | |
| | Wait for 24 hours, and assess client's skin for redness or other responses. | | | |
| 3. | **Remove hair.** | | | |
| *Depilitory:* | | | | |
| | If client's skin remains normal after skin test, apply depilatory and follow above steps for hair removal. | | | |
| *Clipping:* | | | | |
| | Make sure area is dry. | | | |
| | Remove hair with clippers; do not apply pressure. | | | |

| Procedure | S | U | Comments |
|---|---|---|---|
| *Wet shave:* | | | |
| Don gloves and place moisture-proof towel under area to be prepared. | | | |
| Lather skin well with soap solution. | | | |
| Stretch skin taut, and hold razor at about 45° angle to skin. | | | |
| Shave in direction in which hair grows. | | | |
| Wipe off excess hair off skin with sponges. | | | |
| 4. **Clean and disinfect surgical area according to agency practice.** | | | |
| Clean any body crevices with applicators and solutions. Dry with swabs. | | | |
| If antimicrobial solution is used, apply to area immediately after it is clipped. Check agency policy as to how long to leave on. | | | |
| 5. **Inspect skin after hair removal.** | | | |
| Closely observe for reddened or broken areas. Report to nurse in charge any skin lesions. | | | |
| 6. **Dispose of used equipment appropriately.** | | | |
| 7. **Document all relevant information.** | | | |

## Procedure 45-2
## Applying Antiemboli Stockings

| Procedure | S | U | Comments |
|---|---|---|---|
| 1. **Select an appropriate time to apply stockings.** | | | |
| Apply in morning or remove and replace at least twice a day if possible. | | | |
| Wash legs and feet daily. | | | |
| Assist client who has been ambulating to lie down for 15 to 30 minutes before applying stockings. | | | |
| 2. **Apply elastic stocking to foot.** | | | |
| Assist client to lying position in bed. | | | |
| Dust ankle with talcum powder, and ask client to point toes. | | | |
| Turn stocking inside out by inserting hand into stocking from top and grabbing heel pocket from inside. Foot portion should now be inside stocking leg. | | | |

| Procedure | S | U | Comments |
|---|---|---|---|
| Remove hand, and with heel pocket downward, hook index and middle fingers of both hands into foot section. | | | |
| Face client, and slip foot portion of stocking over client's foot, toes, and heel. Move up foot, stretching stocking sideways. | | | |
| Support client's ankle with one hand while using other hand to pull heel pocket under heel. | | | |
| Center heel in pocket. | | | |
| **3. Apply remaining inverted portion of stocking.** | | | |
| Gather remaining portion of stocking up to toes, and pull only this part over heel. | | | |
| At ankle, grasp gathered portion between index and middle fingers, and pull stocking up leg to knee. | | | |
| For thigh- or waist-length stocking, ask client to straighten leg while stretching rest of stocking over knee. | | | |
| Ask client to flex knee while pulling stocking over thigh. Stretch stocking from top to distribute evenly over thigh. Top should rest 2.5 to 7.5 cm ( 1 to 3 in) below gluteal fold. | | | |
| For waist-length stocking, ask client to stand and continue extending stocking up to top of gluteal fold. | | | |
| Apply adjustable belt and adjust foot section to ensure toe comfort. | | | |
| **4. Document application of antiemboli stockings.** | | | |

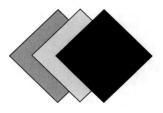

# Appendix
# Universal Precautions

Universal precautions apply to blood and body fluids containing visible blood. They also apply to body tissues and to the following specific body fluids: Vaginal secretions, seminal secretions, cerebrospinal fluid, synovial fluid, pleural fluid, peritoneal fluid, amniotic fluid, saliva in dental procedures, and body fluids in situations where it is difficult to differentiate among body fluids. Universal precautions *do not* apply to feces, urine, nasal secretions, sputum, saliva, sweat, tears, or vomitus unless they contain visible blood.

Health care workers are at risk of exposure to bloodborne pathogens, i.e., hepatitis B virus (HBV), hepatitis C virus (HCV), and human immunodeficiency virus (HIV). Health care workers should consider *all* clients as potentially infected with bloodborne pathogens and must follow the infection control precautions for *all* clients.

The Centers for Disease Control recommend the following specific precautions to reduce the risk of exposure to potentially infective materials:

### Handwashing

• Wash your hands thoroughly with warm water and soap (a) immediately, if contaminated with blood or other body fluids to which universal precautions apply, or potentially contaminated articles; (b) between clients; and (c) immediately after gloves are removed, even if the gloves appear to be intact. When hand washing facilities are not available, use a waterless antiseptic hand cleaner in accordance with the manufacturer's directions.

• If you have an exudative lesion or weeping dermatitis, refrain from all direct client care and from handling client care equipment until the condition resolves.

### Gloves

• Wear gloves when touching blood and body fluids containing blood, as well as when handling items or surfaces soiled with blood or body fluids as mentioned above.

• Wear gloves for all invasive procedures (i.e., any surgical entry into tissues, cavities, or organs or repair of major traumatic injuries).

• Change gloves after client contact.

• Wear gloves (a) if you have cuts, scratches, or other breaks in the skin; (b) in situations where hand contamination with blood may occur, e.g., with an uncooperative client; and (c) when you are performing venipuncture and other vascular procedures.

### Other Protective Barriers

• Wear masks and protective eyewear (glasses, goggles) or face shields to protect the mucous membranes of your mouth, nose, and eyes during all *invasive* procedures and/or any procedure that is likely to generate droplets of blood or other body fluid to which universal precautions apply.

• Wear a disposable plastic apron or gown during procedures that are likely to generate splatters of blood or other body fluids (e.g., peritoneal fluid) and soil your clothing.

**Needles and Sharps Disposal** To prevent injuries, place used disposable needle-syringe units, scalpel blades, and other sharp items in puncture-resistant containers for disposal. Discard used needle-syringe units *uncapped* and *unbroken*. Place puncture-resistant containers as close as practicable to use areas.

**Laundry** Handle soiled linen as little as possible and with minimum agitation to prevent gross microbial contamination of the air and of persons handling the linen. Place linen soiled with blood or body fluids in leakage-resistant bags at the location where it is used.

**Specimens** Put all specimens of blood and listed body fluids in well-constructed containers with secure lids to prevent leakage during transport. When collecting specimens, take care to avoid contaminating the outside of the container.

**Blood Spills** Use a chemical germicide that is approved for use as a hospital disinfectant to decontaminate work surfaces after there is a spill of blood or other applicable body fluids. In the absence of a commercial germicide, a solution of sodium hypochlorite (household bleach) in a 1:100 dilution is effective.

### Infective Wastes

• Follow agency policies for disposal of infective waste, both when disposing of, and when decontaminating, contaminated materials.

• Carefully pour bulk blood, suctioned fluids, and excretions containing blood and secretions, down drains that are connected to a sanitary sewer.

**Sources** U.S. Department of Health and Human Services, Public Health Service, Update: Universal precautions for prevention of transmission of human immunodeficiency virus, hepatitis B virus, and other bloodborne pathogens in health care settings, *Morbidity and Mortality Weekly Report*, June 24, 1988; 37: 377–382, 387–388; *Morbidity and Mortality Weekly Report*, June 23, 1989, 38/No. S–6: 9–18.

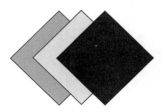

# References Cited in Text*

American Red Cross CPR for the Professional Rescuer. 1993. American National Red Cross.

Guidelines for Cardiopulmonary Resuscitation and Emergency Cardiac Care. 1992. *Journal of the American Medical Association* 286(16): 2171–97.

Hogan, L., and Beland, I. July 1976. Cervical neck syndrome. *American Journal of Nursing* 76:1104–7

Holder, G., Alexander, J. February 1990. A new and improved guide to I.V. therapy . . . protocols for intravenous therapy. *American Journal of Nursing* 90:43–47.

Luce, J.M.; Tyler, M.L.; and Pierson, D.J. 1984. *Intensive respiratory care*. Philadelphia: W.B. Saunders Co.

Maier, P. September 1986. Take the work out of range-of-motion exercises with continuous passive motion machine. *RN* 49: 46–49.

Olds, S.B.; London, M.L.; and P.W. Ladewig. 1992. *Maternal-newborn nursing: A family centered approach*, 4th ed. Redwood City, CA: Addison-Wesley Nursing.

Palau, D. and Jones, S. October 1986. Test your skill at trouble shooting chest tubes. *RN* 49: 43–45.

Quinn, A. September 1986. Thora-Drain III: Closed chest drainage made simpler and safer. *Nursing 86* 16: 46–51.

Smith, A.J., and Johnson, J.Y. 1990. *Nurses guide to clinical procedures*. Philadelphia: J.B. Lippincott Co.

*Additional references can be found in the corresponding chapter of *Fundamentals of Nursing, fifth edition*.